ANNUAL REVIEW OF NURSING RESEARCH

Volume 20, 2002

ANNUAL REVIEW OF NURSING RESEARCH

Volume 20, 2002

Geriatric Nursing Research

Joyce J. Fitzpatrick, PhD, RN, FAAN
Series Editor

Patricia G. Archbold, DNSc, RN, FAAN
Barbara J. Stewart, PhD
Volume Editors

Karen S. Lyons, RN, PhD
Associate Editor

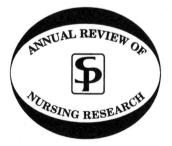

SP SPRINGER PUBLISHING COMPANY
New York

Order ANNUAL REVIEW OF NURSING RESEARCH, Volume 21, 2003, prior to publication and receive a 10% discount. An order coupon can be found at the back of this volume.

Springer Publishing Company, Inc.
536 Broadway
New York, NY 10012

02 03 04 05 06 / 5 4 3 2 1

ISBN-0-8261-4132-3
ISSN-0739-6686

ANNUAL REVIEW OF NURSING RESEARCH is indexed in *Cumulative Index to Nursing and Allied Health Literature* and *Index Medicus*.

Printed in the United States of America by Maple Vail.

Advisory Committee for Volume 20

Contents

Preface   *ix*
    Joyce J. Fitzpatrick
Introduction   *xi*
    Patricia G. Archbold, Barbara J. Stewart, and Karen S. Lyons
Contributors   *xv*

Part I: Managing Common Conditions in Elders

1   Maintaining and Improving Physical Function in Elders   3
    JILL A. BENNETT
2   Pressure Ulcer Prevention and Management   35
    COURTNEY H. LYDER
3   Pain in Older Adults   63
    LOIS L. MILLER AND KAREN AMANN TALERICO
4   Interventions for Persons with Irreversible Dementia   89
    SANDY C. BURGENER AND PRUDENCE TWIGG

Part II: Settings for Elder Care

5   Transitional Care of Older Adults   127
    MARY D. NAYLOR
6   Interventions for Family Members Caring for an Elder   149
      with Dementia
    GAYLE J. ACTON AND MARY A. WINTER
7   End-of-Life Care for Older Adults in ICUs   181
    JUDITH GEDNEY BAGGS
8   Nursing Homes and Assisted Living Facilities As Places   231
      for Dying
    JULIANA C. CARTWRIGHT

Part III: Public Health, Social, and Scientific Trends

9   Home Health Services Research   267
    ELIZABETH A. MADIGAN, SUSAN TULLAI-MCGUINNESS, AND
      DONNA FELBER NEFF
10 Telehealth Interventions to Improve Clinical Nursing   293
      of Elders
    JOSETTE F. JONES AND PATRICIA FLATLEY BRENNAN
11 Genetics and Gerontological Nursing: 323
      A Need to Stimulate Research
    LORRAINE FRAZIER AND SHARON K. OSTWALD

Part IV: Neglected Areas of Research in Gerontological Nursing

12 Hearing Impairment   341
    MARGARET I. WALLHAGEN
13 Elder Mistreatment   369
    TERRY FULMER

Index   397

Contents of Previous Volumes   415

Preface

This volume of the *Annual Review of Nursing Research* marks the conclusion of two decades of the *ARNR* series. Begun in 1983, under the visionary leadership of Harriet Werley, the Series has reflected the development of nursing science from infancy to its present maturity. During its 20-year history the Series has gone through three distinct phases. Early on, in Volumes 1 through 14, we included chapters in four key areas: clinical nursing, nursing care delivery, nursing education, and professional nursing issues. The second phase, Volumes 15 through 17, included research review chapters in two areas: clinical nursing and nursing care delivery. This change coincided with the development of a national research agenda focused principally on clinical nursing research. Beginning with Volume 18, the *ARNR* series moved to topic-focused volumes, with content experts serving as volume editors. Topic areas to include were selected in concert with representatives of the National Institutes of Health, National Institute of Nursing Research, and the *ARNR* series Advisory Board. Volume 18 focused on chronic illness; Volume 19 focused on women's health. These two recent volumes have been well received by the scientific community. Volume 20, focused on geriatric nursing research, is especially timely as attention to geriatric nursing care is increasing in both the development of our science and professional practice.

To mark the completion of two decades of publication, we will include a special chapter reviewing 10 years of the state of the science of nursing. This retrospective will appear in Volume 21.

We plan to dedicate future volumes to specific topics as well. Those content areas targeted for inclusion in future volumes include: nursing research on child health, vulnerable populations, and addictions. Within the next year, the Advisory Board members will seek additional input from the scientific community to determine future content areas.

This *ARNR* series is successful as a result of the contributions of several members of the nursing research community. First, I would like to thank the editors of Volume 20, Drs. Archbold, Stewart, and Lyons, for the excellent work included in this volume. They were able to draw on the expertise of their colleagues, many of whom contributed as reviewers, Volume 20 Advisory Committee members, and chapter authors. We owe a debt of thanks to all of these geriatric nurse experts for their individual and collective contributions to Volume 20.

I also wish to thank the Series Advisory Board members, some of whom are completing their term of service with the conclusion of Volume 20. Your advice and input over the years has been very valuable to me in my role as Series Editor. And, lastly, but importantly, I would like to acknowledge the publisher of the *ARNR* Series, Dr. Ursula Springer, and the Springer Editor, Ruth Chasek. Thank you for your assistance in advancing nursing research.

JOYCE J. FITZPATRICK, PhD, RN, FAAN
ARNR Series Editor

Introduction

It is timely for the *Annual Review of Nursing Research* series to focus on research in gerontological nursing for a number of reasons. As is now common knowledge, the actual number and relative percentage of elders are increasing rapidly throughout the world. The need for high-quality gerontological nursing care has never been as great as it is today—and this need will increase in the foreseeable future. A significant amount of research in specific areas of gerontological nursing—notably the management of common conditions in elders and settings of care—has been completed over the past two decades. Thus, it is a good time to look back at what has been done using systematic research syntheses to serve as a basis for our next steps. Current trends in public health and science call for rethinking traditional approaches to the care of elders by gerontological nurses. Finally, there are areas of research that, although acknowledged as important in gerontological nursing, have not received the attention they deserve from researchers. Volume 20, therefore, looks back to summarize our knowledge from research over the past two decades and looks forward by projecting new directions for gerontological nursing and gerontological nursing research.

For methods we leaned heavily on Cooper and Hedges (1994, p. 5) who state, "The integrative research review can be defined as the conjunction of a particular focus and goal: Research syntheses attempt to integrate empirical research for the purpose of creating generalizations. Implicit in this definition is the notion that seeking generalizations also involves seeking the limits and modifiers of generalizations." Cooper and Hedges' approach to problem formulation, data collection, data evaluation, analysis and interpretation was helpful in developing Volume 20 and specific chapters within it.

All chapters are organized around a question or set of questions that focused the review and synthesis. Each of the authors described his or her approach to selecting and reviewing the literature included in their review.

We wish to thank each of the authors of this volume. All are thoughtful scholars who were wonderful to work with.

To a great degree, the content of this volume was determined by the Volume 20 Advisory Committee. Members are experts in gerontological nursing, who have dedicated their careers to improving nursing care for older persons through research. We are indebted to Drs. Terry Fulmer, Jeannie Kayser-Jones, Toni Tripp-Reimer, and Thelma Wells for their wisdom, advice, and time. The Advisory Committee worked with us to identify topics and authors for chapters in this volume.

It is clear that gerontological nursing has reached a new stage of development. Two factors contributing to its maturation are the increase in well-trained gerontological nurse researchers and the boost in resources to the field from the John A. Hartford Foundation, Inc. For the past 6 years, the Hartford Institute of Geriatric Nursing at New York University has supported advanced research training for fellows and scholars in geriatric nursing in a Summer Institute. Three of the chapters in this volume were authored by Fellows in the Summer Institute (Drs. Bennett, Cartwright, and Wallhagen) and one by a Scholar (Dr. Miller).

This volume is presented in four parts: Managing Common Conditions in Elders; Settings for Elder Care; Public Health, Social and Scientific Trends; and Neglected Areas of Research in Gerontological Nursing. In Part I, Managing Common Conditions in Elders, four areas of research focus are included: maintaining and improving physical function (Bennett), pressure ulcer prevention and management (Lyder), pain in older adults (Miller & Talerico), and interventions to support persons with irreversible dementia (Burgener & Twigg). These content areas seemed ready for information synthesis, yet at the time we planned the volume, recent information syntheses had not been published. Recent reviews of research in important areas such as cognitive interventions among older adults (McDougall, 1999), health promotion in old age (Heidrich, 1998), and wandering in dementia (Algase, 1999) led to our decision not to include them. Part II includes research on Settings for Elder Care. In this section, chapters are focused on transitional care across care settings, in-home interventions for families caring for a person with dementia, and end-of-life care within two specific settings—intensive care units and nursing home and assisted living facilities. The research base in the areas of transitional care (Naylor) and interventions for family members caring for an elder with dementia in the home (Acton & Winter) is extensive. There has been little work in the area of end-of-life care in nursing homes and assisted living facilities (Cartwright), however. Likewise, despite a great deal of research on end-of-life care in ICUs, very little has focused on elders in these settings (Baggs). Part III includes chapters focused on public health, social, and scientific trends. Three chapters related to trends outside gerontological nursing that influence, or are expected to influence, gerontological nursing in the future are included. Madigan, Tullai-McGuinness, and Neff analyze the social and political trends that have shaped home health care in the past decade and identify critical areas for health services research. Jones and Brennan provide a research synthesis of telehealth interventions in gerontological nursing. Finally, Frazier and Ostwald discuss the potential impact of developments in genetics for gerontological nursing. Part IV includes two chapters focused on neglected areas of research in gerontological nursing—hearing impairment in elders (Wallhagen) and elder mistreatment (Fulmer). Both authors call for more nursing research in these areas.

In conclusion, we are impressed with the vast amount of gerontological nursing research that has been done in such a short span of time. There are many exciting findings summarized in the chapters that could influence practice, education, future research, and public policy. Although the volume reflects the breadth of gerontological nursing, many important areas of the field were not included—and remain to be summarized in a future volume of the *Annual Review*. The information syntheses included in the volume will assist future nurse researchers to gain insight into the state of the research and ways in which research can be strengthened (e.g., larger sample sizes, longitudinal research designs, better conceptualizations, theoretical paradigms, and movement toward interventions). The volume also highlights how much areas can overlap (e.g., pain and dementia), and this can be an enormous benefit in understanding complex problems. Finally, it is clear that much gerontological nursing research is interdisciplinary in nature, and much of the research summarized in the volume, because it is relevant to nursing, is based on findings from other disciplines. We hope that the volume will provide a foundation for moving forward in gerontological nursing research. Future nurse researchers will be able to build on what has been done and move forward with more rigorous methods, pushing the field forward into the new century.

Patricia G. Archbold
Barbara J. Stewart
Karen S. Lyons

Editors

REFERENCES

Algase, D. L. (1999). Wandering in dementia. In J. J. Fitzpatrick (Ed.), *Annual review of nursing research* (Vol. 18, pp. 185–218). New York: Springer Publishing Co.

Cooper, H., & Hedges, L. V. (1994). *The handbook of research synthesis.* New York: Russell Sage Foundation.

Heidrich, S. M. (1998). Health promotion in old age. In J. J. Fitzpatrick (Ed.), *Annual review of nursing research* (Vol. 17, pp. 173–196). New York: Springer Publishing Co.

McDougall, G. J. (1999). Cognitive interventions among older adults. In J. J. Fitzpatrick (Ed.), *Annual review of nursing research* (Vol. 18, pp. 219–240). New York: Springer Publishing Co.

Contributors

Gayle J. Acton, PhD, RN
Assistant Professor
School of Nursing
The University of Texas at Austin

Judith Gedney Baggs, PhD, RN
Associate Professor and Associate
    Dean for Academic Affairs
School of Nursing
University of Rochester

Jill A. Bennett, PhD, RN
Assistant Professor and Project
    Director
John A. Hartford Center of
    Geriatric Nursing Excellence
School of Nursing
University of California at San
    Francisco

**Patricia Flatley Brennan, PhD,
    RN, FAAN, FACMI**
Moehlman Bascom Professor
School of Nursing and College of
    Engineering
University of Wisconsin–Madison

Sandy C. Burgener, PhD, RNC
Associate Professor
College of Nursing at Urbana
University of Illinois

Juliana C. Cartwright, PhD, RN
Associate Professor
School of Nursing
Oregon Health & Science
    University

**Lorraine Frazier, DSN, RN,
    GNP**
Postdoctoral Fellow
Institute of Molecular Medicine
Associate Professor
School of Nursing
The University of Texas Health
    Science Center at Houston

Terry Fulmer, PhD, RN, FAAN
Professor
Co-director of the Hartford
    Institute for Geriatric Nursing
Division of Nursing
New York University

Josette F. Jones, RN
Doctoral Candidate
School of Nursing
University of Wisconsin–Madison

Courtney H. Lyder, ND, GNP, FAAN
Associate Professor
Director, Adult, Family,
    Gerontological, and Women's
    Health Division
School of Nursing
Yale University

Elizabeth A. Madigan, PhD, RNB
Associate Professor
Assistant Dean for International
    Health Programs
Frances Payne Bolton School of
    Nursing
Case Western Reserve University

Lois L. Miller, PhD, RN
Associate Professor and Scientist
School of Nursing
Oregon Health & Science
    University

Mary D. Naylor, PhD, FAAN
Marian S. Ware Professor in
    Gerontology
School of Nursing
University of Pennsylvania

Donna Felber Neff, PhD, RN
Assistant Professor
College of Nursing
University of Akron

Sharon K. Ostwald, PhD, RN, GNP
Professor and Isla Carroll Turner
    Chair in Gerontological
    Nursing
Director, Center on Aging
School of Nursing
University of Texas Health
    Science Center at Houston

Karen Amann Talerico, PhD, RN, CS
Assistant Professor and Scientist
School of Nursing
Oregon Health & Science
    University

Susan Tullai-McGuinness, MSN, MPA, RN
Doctoral Student and Project
    Manager
Frances Payne Bolton School of
    Nursing
Case Western Reserve University

Prudence Twigg, MS, RNC
Doctoral Student
School of Nursing
Indiana University at Indianapolis

Margaret I. Wallhagen, PhD, RN, CS, GNP
Associate Professor
Associate Director
John A. Hartford Foundation
    Center of Geriatric Nursing
    Excellence
School of Nursing
University of California at San
    Francisco

**Mary A. Winter, MSN, RN,
  LNFA**
Project Director
Caregiver Intervention Study
School of Nursing
The University of Texas at Austin

PART I

Managing Common Conditions in Elders

Chapter 1

Maintaining and Improving Physical Function in Elders

JILL A. BENNETT

ABSTRACT

This chapter reviews 60 published research reports about maintaining and improving physical function in elders. Reports were identified through searches of MEDLINE and CINAHL using the following search terms: *Activities of Daily Living, aged, nursing care, nurse-patient relations, geriatric nursing, nursing assessment, geriatric assessment, behavior therapy, disability evaluation, exercise,* and *physical.* Reports were included if published in English between 1985 and 2000, if conducted in adults over age 60, and if the first author was a nurse or the reported intervention was implemented by nurses. Descriptive and experimental studies of physical function in elders were included. The results of this synthesis showed that nurse scientists have developed new instruments to measure physical function, including scales sensitive to changes in physical function caused by dementia. Nursing studies have described many of the physical and psychological factors associated with poor physical function in elders, though environmental factors and ethnic differences in physical function merit further study. Many nurse scientists are currently investigating behavioral interventions, exercise interventions, and changes in nursing care that could improve the physical function of both community-dwelling elders and those who live in residential facilities.

Keywords: aged, activities of daily living, functional status, disability

Physical function in elders is usually defined as ability to perform Activities of Daily Living (ADL), such as bathing, dressing, toileting, feeding, and

3

transferring from a bed or chair. Physical function can also be measured by mobility tasks, such as walking, stooping, reaching, or climbing stairs. In independent elders—those who can perform all ADL independently— physical function may be measured by Instrumental Activities of Daily Living (IADL), which include telephoning, managing money, shopping, housekeeping, and managing medications. The common factor underlying these different definitions of physical function is that all are measured by a person's ability to perform tasks that require physical strength and/ or dexterity.

Many elders have chronic medical conditions that lead to poor physical function (National Academy on an Aging Society, 1999). Approximately 11% of adults over age 85 receive help with two or more ADL, and many (79%) of those needing help are elderly women (Kassner & Bectel, 1998). This group of "oldest old," now about 4 million people, is growing rapidly. By 2050, there will be 18 million Americans over age 85 and many will be older women with chronic conditions, little money, and poor physical function that is not sufficient to maintain safety, independence, or good quality of life without assistance (Rice, 2001).

There is little doubt that poor physical function has adverse consequences for each elder, for his or her family, and for the community. An elder who is unable to function independently may suffer a loss of self-esteem (Blair, 1999), or may be more socially isolated than if he or she were mobile (Simonsick, Kasper, & Phillips, 1998). Families often bear the burden of care if an elder needs help with ADL and remains at home; 67% of low-functioning elders rely completely on unpaid caregivers, mostly wives or daughters (Kassner & Bectel, 1998). Difficulty with ADL is a common reason for entering a long-term care facility; 96% of people who enter nursing homes need help with bathing and 87% need help with dressing (Kassner & Bectel, 1998). Transitioning to a long-term care facility is not only emotionally difficult for an elder, it is very expensive for the individual, family, and community.

Physical function is measured by an individual's ability to perform ADL, IADL, or mobility tasks. Poor physical function may be an acute, temporary result of an illness or other stressful event or, in contrast, physical function may decline slowly, a result of frailty, chronic medical conditions, or dementia. Prevention of decline in physical function should be part of routine health maintenance for elders, and nurses are often in a position to notice and intervene when an elder's physical or cognitive health is changing. Thus, nurse clinicians and scientists are interested in precise methods for assessing physical function and efficacious interventions to maintain or improve physical function in elders.

The purpose of this chapter is to review the nursing research literature devoted to physical function in elders. The methods for the review are described and the findings from nursing research studies are synthesized to answer five questions that are critical to understanding the ways in which nurses can help elders maintain or improve physical function,

1.   How is physical function conceptualized?
2.   How is physical function measured?
3.   What personal, environmental, and psychological factors are associated with poor physical function in elders?
4.   How does nursing care affect physical function in elders?
5.   What nursing interventions are effective for maintaining or improving physical function in independent elders and in elders who are dependent on caregivers?

METHOD

For this review of the literature, physical function was defined as ability to perform ADL, IADL, and mobility tasks such as walking, climbing stairs, stooping, reaching, and other similar tasks. Therefore, other concepts that are sometimes called measures of function were not included in this review, such as number of falls, cognitive function, and various physiological functions such as cardiac function. In order to synthesize the knowledge about physical function that was applicable to the largest population of elders, the review focused on the gradual changes in physical function that occur in elders with chronic medical conditions, dementia, or sedentary lifestyle, rather than temporary, short-term loss of physical function due to hospitalization, recovery from surgery, or acute illness.

The primary purpose of the search of the literature was to identify studies of physical function in elders that were designed by nurse scientists. Research articles published from 1985-2000 were reviewed for this chapter. The searches were conducted with sets of Medical Subject Headings (MeSH) terms in MEDLINE and the Cumulative Index of Nursing and Allied Health (CINAHL). Each set of terms was searched first in nursing journals, and second in nonnursing journals, if the first author had an affiliation with a school of nursing. All MeSH terms were prefixed with

SU (subject) so the search would identify articles in which the term was designated as a major topic of the article. A base set of terms was searched first: "SU *Activities of Daily Living* and SU *aged*." Subsequent searches were conducted with sets to which one of the following terms was added to the base set: (a) *nursing care*, (b) *nurse-patient relations*, (c) *geriatric nursing*, (d) *nursing assessment*, (e) *geriatric assessment*, (f) *behavior therapy*, (g) *disability evaluation*, (h) *exercise*, and (i) *physical*. Terms (h) and (i) were prefixed with KW (keyword) rather than SU, because they were not MeSH terms. Terms (e), (f), and (g) were also searched in nonnursing journals with authors who did not have a school of nursing affiliation; articles from this search were retrieved for review if the study abstract described nursing interventions, even if the authors were not nurses.

The search process identified approximately 900 article abstracts. Articles were included in this synthesis if the research was about changes in long-term physical function in elders and the first author of the article was a nurse. Articles were also included if the study evaluated an intervention to improve physical function that was implemented by nurses, even if the authors were not nurses, because such studies add to knowledge about nursing care and nursing interventions. During the process of reading abstracts and articles, the decision was made to include articles by nurses about exercise and physical activity in elders, even if outcomes were not measured in terms of ADL, IADL, or mobility tasks. The rationale for the decision to expand the focus of the synthesis was the realization that many nurses were adding to knowledge about physical activity and exercise in elders and eliminating these articles would leave out an important area of research that is very closely related to physical function. Abstracts were excluded if they were duplicates, if the definition of function was not ADL, IADL, or mobility, or if loss of physical function was a temporary condition resulting from surgery, hospitalization, or acute illness. After reviewing the abstracts, a final sample of 60 studies was read and synthesized.

The sample contained studies about physical function and physical activity in elders. The age ranges of the study participants were as broad as 33–91 (Oka, Gortner, Stotts, & Haskell, 1996) or 40–84 (Narsavage & Weaver, 1994; Weaver & Narsavage, 1992), though most studies were of individuals over age 60. The studies with wider age ranges were included in the review if the participants in those studies suffered from chronic conditions common in elders, and if the study samples included many individuals over age 60.

RESULTS AND DISCUSSION

How Is Physical Function Conceptualized?

The study of physical function as a separate concept, rather than as a simple clinical measurement, is relatively new in all health fields. Though the first measurement tools for ADL were designed in the 1960s, for many years their use was limited to that of a clinical measure used by health providers to rate the activity level of institutionalized patients (Katz, Ford, Moskowitz, Jackson, & Jaffe, 1963). Gradually, clinicians recognized the need to measure function in independent adults who were managing chronic conditions, and the ADL tools were used to ask patients about their own perceptions of difficulty in functional tasks. Since the 1980s, new self-report tools have been developed that purport to measure physical function either as a global concept that is experienced similarly by all elders, or as a concept that varies according to the presence of a particular chronic condition. In the 1990s, new conceptual models, such as The Disablement Process (Verbrugge & Jette, 1994), were developed that included individual and environmental predictors of decline in function. Because these models do not assume that age or physical health are the only factors that affect physical function, they are appropriate frameworks for nursing studies that investigate the personal, environmental, or social reasons for changes in physical function.

Nurse scientists have also developed theoretical models of physical function that contribute to interdisciplinary knowledge. Leidy developed a model of functional status, defined as ability to perform normal activities, with four dimensions: capacity, performance, reserve, and capacity utilization. This model has not only clarified the dimensions that should be measured as outcomes in studies, but also the distinct measures that should be used to assess each dimension. The model is applicable to elders with chronic conditions and it has been used in studies to differentiate the functional outcomes of patients with chronic obstructive pulmonary disease (Leidy, 1994, 1999).

Rush and Ouellet (Ouellet & Rush, 1996; Rush & Ouellet, 1998) have initiated the development of a conceptual model of physical function for nursing assessment by comparing the perceptions of nurses and elders about the underlying dimensions of mobility. A theoretical model of mobility with four dimensions—physical, cognitive, emotional, and social—was tested in qualitative interviews with nurses and elders: In the physical dimension, a person's movement or physiology affects mobility; in the cognitive dimension, the person's coping with the environment affects mobility; in the emotional dimension, the person's inner resources allow him/her to manage stress and maintain mobility; and in the social dimension, the person's ability to manage social interactions affects mobility. Study results showed that both nurses and elderly residents described the physical, cognitive, and social dimensions of mobility, but neither the nurses nor the residents perceived an emotional dimension of mobility. This exploratory study may be a first step in the development of a theory of physical function that relates specifically to nursing practice.

How Is Physical Function Measured?

Physical function in elders has been traditionally measured by ADL or IADL questions that are answered by the elder, or rated by a health care provider (McDowell & Newell, 1996; Pearson, 2000). The physical function of nursing home residents is usually rated by nursing aides, whose ratings have been shown to correlate with those of nurse practitioners (Hartig, Engle, & Graney, 1997). However, it is possible that both nurse practitioners and nursing aides may perceive an individual's function differently than does the individual himself or herself. Thus, it is possible that the concept of poor physical function is different when it is measured by self-report of the elder than when it is measured by the rating of a nurse or aide. Nursing studies that explore this issue were done in nursing homes, where many residents have difficulty with ADL. One survey of residents and nurses found that there was considerable agreement on the rating of each resident's need for assistance in ADL, though there were differences in two of the ADL tasks; residents thought they needed more help with bathing and less help with grooming than did nurses (Lindgren & Linton, 1991). It is possible that these differences were due to different interpretations of "assistance," rather than to different perceptions of each resident's physical function. This study illustrates how difficult it is to accurately measure physical function when the related concepts, such as assistance, have not been clearly defined.

Measuring physical function in some elders is more complicated than simply measuring ADL and IADL. For example, different measures of physical function may be needed for patients with dementia who cannot report changes in their ability to perform ADL. A traditional ADL scale in which a nurse rates a patient as either "needs assistance" or "independent" for each task may be sufficient if the purpose of the functional assessment is to plan for level of care, but a more sensitive scale is needed to measure the small changes in physical function that occur with the progression of dementia (Patterson et al., 1992). Nurses have developed scales that break the ADL tasks into smaller measurable parts that are more precise for measuring changes in physical function due to dementia. For example, The Beck Dressing Performance Scale (Beck, 1988) measures seven distinct levels of caregiver assistance for each of 45 separate steps of dressing. A similar approach was used to develop The Refined ADL Scale for patients with dementia (Tappen, 1994a), which measures 14 tasks within the 5 traditional ADL tasks. This scale also specifically defines level of assistance in terms of verbal, nonverbal, and physical levels of assistance. Likewise, The Cleveland Scale for Activities of Daily Living (Patterson et al., 1992) includes 16 tasks, some broken down into component behaviors, for a total of 66 items. This scale is designed to be sensitive to changes in physical function caused by progression of dementia, even in elders who are in the early stages of dementia and still living at home.

Nurses have also explored the problem of measuring physical function in elders who live in the community. The traditional ADL and IADL scales have ceiling effects with this population, because high functioning elders adapt to early functional changes and thus report no difficulty, even if physical function has declined. Leidy and Haase (Leidy, 1994, 1999; Leidy & Haase, 1996) addressed this issue by developing a model of functional status that differentiates between the maximum functional capacity of which a person is capable, and the functional performance that the person chooses to do. The Functional Performance Inventory was designed to specifically measure the performance dimension of this model (Leidy & Haase, 1999). Porter (1995) has suggested that ADL and IADL scales may not reflect the lived experience of older women and thus phenomenological inquiry may be better than traditional ADL for understanding the physical function of women.

Some nurses have suggested that the physical function of independent elders may be measured better by performance tests of function than by self-report of the elder (Bennett, 1999) or by a variety of functional assessments, including both performance and self-report (Brown, 1988). Kinugasa and Nagasaki (1998) developed a self-report instrument, The Motor Fitness Scale, that measures motor capability by asking questions that are similar to the tasks in a performance test. Another scale designed to screen independent elders for functional decline combines questions about household ability (HHA) with ADL questions. Examples of HHA questions are "Are you able to make a bed?" or "Are you able to do the laundry?" The seven HHA questions ask about "ability" and the six ADL questions ask about the need for help (Frederiks, te Wierik, Visser, & Sturmans, 1991).

In summary, nurses have designed a variety of measures that target different issues in the assessment of physical function in elders, such as the small changes in task performance that occur as dementia progresses or the problems associated with measuring physical function in independent elders. However, there are few studies reported in the literature that actually used these nurse-designed measures in research or clinical practice. To ascertain whether these measures are valid, reliable, and precise measures of physical function, it would be helpful if nurses conducting descriptive and experimental studies adopted some of these new measures and reported on their utility for research and clinical practice. Instead, most nursing studies use the traditional ADL and IADL measures of physical function.

What Factors Are Associated with Poor Physical Function in Elders?

An elder's physical function may be determined by personal characteristics, such as the presence of chronic medical conditions, motivation, perception of ability, and other factors. In addition to personal characteristics, environmental factors may affect physical function. For example, the arrangement of an elder's furniture, or the elder's ability to acquire assistive devices may affect performance of ADL.

In the last 10 years, researchers in many disciplines have worked to identify the factors associated with poor physical function in elders. Studies by nurse researchers who have contributed to the scientific knowledge in this area are shown in Table 1.1. Most nursing studies identified factors that could cause poor function in elders who lived in the community, though three articles reported on difficulty in ADL in nursing home residents (Engle & Graney, 1995; Marx, Werner, Cohen-Mansfield, & Feldman, 1992; Stegbauer, Engle, & Graney, 1995).

All nursing studies of factors associated with poor physical function used descriptive, cross-sectional designs that were appropriate to identify

TABLE 1.1   Factors Associated with Poor Physical Function in Elders: Nursing Studies 1985–2000

Study	Methods	Selected findings relevant to identifying risk factors for poor function in elders
Belza, B. L., Henke, C. J., Yelin, E. H., Epstein, W. V., & Gilliss, C. L. (1993).	Design: Descriptive Measure of function: HAQ (McDowell & Newell, 1996) Sample: 133 community-living elders age 56–86 75% female, 84% White	Poor function associated with fatigue
Dayhoff, N. E., Suhrheinrich, J., Wigglesworth, J., Topp, R., & Moore, S. (1998).	Design: Descriptive Measure of function: WHO Assessment of Functional Capacity (Ferrucci, L., Guralnik, J. M., Baroni, A., Tesi, G., Antonini, E., & Marchionni, N., 1991). Sample: 84 community-living elders age 60–88 86% female, ethnicity not reported	Poor function associated with • poor balance • poor dorsiflexion strength Balance and strength were not associated with age in this sample.
Duffy, M. E., & MacDonald, E. (1990).	Design: Descriptive Measure of function: OMFAQ (McDowell & Newell, 1996) Sample: 179 community-living elders aged 65–99 56% female, 76% White	Poor function associated with • older age • low income • low perceived health • others control of health • poor nutrition

(continued)

TABLE 1.1   *(continued)*

Study	Methods	Selected findings relevant to identifying risk factors for poor function in elders
Engle, V. F., & Graney, M. J. (1995).	Design: Descriptive Measure of function: ADL reported by nursing assistants Sample: 358 nursing home residents mean age approx. 81 (range not reported) 100% female, 73% White	Black women had lower ADL function on admittance to nursing home. White women improved in hygiene and dressing after admittance to nursing home, but Black women's ADL remained stable.
Martin, J. C. (1996).	Design: Descriptive Measure of function: Arthritis Impact Measurement Scales 2 (AIMS2) (McDowell & Newell, 1996) and a timed 8-foot walk Sample: 100 community-living elders age 60–92 100% female, 100% Black	Black women's scores on AIMS2 and 8-foot walk were correlated. In Black women, depression and number of arthritic joints were strongly associated with AIMS2 score.
Marx, M. S., Werner, P., Cohen-Mansfield, J., & Feldman, R. (1992).	Design: Descriptive Measure of function: ADL Sample: 103 nursing home residents age 66–98 80% female, ethnicity not reported	Elders with poor vision were significantly worse than those with good vision in • toileting • transferring • washing • dressing

TABLE 1.1 *(continued)*

Study	Methods	Selected findings relevant to identifying risk factors for poor function in elders
Narsavage, G. L., & Weaver, T. E. (1994).	Design: Descriptive Measure of function: Pulmonary Functional Status Scale (by the authors) Sample: 96 community-living elders age 40–84 18% female, 92% White	Poor function associated with • low exercise capacity • low hardiness (commitment component)
Oka, R. K., Gortner, S. R., Stotts, N. A., & Haskell, W. L. (1996).	Design: Descriptive Measure of function: Duke Activity Status Index (Hlatky et al., 1989) Sample: 43 community-living elders with heart failure age 33–91 19% female, 56% White	Poor function was associated with low self-efficacy.
Stegbauer, C. C., Engle, V. F., & Graney, M. J. (1995).	Design: Descriptive Measure of function: ADL reported by nursing assistants Sample: 134 newly admitted nursing home residents mean age 80 (range not reported) 71% female, 40% White	Blacks had lower levels of self-care ADL. Blacks and Whites had similar levels of mobility ADL.

(continued)

TABLE 1.1   *(continued)*

Study	Methods	Selected findings relevant to identifying risk factors for poor function in elders
Weaver, T. E., & Narsavage, G. L. (1992).	Design: Descriptive Measure of function: Pulmonary Functional Status Scale (by the authors) Sample: 104 community-living elders age 40–84 18% female, 92% White	Poor function associated with • asking "why me?" • low exercise capacity • depression
Weaver, T. E., Richmond, T. S., & Narsavage, G. L. (1997).	Design: Descriptive Measure of function: Pulmonary Functional Status Scale (by the authors) Sample: 104 community-living elders age 40–84 18% female, 92% White	Poor function associated with • low exercise capacity • dyspnea • depressed mood • anxiety • low self-esteem
Yu, S. (1995).	Design: Descriptive Measure of function: a questionnaire by the authors, not included in article Sample: 247 community-living elders age > 65 (range not reported) 47% female, study conducted in Taiwan, but ethnicity of sample not reported	Poor function associated with • low physical activity • chronic diseases • older age • high need for health care

Note. OMFAQ = Older Americans Resources and Services Multidimensional Functional Assessment Questionnaire; ADL = activities of daily living; HAQ = Health Assessment Questionnaire; WHO = World Health Organization.

associations, but not sufficient to establish causality. Factors that were associated with poor function were older age (Duffy & MacDonald, 1990; Yu, 1995), chronic disease (Yu, 1995), dyspnea (Weaver, Richmond, & Narsavage, 1997), poor vision (Marx et al., 1992), and poor balance and muscle strength (Dayhoff, Suhrheinrich, Wigglesworth, Topp, & Moore, 1998). Some factors associated with poor physical function could be either a cause or an outcome of difficulty with functional tasks, such as low level of physical activity (Yu, 1995), low exercise capacity (Narsavage & Weaver, 1994; Oka, Gortner, Stotts, & Haskell, 1996; Weaver & Narsavage, 1992; Weaver et al., 1997), and poor nutrition (Duffy & MacDonald, 1990).

Nurse researchers have also identified psychological factors associated with poor physical function, such as depression (Martin, 1996; Weaver & Narsavage, 1992; Weaver et al., 1997), fatigue (Belza, Henke, Yelin, Epstein, & Gilliss, 1993), low self-efficacy (Oka et al., 1996), low self-esteem and anxiety (Weaver et al., 1997), low hardiness (Narsavage & Weaver, 1994), and lack of control over health and low perceived health (Duffy & MacDonald, 1990). However, it is also possible that some or all of these psychological factors were outcomes, rather than causes, of poor physical function. Therefore, testing these associations in longitudinal studies or nursing intervention studies would be a useful future direction for nurse scientists. Such studies could establish the causes for poor physical function that are amenable to nursing interventions.

Some gaps in nursing knowledge about the factors associated with poor physical function may point the way toward useful areas for new research. Though the earliest nursing study reviewed here (Duffy & MacDonald, 1990) showed that low income was associated with poor physical function, no other nursing studies have identified environmental factors associated with physical function. For example, living in a second-story apartment or a dangerous neighborhood may restrict an individual's mobility, leading to decline in physical function due to lack of physical activity. Though researchers in other disciplines have studied the association between environment and physical function in elders, nurses could make important contributions to knowledge of environments surrounding nursing care, such as the noise in nursing homes that prevents sleep, resulting in tiredness that affects physical function.

There is a need for more research on ethnic and cultural influences on physical function in elders. Nurse researchers have found that African American nursing home residents had poorer physical function than White residents (Engle & Graney, 1995; Stegbauer et al., 1995). Martin (1996) has reported on the cultural determinants of physical function in low-income African American women with osteoarthritis. However, nursing research into ethnic factors in physical function should be expanded to increase knowledge about elders who are members of other ethnic populations that are increasing rapidly. For example, the Latino population over age 65 is growing 5 times faster than the White population over age 65 (National Center for Health Statistics, 1999). Thus, it is essential to understand any differences in functional ability, perceptions of function, and risk factors that affect Latinos, African Americans, Asians, and other ethnic groups. Some nursing studies reviewed for this paper did not report the ethnicity of the participants. This information should be considered essential in any nursing research report in the future. Until these data are part of the nursing knowledge about function in elders, nurses cannot design interventions that will be useful to maintain or improve physical function in elders of all ethnicities.

How Does Nursing Care Affect Physical Function in Elders?

Physical function in elders who are hospitalized or who live in an institutional setting may be affected not only by personal and environmental factors, but also by the nursing care they receive. Nurse researchers have explored ways of understanding which functional tasks are most difficult, when and how the nursing staff should offer assistance, and how to encourage elders' autonomy and independence in functional tasks. Nursing research on these issues reflects one of the core perspectives of the discipline of nursing; that the purpose of knowledge development is to shape nursing practice to empower individuals to care for themselves, thereby encouraging self-respect, autonomy, and well-being (Meleis, 1997). Thus, this particular group of studies reflects the unique perspective of nursing within the interdisciplinary field of research on physical function and these studies may lead directly to changes in clinical nursing practice.

In other disciplines, most research on physical function focuses on the self-care ADL or mobility tasks. In contrast, some nurse researchers have attempted to determine which specific parts of each ADL task are most difficult for frail or dependent elders. The goal of the research is to determine when assistance is needed and when an individual may be able to function independently. For example, one research team found that in the dressing task, residents reported having the most difficulty tying shoelaces, fastening pants, and buttoning shirts. In grooming, residents reported the most difficult areas were applying toothpaste and combing hair at the top and back of the head. Other ADL tasks were analyzed in a similar manner (Johnson, Stone, Larson, & Hromek, 1992). Descriptive studies such as this provide the groundwork for intervention studies of how and when nursing staff should offer assistance, which are discussed later in this chapter.

Nursing care may affect physical function in elders by causing individuals to give up individual control over their performance of tasks. One qualitative study of nursing home residents found that elders performed ADL tasks, but not to the full extent of their abilities. When asked why, residents expressed frustration at not knowing about scheduling and not being able to anticipate the timing of care events. They also reported that they could not predict each time whether the nurse would perform the ADL or the resident him- or herself would be expected to do it. Residents also perceived that nurse permission was necessary before proceeding with ADL (Brubaker, 1996). These findings suggest that individual control over the timing of ADL and ability to choose to perform ADL may be important determinants of level of physical function in residents of nursing homes.

What Nursing Interventions Are Effective for Maintaining or Improving Physical Function?

The nursing literature contains many descriptive studies that have identified important risk factors for poor physical function in elders, but nurses have conducted few studies to test interventions to prevent decline in physical function. More nursing intervention studies directed at maintaining or improving physical function in elders were published after 1993 ($n = 9$) than from 1985–1993 ($n = 4$). The number of nursing intervention studies may increase and it is likely that those studies will test interventions to address the factors associated with poor physical function that were identified in earlier descriptive studies.

Descriptive studies conducted by nurses have shown that individual factors and psychological factors may be associated with poor physical function in elders. No nursing intervention studies were found that addressed these risk factors. Descriptive studies have also shown that nursing care, such as the timing and type of assistance offered to residents of nursing homes, may affect physical function. Nursing interventions in staff behavior and changes to nursing care have been tested and reported. Published nursing intervention studies, shown in Table 1.2, generally fall into three categories: behavioral interventions, exercise interventions and strategies, and evaluations of multifactorial programs to improve function. Table 1.2 includes some studies conducted by researchers who are not nurses, but whose findings are important to nursing knowledge because the researchers evaluated functional outcomes of interventions conducted by nurses. The studies conducted by nurse researchers are labeled "nurse researcher" in order to identify knowledge developed within the discipline of nursing.

Nursing studies conducted in nursing homes have focused on behavioral strategies to improve physical function in residents. Blair, Lewis, Vieweg, and Tucker (Blair, 1995; Blair et al., 1996) found that training nursing home staff in behavior management skills, such as prompting, shaping, and positive reinforcement, improved the ADL performance of cognitively intact residents who were cared for by trained staff. Though this behavioral intervention was aimed at nursing staff, behavioral techniques to improve physical function have also been applied directly to elders with dementia. For example, Tappen's (1994b) research on improving physical function in nursing home residents with dementia demonstrated that daily practice of ADL, guided by minimal help from nursing assistants, significantly improved ADL performance measured by a rating scale (presumably completed by staff or research assistants), but did not improve ADL performance measured by a test in which residents actually performed the tasks. This paradoxical finding may have been caused by the measurement methods, each of which measured different tasks. Behavioral techniques to improve the dressing skills of elders with dementia were also tested by Beck and colleagues (1991; 1997), who showed that individualized prescriptions for minimal assistance, behavior and communication strategies, and problem solving strategies, all administered by trained nursing assistants, improved dressing skills in cognitively impaired nursing home residents and home care clients.

Nursing studies have shown that personal characteristics, such as balance, muscle strength, level of physical activity, and exercise capacity were associated with level of physical function in elders. Even so, few nurses have measured ADL or IADL outcomes in their exercise intervention studies, though some have reported outcomes that are similar to

TABLE 1.2   Interventions to Maintain or Improve Physical Function in Elders: Selected Research Studies 1985–2000

Study	Methods	Selected findings relevant to maintaining and improving function in elders
Beck, C., Heacock, P., Mercer, S., Walton, C. G., & Shook, J. (1991). nurse researcher	Design: Descriptive Measure of function: Dressing Sample: 5 elders with Alzheimer's in home setting and 16 elders with Alzheimer's in nursing home	Elders with dementia needed less assistance in dressing after their caregivers implemented behavioral strategies.
Beck, C., Heacock, P., Mercer, S. O., Walls, R. C., Rapp, C. G., & Vogelpohl, T. S. (1997). nurse researcher	Design: Quasi-experimental Measure of function: Beck Dressing Performance Scale (Beck, 1988) Sample: 90 residents of nursing homes age 60–100, 83% female, 83% White Intervention: Behavioral Strategies to Promote Independence in Dressing (SPID)	Cognitively impaired residents improved independence (needed less assistance dressing) after 6 weeks.
Blair, C. E. (1995). nurse researcher	Design: Experimental Measure of function: ADL Sample: • Nursing Home 1: Staff trained in behavior modification and goal setting • Nursing Home 2: Staff trained in goal setting only • Nursing Home 3: Routine care	Residents in Nursing Homes 1 and 2 improved their ADL compared with nursing home 3. Only residents in Nursing Home 1 retained ADL skills in follow-up period (an additional 8 weeks).

(continued)

TABLE 1.2 *(continued)*

Study	Methods	Selected findings relevant to maintaining and improving function in elders
Blair, C. E., Lewis, R., Vieweg, V., & Tucker, R. (1996). nurse researcher	Design: Experimental Measure of function: ADL Sample: 15 residents of a nursing home age 64–96, 73% female, and staff caring for them • T1: Staff trained in behavior modification and goal setting • T2: Staff trained in goal setting only • C: Routine care	T1 improved in ADL compared with T2 and C.
Bula, C. J., Berod, A. C., Stuck, A. E., Alessi, C. A., Aronow, H. R., Santos-Eggimann, B., Rubenstein, L. Z., & Beck, J. C. (1999).	Design: Randomized controlled trial Measure of function: ADL Sample: 414 community-living elders age 75+, 68% female • T: Annual preventive in-home geriatric assessment, with quarterly visits by gerontologic nurse practitioners for 3 years • C: usual care	Subgroup analysis of subjects without ADL impairment at baseline showed that T spent fewer days dependent in ADL than did C during the 3 years.

TABLE 1.2 *(continued)*

Study	Methods	Selected findings relevant to maintaining and improving function in elders
Dungan, J. M., Brown, A. V., & Ramsey, M. A. (1996). nurse researcher	Design: Descriptive Measure of physical well-being: hand strength, ROM, and BP sample: 44 community-living elders age 61–93 66% female, 46% White, 36% Japanese, 12% Chinese Intervention: 6 months of health program that included support groups, teaching, exercise	• Systolic BP improved. • Diastolic BP did not improve. • ROM in right ankle improved. • Hand strength did not improve.
Garrard, J., Kane, R. L., Radosevich, D. M., Skay, C. L., Arnold, S., Kepferle, L., Mc-Dermott, S., & Buchanan, J. L. (1990).	Design: Quasi-experimental Measure of function: ADL Sample: • T: 525 residents in 5 nursing homes with a GNP • C: 323 residents in 5 nursing homes without a GNP	There were no differences in ADL between T and C.
Kane, R. L., Garrard, J., Skay, C. L., Radosevich, D. M., Buchanan, J. L., McDermott, S. M., Arnold, S. B., & Kepferle, L. (1989).	Design: Quasi-experimental Measure of function: ADL Sample: • T: 30 nursing homes with geriatric nurse practitioner (GNP) • C: 30 control nursing homes with no GNP	Compared with C, T improved transferring and dressing, but did not improve ambulation, feeding, or toileting.

(continued)

TABLE 1.2 *(continued)*

Study	Methods	Selected findings relevant to maintaining and improving function in elders
Mills, E. M. (1994). nurse researcher	Design: Experimental Measures: Muscle strength, flexibility, and balance Sample: • T: 20 community-living elders age 65–88, 100% female, attended classes of strengthening and stretching lower extremities • C: 27 community-living elders age 65–88, 97% female, did not exercise	T improved flexibility compared with C. No difference between T and C in balance or muscle strength.
Roberts, B. L. (1990). nurse researcher	Design: Quasi-experimental Measure of function: Reaction time and movement Sample: • T: 31 community-living elders mean age 71. 8 (range not reported) 84% female, ethnicity not reported, walked for exercise • C: 30 community-living elders mean age 71. 8 (range not reported) 87% female, did not exercise	No differences in reaction time or movement between T and C.

TABLE 1.2 *(continued)*

Study	Methods	Selected findings relevant to maintaining and improving function in elders
Tappen, R. M. (1994b) nurse researcher	Design: Experimental Measure of function: The Physical Self-Maintenance Scale (McDowell & Newell, 1996) and a performance test of ADL Sample: 63 elders with dementia who resided in a nursing home, age 59–102 75% female • T 1: Daily practice of ADL • T 2: General stimulation playing recreational games such as ball toss • C: usual care	T 1 improved scores on the Physical Self-Maintenance Scale compared with C, but T 2 was not significantly different from C. There was no difference between T 1, T 2, and C on the ADL performance test.
Topp, R., & Stevenson, J. S. (1994). nurse researcher	Design: Quasi-experimental Measure of Function: Cycle exercise test Sample: 66 community-living elders age 60–81 attended 9 mos. of cycle exercise classes. Gender and ethnicity not reported • Group 1: above-average attendance and effort during exercise sessions • Group 2: below-average attendance and effort during exercise sessions	• VO2max improved in both groups, groups not significantly different. • Maximum exercise improved in both groups. Group 1 improved significantly more than Group 2. • Maximum workload improved in both groups. Group 1 improved significantly more than Group 2.

Note. T = treatment group; C = control group; ADL = activities of daily living; GNP = geriatric nurse practitioner; ROM = range of motion; BP = blood pressure.

measures of physical function, such as improved exercise capacity (Topp & Stevenson, 1994; Potempa et al., 1995), improved flexibility and balance (Mills, 1994), and reaction time and movement (Roberts, 1990).

Though ADL, IADL, and mobility outcomes have not been included in many exercise studies, nurse researchers are making important additions to knowledge about exercise. Gueldner and colleagues (1997) have studied the association between immune function and long-term exercise, and Talbot, Metter, and Fleg (2000) have reported a relationship between physical activity and cardiorespiratory fitness. Potempa and colleagues (1995) showed that endurance exercise improved maximal oxygen consumption in hemiparetic individuals. Other nurse scientists have added to our understanding about why elders do or don't exercise (Conn, 1998a; McBride, 1994; Melillo et al., 1996; Lucas, Orshan, & Cook, 2000), the association of self-efficacy with exercise behavior (Conn, 1998b; Resnick, 1999b; Resnick & Jenkins, 2000; Resnick, Palmer, Jenkins, & Spellbring, 2000; Resnick, 2000) and ethnic differences in exercise beliefs (Jones & Nies, 1996; Laffrey, 2000; Brady & Nies, 1999; Gonzalez & Jirovec, 2001). Understanding why people exercise and demonstrating the benefits of regular physical activity for elders is an important area of research in nursing and other disciplines. However, there is little empirical evidence in the current nursing literature for an association between an exercise intervention and improvement in physical function in elders. This knowledge gap could be filled if nurse researchers included measures of function, such as ADL, IADL, or mobility tasks, in exercise studies along with other outcomes of interest.

Researchers who implemented multifactorial intervention programs to prevent functional decline in residents of nursing homes have reported mixed results. For example, one study showed no improvement in the ADL function of nursing home residents after a geriatric nurse practitioner (GNP) was added to the staff (Garrard et al., 1990). Another study showed that residents improved transferring and dressing skills when a GNP was on the staff, though they did not improve in ambulation, feeding, or toileting (Kane et al., 1989).

Some researchers have evaluated the role of multifactorial intervention programs in preventing functional decline in community-dwelling elders. A study that evaluated an annual in-home geriatric assessment by a GNP found that elders who had no ADL difficulties, but some IADL difficulties, at baseline were more likely to remain free of ADL difficulties 3 years later than were elders without the annual assessment. However, there was no significant benefit of the annual assessment for elders who had no ADL or IADL impairment at baseline (Bula et al., 1999). Another community-based program showed an improvement only in right ankle range-of-motion after 6 months of participation in a multifactorial health program that included support groups run by nurses or social workers, exercise classes, and health education groups (Dungan, Brown, & Ramsey, 1996).

These studies showed that only small improvements in physical function resulted from nurse-centered multifactorial programs focused on improving physical function in nursing home residents and community-living elders. Because these programs were each different in approach, it is difficult to synthesize the knowledge gained from these studies. However, they are included here because these studies are among the few that evaluate the influence of the GNP and/or nursing care in preserving physical function in elders. Because the roles of nurses were different in each program, and each program had different effects on physical function, these studies are not adequate evidence for or against the ability of GNPs or nurses to affect physical function within a multifactorial program.

The most clinically relevant nursing intervention studies have been done in behavioral techniques to improve ADL function in patients with dementia (Beck et al., 1991; Beck et al., 1997; Tappen, 1994b) and there is also potential for the use of behavioral techniques to improve the physical function of cognitively intact nursing home residents (Blair, 1995; Blair et al., 1996). Exercise interventions may improve physical function in active elders, but many exercise studies by nurses have not measured functional outcomes, such as ADL, IADL, or mobility tasks. Evaluations of the effect of GNPs and nurses in multifactorial programs are few and it is difficult to distinguish whether the nurses or the program designs have been the cause of the small improvements in physical function of the participants in those studies.

CONCLUSIONS

Maintaining and improving physical function in elders is an important area of scientific inquiry because adequate physical function may be a key factor in an elder's sense of self, quality of life, and independence. Nurse scientists are approaching the problem of maintaining and improving physical function in elders from many research directions.

The conceptualization of physical function is an interdisciplinary effort that includes the work of nurse theorists, such as Leidy and Haase

(Leidy, 1994; Leidy, 1999; Leidy & Haase, 1996; Leidy & Haase, 1999), who developed a model of function that differentiates physiological capacity from actual performance. This model uses concepts that many nurses understand from clinical practice and places those concepts in a theoretical model that provides a rationale for many nursing interventions. For example, an elder whose physical performance is close to his or her full capacity has little reserve capacity and may not be able to survive unexpected adverse events. Thus, nurses should intervene to help patients build physiological capacity, such as muscle strength, so they can continue to function during periods of illness or stress. Leidy's model, and the four-dimensional model of Rush and Ouelett (Ouellet & Rush, 1996; Rush & Ouelett, 1998) contribute to a broad interdisciplinary area of inquiry from which nurse researchers can draw theoretical frameworks for studies. Much work remains to be done in modeling the antecedents and outcomes of physical function in elders and it is hoped that nurses will continue to contribute to the research.

Nurse scientists have shown that the measurement of physical function in elders should go beyond the traditional ADL and IADL scales. Nurses have raised questions about gender bias (Porter, 1995) in ADL scales and whether traditional ADL scales are useful to measure physical function in patients with dementia (Beck, 1988; Patterson et al., 1992). Nursing studies have found discrepancies between individual self-report of ADL and proxy report by nurses (Lindgren & Linton, 1991), findings that may have implications for the accuracy of Minimum Data Set records and other documents. In the future, nurses in clinical practice and nurse researchers should be aware that the traditional ADL and IADL self-report scales may not be the best measures of physical function for all elders. Nurses have developed new scales for measuring physical function of independent elders (Frederiks, te Wierik, Visser, & Sturmans, 1991; Kinugasa & Nagasaki, 1998) and elders with dementia (Beck, 1988; Patterson et al., 1992; Tappen, 1994a). Unfortunately, few studies have adopted these scales to measure physical function in elders. It would be especially interesting see published reports from nurses in clinical practice about their use of the new ADL scales to assess changes in a patient's physical function as dementia progresses; perhaps such reports will be published in the future.

Nurse researchers have made important contributions to knowledge about the factors associated with poor physical function in elders. The identification of psychological factors associated with poor physical function, such as fatigue (Belza, Henke, Yelin, Epstein, & Gilliss, 1993), depression (Martin, 1996; Weaver & Narsavage, 1992; Weaver, Rich-mond, & Narsavage, 1997), low self-efficacy (Oka et al., 1996), and anxiety (Weaver et al., 1997) are especially interesting for clinical nursing practice because nurses often assess for these factors in elders. Therefore, nursing assessments and interventions may improve not only psychological well-being, but also physical function, though this has not yet been verified in a nursing intervention study. Environmental factors may also be im-portant for maintaining or improving physical function in elders, but nurs-ing studies have provided little empirical data to support this association. A critically important future direction for nurse researchers is to design longitudinal or experimental studies to demonstrate that nursing interven-tions that focus on psychological or environmental factors can actually improve physical function.

In the future, descriptive and experimental nursing studies that explore ethnic and gender differences in physical function will be needed so nurses in clinical practice can design care that meets the needs of elders from other cultures. Though some studies have focused on African American or Latino elders (Engle & Graney, 1995; Gonzalez & Jirovec, 2001; Martin, 1996; Stegbauer, Engle, & Graney, 1995), much more research is needed. Some nursing studies included in this review did not report the ethnicity of the sample. This should be reported in all nursing studies in the future, and efforts to recruit participants from diverse populations should increase. It would be useful if nurse researchers reported on methods of recruitment and retention of diverse participants, so other researchers can benefit from the lessons learned.

Few intervention studies to improve physical function in elders have been conducted by nurses, though perhaps this will be a new growth area in nursing research. Indeed, the intervention studies that do exist have been published quite recently, so more may be under review or in press. In recent years, nurse scientists have conducted exercise intervention stud-ies, but few have measured the effect of exercise on ADL, IADL, or mobility outcomes. Researchers in other disciplines are investigating the effect of exercise on physical function in elders and this association should be included in exercise intervention studies conducted by nurses.

A serious gap in the literature is the lack of studies conducted by nurse researchers to evaluate the effect of GNPs on physical function in elders. It is possible that a GNP can implement interventions to improve physical function and, at the same time, lower costs by decreasing hospital visits or postponing admissions to nursing homes. Scientific evidence of the efficacy of GNP practice is essential to justify the existence of this advanced practice specialty. Studies will have to be carefully designed so the effect of the GNP can be differentiated from other aspects of the program within which the GNP works.

Nursing knowledge about physical function in elders will be augmented by the continuing work of nurse scientists who have developed programs of research in this area (Beck, 1988; Beck et al., 1991; Beck et al., 1997; Leidy, 1994, 1999; Leidy & Haase, 1996, 1999; Ouellet & Rush, 1996; Resnick, 1999a, 1999b; Resnick & Jenkins, 2000; Resnick et al., 2000; Rush & Ouellet, 1998; Weaver & Narsavage, 1992; Weaver et al., 1997). These nurse scientists have conducted sequential studies to build a body of empirical evidence to increase our knowledge about physical function in elders. It is likely that other researchers cited in this paper are in the process of building programs of research that will contribute to deeper understanding of the factors that influence the maintenance of physical function in elders.

In summary, nursing research that focuses on physical function in elders is a growing area of inquiry. A review of nursing studies published from 1985 to 2000 revealed that most nursing research studies have been descriptive studies that identified factors associated with poor physical function in elders. Recently, intervention studies conducted by nurses have appeared more frequently in the literature. This progression from descriptive to experimental studies supports an expectation that the number of experimental nursing studies will increase. These studies should focus on maintaining and improving physical function in elders by testing interventions that are useful for clinical nursing practice.

REFERENCES: PRIMARY STUDIES

Beck, C. (1988). Measurement of dressing performance in persons with dementia. *American Journal of Alzheimer's Care and Related Disorders and Research,* *3*(3), 21–25.

Beck, C., Heacock, P., Mercer, S., Walton, C. G., & Shook, J. (1991). Dressing for success. Promoting independence among cognitively impaired elderly. *Journal of Psychosocial Nursing and Mental Health Services, 29*(7), 30–35.

Beck, C., Heacock, P., Mercer, S. O., Walls, R. C., Rapp, C. G., & Vogelpohl, T. S. (1997). Improving dressing behavior in cognitively impaired nursing home residents. *Nursing Research, 46,* 126–132.

Belza, B. L., Henke, C. J., Yelin, E. H., Epstein, W. V., & Gilliss, C. L. (1993). Correlates of fatigue in older adults with rheumatoid arthritis. *Nursing Research, 42,* 93–99.

Bennett, J. A. (1999). Activities of daily living. Old-fashioned or still useful? *Journal of Gerontological Nursing, 25*(5), 22–29.

Blair, C. E. (1995). Combining behavior management and mutual goal setting to reduce physical dependency in nursing home residents. *Nursing Research, 44,* 160–165.

Blair, C. E. (1999). Effect of self-care ADLs on self-esteem of intact nursing home residents. *Issues in Mental Health Nursing, 20,* 559–570.

Blair, C. E., Lewis, R., Vieweg, V., & Tucker, R. (1996). Group and single-subject evaluation of a programme to promote self-care in elderly nursing home residents. *Journal of Advanced Nursing, 24,* 1207–1213.

Brady, B., & Nies, M. A. (1999). Health-promoting lifestyles and exercise: A comparison of older African American women above and below poverty level. *Journal of Holistic Nursing, 17,* 197–207.

Brown, M. D. (1988). Functional assessment of the elderly. *Journal of Gerontological Nursing, 14*(5), 13–17.

Brubaker, B. H. (1996). Self-care in nursing home residents. *Journal of Gerontological Nursing, 22*(7), 22–30.

Bula, C. J., Berod, A. C., Stuck, A. E., Alessi, C. A., Aronow, H. U., Santos-Eggimann, B., Rubenstein, L. Z., & Beck, J. C. (1999). Effectiveness of preventive in-home geriatric assessment in well functioning, community-dwelling older people: Secondary analysis of a randomized trial. *Journal of the American Geriatrics Society, 47,* 389–395.

Conn, V. S. (1998a). Older women's beliefs about physical activity. *Public Health Nursing, 15,* 370–378.

Conn, V. S. (1998b). Older adults and exercise: Path analysis of self-efficacy related constructs. *Nursing Research, 47,* 180–189.

Dayhoff, N. E., Suhrheinrich, J., Wigglesworth, J., Topp, R., & Moore, S. (1998). Balance and muscle strength as predictors of frailty among older adults. *Journal of Gerontological Nursing, 24*(7), 18–27.

Duffy, M. E., & MacDonald, E. (1990). Determinants of functional health of older persons. *Gerontologist, 30,* 503–509.

Dungan, J. M., Brown, A. V., & Ramsey, M. A. (1996). Health maintenance for the independent frail older adult: Can it improve physical and mental well-being? *Journal of Advanced Nursing, 23,* 1185–1193.

Engle, V. F., & Graney, M. J. (1995). Black and white female nursing home residents: Does health status differ? *Journals of Gerontology. Series A, Biological Sciences and Medical Sciences, 50,* M190–M195.

Frederiks, C. M., te Wierik, M. J., Visser, A. P., & Sturmans, F. (1991). A scale for the functional status of the elderly living at home. *Journal of Advanced Nursing, 16,* 287–292.

Garrard, J., Kane, R. L., Radosevich, D. M., Skay, C. L., Arnold, S., Kepferle, L., McDermott, S., & Buchanan, J. L. (1990). Impact of geriatric nurse practitioners on nursing-home residents' functional status, satisfaction, and discharge outcomes. *Medical Care, 28,* 271–283.

Gonzalez, B., & Jirovec, M. (2001). Elderly Mexican women's perceptions of exercise and conflicting role responsibilities. *International Journal of Nursing Studies, 38*(1), 45–49.

Gueldner, S. H., Poon, L. W., La Via, M., Virella, G., Michel, Y., Bramlett, M. H., Noble, C. A., & Paulling, E. (1997). Long-term exercise patterns and immune function in healthy older women. A report of preliminary findings. *Mechanisms of Ageing and Development, 93,* 215–222.

Hartig, M. T., Engle, V. F., & Graney, M. J. (1997). Accuracy of nurse aides' functional health assessments of nursing home residents. *Journals of Gerontology. Series A, Biological Sciences and Medical Sciences, 52,* M142–M148.

Johnson, P. A., Stone, M. A., Larson, A. M., & Hromek, C. A. (1992). Applying nursing diagnosis and nursing process to activities of daily living and mobility. *Geriatric Nursing, 13,* 25–27.

Jones, M., & Nies, M. A. (1996). The relationship of perceived benefits of and barriers to reported exercise in older African American women. *Public Health Nursing, 13,* 151–158.

Kane, R. L., Garrard, J., Skay, C. L., Radosevich, D. M., Buchanan, J. L., McDermott, S. M., Arnold, S. B., & Kepferle, L. (1989). Effects of a geriatric nurse practitioner on process and outcome of nursing home care. *American Journal of Public Health, 79,* 1271–1277.

Kinugasa, T., & Nagasaki, H. (1998). Reliability and validity of the Motor Fitness Scale for older adults in the community. *Aging, 10,* 295–302.

Laffrey, S. C. (2000). Physical activity among older Mexican American women. *Research in Nursing and Health, 23,* 383–392.

Leidy, N. K. (1994). Functional status and the forward progress of merry-go-rounds: Toward a coherent analytical framework. *Nursing Research, 43,* 196–202.

Leidy, N. K. (1999). Psychometric properties of the functional performance inventory in patients with chronic obstructive pulmonary disease. *Nursing Research, 48,* 20–28.

Leidy, N. K., & Haase, J. E. (1996). Functional performance in people with chronic obstructive pulmonary disease: A qualitative analysis. *Advances in Nursing Science, 18*(3), 77–89.

Leidy, N. K., & Haase, J. E. (1999). Functional status from the patient's perspective: The challenge of preserving personal integrity. *Research in Nursing and Health, 22,* 67–77.

Lindgren, C. L., & Linton, A. D. (1991). Problems of nursing home residents: Nurse and resident perceptions. *Applied Nursing Research, 4*(3), 113–121.

Lucas, J. A., Orshan, S. A., & Cook, F. (2000). Determinants of health-promoting behavior among women ages 65 and above living in the community. *Scholarly Inquiry for Nursing Practice, 14*(1), 77–100.

Martin, J. C. (1996). Determinants of functional health of low-income black women with osteoarthritis. *American Journal of Preventive Medicine, 12,* 430–436.

Marx, M. S., Werner, P., Cohen-Mansfield, J., & Feldman, R. (1992). The relationship between low vision and performance of activities of daily living in nursing home residents. *Journal of the American Geriatrics Society, 40,* 1018–1020.

McBride, S. (1994). Patients with chronic obstructive pulmonary disease: Their beliefs about measures that increase activity tolerance. *Rehabilitation Nursing, 19*(1), 37–41.

Melillo, K. D., Futrell, M., Williamson, E., Chamberlain, C., Bourque, A. M., MacDonnell, M., & Phaneuf, J. P. (1996). Perceptions of physical fitness and exercise activity among older adults. *Journal of Advanced Nursing, 23,* 542–547.

Mills, E. M. (1994). The effect of low-intensity aerobic exercise on muscle strength, flexibility, and balance among sedentary elderly persons. *Nursing Research, 43,* 207–211.

Narsavage, G. L., & Weaver, T. E. (1994). Physiologic status, coping, and hardiness as predictors of outcomes in chronic obstructive pulmonary disease. *Nursing Research, 43,* 90–94.

Oka, R. K., Gortner, S. R., Stotts, N. A., & Haskell, W. L. (1996). Predictors of physical activity in patients with chronic heart failure secondary to either ischemic or idiopathic dilated cardiomyopathy. *American Journal of Cardiology, 77,* 159–163.

Ouellet, L. L., & Rush, K. L. (1996). A study of nurses' perceptions of client mobility. *Western Journal of Nursing Research, 18,* 565–579.

Patterson, M. B., Mack, J. L., Neundorfer, M. M., Martin, R. J., Smyth, K. A., & Whitehouse, P. J. (1992). Assessment of functional ability in Alzheimer disease: A review and a preliminary report on the Cleveland Scale for Activities of Daily Living. *Alzheimer Disease and Associated Disorders, 6,* 145–163.

Porter, E. J. (1995). A phenomenological alternative to the "ADL research tradition." *Journal of Aging and Health, 7,* 24–45.

Potempa, K., Lopez, M., Braun, L. T., Szidon, J. P., Fogg, L., & Tincknell, T. (1995). Physiological outcomes of aerobic exercise training in hemiparetic stroke patients. *Stroke, 26,* 101–105.

Resnick, B. (1999a). Motivation to perform activities of daily living in the institutionalized older adult: Can a leopard change its spots? *Journal of Advanced Nursing, 29,* 792–799.

Resnick, B. (1999b). Reliability and validity testing of the Self-Efficacy for Functional Activities Scale. *Journal of Nursing Measurement, 7,* 5–20.

Resnick, B. (2000). Functional performance and exercise of older adults in long-term care settings. *Journal of Gerontological Nursing, 26*(3), 7–16.

Resnick, B., & Jenkins, L. S. (2000). Testing the reliability and validity of the Self-Efficacy for Exercise Scale. *Nursing Research, 49,* 154–159.

Resnick, B., Palmer, M. H., Jenkins, L. S., & Spellbring, A. M. (2000). Path analysis of efficacy expectations and exercise behaviour in older adults. *Journal of Advanced Nursing, 31,* 1309–1315.

Roberts, B. L. (1990). Effects of walking on reaction and movement times among elders. *Perceptual and Motor Skills, 71,* 131–140.

Rush, K. L., & Ouellet, L. L. (1998). An analysis of elderly clients' views of mobility. *Western Journal of Nursing Research, 20,* 295–308.

Stegbauer, C. C., Engle, V. F., & Graney, M. J. (1995). Admission health status differences of black and white indigent nursing home residents. *Journal of the American Geriatrics Society, 43,* 1103–1106.

Talbot, L. A., Metter, E. J., & Fleg, J. L. (2000). Leisure-time physical activities and their relationship to cardiorespiratory fitness in healthy men and women 18–95 years old. *Medicine and Science in Sports and Exercise, 32,* 417–425.

Tappen, R. M. (1994a). Development of the Refined ADL Assessment Scale for patients with Alzheimer's and related disorders. *Journal of Gerontological Nursing, 20*(6), 36–42.

Tappen, R. M. (1994b). The effect of skill training on functional abilities of nursing home residents with dementia. *Research in Nursing and Health, 17,* 159–165.

Topp, R., & Stevenson, J. S. (1994). The effects of attendance and effort on outcomes among older adults in a long-term exercise program. *Research in Nursing and Health, 17,* 15–24.

Weaver, T. E., & Narsavage, G. L. (1992). Physiological and psychological variables related to functional status in chronic obstructive pulmonary disease. *Nursing Research, 41,* 286–291.

Weaver, T. E., Richmond, T. S., & Narsavage, G. L. (1997). An explanatory model of functional status in chronic obstructive pulmonary disease. *Nursing Research, 46,* 26–31.

Yu, S. (1995). A study on functioning for independent living among the elderly in the community. *Public Health Nursing, 12,* 31–40.

References Other Than Primary Studies

AARP. (1996). *A profile of older Americans* (PF3049 (1296).D996). Washington, DC: American Association of Retired Persons.

Ferrucci, L., Guralnik, J. M., Baroni, A., Tesi, G., Antonini, E., & Marchionni, N. (1991). Value of combined assessment of physical health and functional status in community-dwelling aged: A prospective study in Florence, Italy. *Journal of Gerontology, 46*(2), M52–M56.

Hlatky, M. A., Boineau, R. E., Higginbotham, M. B., Lee, K. L., Mark, D. B., Califf, R. M., Cobb, F. R., & Pryor, D. B. (1989). A brief self-administered questionnaire to determine functional capacity (Duke Activity Status Index). *American Journal of Cardiology, 64,* 651–654.

Kassner, E., & Bectel, R. (1998). *Midlife and older Americans with disabilities: Who gets help?* (PPE5635(1198).D16883). Washington, DC: AARP Public Policy Institute.

Katz, S., Ford, A. B., Moskowitz, R. W., Jackson, B. A., & Jaffe, M. W. (1963). Studies of illness in the aged. The Index of ADL: A standardized measure of biological and psychosocial function. *Journal of the American Medical Association, 185,* 914–919.

McDowell, I., & Newell, C. (1996). *Measuring health: a guide to rating scales and questionnaires.* New York: Oxford University Press.

Meleis, A. I. (1997). *Theoretical nursing: Development & progress* (3rd ed.). Philadelphia: Lippincott.

National Academy on an Aging Society. (1999, November). *Chronic conditions: A challenge for the 21st century* (Report Number 1). Washington, DC: Author.

National Center for Health Statistics. (1999). *Health, United States, 1999* (PHS 99–12320). Hyattsville, MD: Public Health Service.

Pearson, V. (2000). Assessment of function in older adults. In R. L. Kane & R. A. Kane (Eds.), *Assessing older persons: Measures, meaning, and practical applications* (pp. 17–48). New York: Oxford University Press.

Pender, N. J. (1996). *Health promotion in nursing practice.* Stamford, CT: Appleton & Lange.

Rice, D. P. (2001). Medicare: A women's issue. In P. Lee & C. Estes (Eds.), *The nation's health* (6th ed., pp. 514–522). Sudbury, MA: Jones and Bartlett.

Simonsick, E. M., Kasper, J. D., & Phillips, C. L. (1998). Physical disability and social interaction: Factors associated with low social contact and home confinement in disabled older women (The Women's Health and Aging Study). *Journals of Gerontology. Series B, Psychological Sciences and Social Sciences, 53,* S209–S217.

Verbrugge, L. M., & Jette, A. M. (1994). The disablement process. *Social Science and Medicine, 38,* 1–14.

Chapter 2

Pressure Ulcer Prevention and Management

Courtney H. Lyder

ABSTRACT

This chapter reviews 218 published and unpublished research reports of pressure ulcer prevention and management by nurse researchers and researchers from other disciplines. The electronic databases MEDLINE (1966–July 2001), CINAHL (1982–June 2001), AMED (1985–July 2001), and EI Compedex*Plus (1980–June 2001) were selected for the searches because of their focus on health and applied research. Moreover, evaluations of previous review articles and seminal studies that were published before 1966 are also included. Research conducted worldwide and published in English between 1930 and 2001 was included for review. Studies using descriptive, correlational, longitudinal, and randomized control trials were included. This review found that numerous gaps remain in our understanding of effective pressure ulcer prevention and management. Moreover, the majority of pressure ulcer care is derived from expert opinion rather than empirical evidence. Thus, additional research is needed to investigate pressure ulcer risk factors of ethnic minorities. Further studies are needed that examine the impact of specific preventive interventions (e.g., turning intervals based on risk stratification) and the cost-effectiveness of comprehensive prevention programs to prevent pressure ulcers. Finally, an evaluation is needed of various aspects of pressure ulcer management (e.g., use of support surfaces, use of adjunctive therapies) and healing of pressure ulcers.

Keywords: pressure ulcer, prevention, pressure ulcer management, wound care

Pressure ulcers are a serious and common health problem affecting approximately 1.5 to 3 million adults (Eckman, 1989). With the increasing aging of the U.S. population, fragmented care, and impending nursing shortage, the incidence of pressure ulcers in elders will most likely continue to rise. The purpose of this chapter is to review current research related to the effective prevention and management of pressure ulcers, as well as identify the gaps in our current knowledge. This chapter will examine the following questions:

1. What is known about pressure ulcer prevention?
2. What are known risk factors for pressure ulcers?
3. What instruments are available to predict pressure ulcers?
4. What is known about skin care and pressure ulcer prevention?
5. What is known about the use of support surfaces in preventing pressure ulcers?
6. What is known about the implementation of comprehensive prevention programs in decreasing the incidence of pressure ulcers?
7. What is known about staging pressure ulcers?
8. What instruments are available to monitor the healing of pressure ulcers?
9. What is known about the comprehensive management of pressure ulcers?
10. What is the role of adjunctive therapies in healing pressure ulcers?

INCIDENCE AND PREVALENCE OF PRESSURE ULCERS

Approximately 70% of all pressure ulcers occur in elders (Barbenel, Jordan, & Nicol, 1977). The cost associated with the treatment of pressure ulcers has been estimated to be between $500 and $40,000 per ulcer (Lyder, Yu, et al., 1998). It is important to note that these costs do not account for the pain and suffering that can also be associated with pressure ulcers.

In elders the incidence of pressure ulcers is believed to be associated with the aging process. With aging, local blood supply to the skin decreases, epithelial layers flatten and thin, subcutaneous fat decreases, and collagen fibers lose elasticity (Basson & Burney, 1982; Mawson, Siddiqui, & Biundo, 1993). Cutaneous pain sensitivity decreases after age 50, perhaps leading to failure to shift weight appropriately (Mawson et al., 1993; Rousseau, 1988). These changes in aging skin and the resultant lowered tolerance to hypoxia may enhance pressure ulcer development (Ek, Lewis, Zetterqvist, & Svensson, 1984). Because pressure is the major physiological factor that leads to soft-tissue destruction, the term "pressure ulcer" is most widely used and preferred over "decubitus ulcer" or "bedsore."

The National Pressure Ulcer Advisory Panel found a wide variation in pressure ulcer incidence rates depending on setting (Cuddigan, Ayello, Sussman, & Baranoski, 2001). Rates of 0.4% to 38% for hospitals; 2.2% to 23.9% for long-term care; and 0% to 17% for home care were reported. Inconsistencies in methods and samples studied hampered comparisons.

Among patients who develop pressure ulcers, 57–60% occur in the acute care hospital (Peterson & Bittman, 1971; Morrison, 1984)—usually within the first 2 weeks of hospitalization (Langemo et al., 1989). With the increased acuity of elders admitted to hospitals, it is estimated that 15% of elderly patients will develop pressure ulcers within the first week of hospitalization (Lyder, Preston, Scinto, Grady, & Ahearn, 1998; Lyder et al., 2001). Pressure ulcers are most likely to develop within the first 4 weeks of an elder's admission to long-term care (Bergstrom & Braden, 1992). This is probably attributed to the higher acuity level of residents being admitted. Mortality is associated with pressure ulcers. Several studies have noted mortality rates as high as 60% for elders with a pressure ulcer within 1 year of hospital discharge (Allman et al., 1995; Thomas, Goode, Tarquine, & Allman, 1996; Lyder, Grady, Mathur, Patrello, & Meehan, in press). Usually, the pressure ulcer does not cause death, rather it develops after a decline in health status of the elder. Thus, the development of pressure ulcers can be used as a predictor of mortality.

The staging of pressure ulcers is used to classify the extent of tissue damage observed. Staging can provide the clinician with estimates of the amount of care and resources needed to manage the ulcer. The Stage I pressure ulcer (persistent erythema) occurs most frequently, accounting for 47% of all pressure ulcers (Kelley & Mobily, 1991). Stage II pressure ulcers (partial skin thickness loss involving only the epidermal and dermal layer) accounted for 33% (Kelly & Mobily, 1991). Stage III (full thickness skin loss involving subcutaneous tissue) and Stage IV (full thickness involving muscle or bone or supporting structures) pressure ulcers make up the remaining 20% (Kelly & Mobily, 1991). Several studies have noted that the incidence of pressure ulcers differs between Blacks and Whites (Fuhrer, Garber, Rintola, Clearman, & Hart, 1993; Spector, Kapp,

Tucker, & Sternberg, 1988). Blacks tend to have a greater incidence of Stage III and Stage IV pressure ulcers than Whites. In a 1998 study, the U.S. Centers for Medicare and Medicaid Services (formerly the Health Care Financing Administration [HCFA]), found that 19% of Black and Hispanic elders developed Stage III and Stage IV pressure ulcers compared with only 9% of Whites (Lyder et al., 1998). These data suggest that Stage I pressure ulcers may be underdiagnosed in darkly pigmented elders, thus prevention interventions may not occur in a timely manner.

Pressure ulcers have now become a national concern. For the first time in U.S. history, the Surgeon General identified pressure ulcers as a national health issue for long-term care (Healthy People 2010, 2000). The Centers for Medicare and Medicaid Services placed pressure ulcers as one of three sentinel events for long-term care (HCFA, 2000). The formation of a pressure ulcer or subsequent deterioration of a pressure ulcer can lead to significant civil monetary penalties for those long-term care facilities assessed as deficient in either the prevention and/or management of pressure ulcers (HCFA, 2000). Thus, in addition to the health-related mandate there are financial and policy incentives to prevent and heal pressure ulcers.

There is little intellectual discord about the main cause of pressure ulcers—it is *pressure* (Kosiak, 1959). A landmark study conducted by Landis (1930) found that capillary blood flow stopped when external pressures between 20 to 40 mmHg were applied to the skin. Kosiak, Kubicek, Olson, Dantz, and Kottke (1958) found an inverse relationship between the amount of time and pressure needed to cause tissue destruction. In fact, Kosiak and colleagues (1958) found that 60 to 70 mmHG of pressure applied to muscle tissue caused damage within 1 to 2 hours. Thus, pressure alone may not cause tissue damage, however sustained pressure to a specific area (i.e., bony prominence) coupled with time can cause tissue damage. Recently scientists have explored other causative factors for pressure ulcers, such as free radicals (Salcido, Donofrio, & Fisher, 1994); however, their causal relationships remain unclear.

METHODS

A systematic review of published research on *pressure ulcer prevention and management* was conducted. Several electronic databases were used to cull the literature. The databases were limited to those that had a focus on *health* and *applied research*. These databases included: MEDLINE

(1966–July 2001), CINAHL (1982–June 2001), AMED (1985–July 2001), EI Compedex*Plus (1980–June 2001).

Articles published between 1930 and 2001 in English were included for review. Seminal studies published before 1966 were also included. The inclusion criteria were: samples age 50 or older, and the article identified a pressure ulcer variable of interest to gerontological nursing. Both nursing and nonnursing research were included. Upon completion of the literature search ($N = 1,245$ abstracts), 345 articles were screened. Of these, 218 reported research findings.

RESULTS

Pressure Ulcer Prevention

WHAT ARE KNOWN RISK FACTORS FOR PRESSURE ULCERS?

The first step in preventing pressure ulcers is the identification of those elders who are at risk. Numerous studies have been conducted in the past 10 years that examine pressure ulcer risk factors. Logistic regression models have been used in causal models of pressure ulcer development in elders. These models illustrate the complex interaction between risk factors and the development of pressure ulcers. One limitation of these models is related to the variables entered (or not entered) in the modeling. Nonetheless, variables found to predict pressure ulcer development include: age $\geq$ 70 years; male gender; White race; current smoking history; low body mass index; impaired mobility; altered mental status (i.e., confusion); urinary and fecal incontinence; malnutrition; physical restraints; malignancy; diabetes mellitus; cerebral vascular accident; pneumonia; heart failure; fever; sepsis; hypotension; renal failure; dry, scaly skin; history of pressure ulcers; anemia; lymphopenia; and hypoalbuminemia (Allman et al., 1986; Allman et al., 1995; Berlowitz & Wilking, 1989; Brandeis, Morris, Nash, & Lipsitz, 1990; Guralnik, Harris, White, & Coroni-Huntley, 1988). While the literature notes that the White race is a predictor of pressure ulcers, the lack of sufficient non-White subjects in most studies makes this finding questionable. The studies that have included sufficient numbers of Black subjects for analysis purposes have found that Blacks have more severe pressure ulcers than non-Blacks (Fuhrer et al., 1993; Lyder, Yu, et al., 1998; Spector et al., 1988) and Blacks have a higher incidence rate of pressure ulcer as compared with Whites (Lyder et al., 1999).

WHAT INSTRUMENTS ARE AVAILABLE TO PREDICT PRESSURE ULCERS?

Tools have been developed to quantify risk categories for pressure ulcer development. Nursing research has taken leadership in developing risk assessment tools. Although no scale has been developed that captures all known risk factors, several scales attempt to capture the main risk factors. The Braden Scale and the Norton Scale are the most widely used scales (Bergstrom et al., 1992). The Braden Scale comprises six subscales: sensory perception (ability to respond to pressure-related discomfort), moisture, activity, mobility, nutrition, and friction and shear (Braden & Bergstrom, 1987). Scores on this scale range from 6 (high risk) to 23 (low risk). When the Braden Scale is completed by a registered nurse rather than licensed practical nurses, its probability to predict pressure ulcers is greatly increased (Bergstrom, Demuth, & Braden, 1987). The Norton Scale comprises five subscales. These subscales include: physical condition, mental condition, activity, mobility, and incontinence (Norton, 1989). The total scores range from 5 (high risk) to 20 (low risk).

Both the Braden and Norton scales are recommended by the Agency for Healthcare Quality and Research. This recommendation is based on extensive support for their validity and reliability. The Braden and Norton Scales have good sensitivity (83%–100% and 73%–92%, respectively) and specificity (64%–77% and 61%–94%, respectively), but have poor positive predictive value (around 40% and 20% respectively) (Bergstrom, Braden, Laguzza, & Holzman, 1987; Norton, McLaren, & Exton-Smith, 1975). The Norton and Braden Scales show a .73 Kappa statistic agreement among at-risk patients, with the Norton Scale tending to classify patients as at risk when the Braden Scale classified them as not at risk (Pang & Wong, 1998). The effect of poor positive predictive value is that many patients who will not develop pressure ulcers may receive expensive and unnecessary treatment.

In recent years, the need to establish optimal cutoff scores depending on setting and patient populations has emerged. In a study of 337 pressure ulcer-free patients undergoing cardiothoracic surgery, Lewicki, Mion, and Secic (2000) found that using a score of ≤ 16 on the Braden Scale to identify risk had poor sensitivity and specificity. In fact, these researchers found that the appropriate cutoff scores on postoperative Days 1, 3, and 5 were 13, 14, and 20, respectively. The use of these optimal cutoff scores yielded 67% pressure ulcer-positive patients on postoperative Day 1, 57% on postoperative Day 3, and 50% on postoperative Day 5 (Lewicki et al., 2000). In another study investigating three distinct health care settings (tertiary care hospitals, Veterans Administration medical centers, and skilled nursing facilities), researchers found that the optimal cutoff score for the Braden Scale was 18 and that risk assessments completed 48 to 72 hours after admission were highly predictive of those patients that would develop pressure ulcers (Bergstrom, Braden, Kemp, Champayne, & Ruby, 1998). These nursing studies suggest that optimal cutoff scores must be evaluated for specific patient populations.

Both the Braden and Norton Scales have been tested in non-White populations. In a study comparing the predictive validity of the Braden Scale, the Norton Scale and the Waterlow Scale (another pressure ulcer scale used widely in the United Kingdom) in a Chinese sample, researchers found that both the Norton and Waterlow Scales had relatively high sensitivity (81% and 95%, respectively), but poor specificity (Pang & Wong, 1998). The Braden Scale had both a high sensitivity (91%) and specificity (62%). In a prospective study of the predictive validity of the Braden Scale in 60 non-White subjects, the scale was found to be highly predictive in Black and Hispanic elders (Lyder et al., 1999). The Braden Scale with a cutoff of 18 was associated with predicting Black elders age ≤ 75 at-risk for pressure ulcers ($p \leq 0.011$). Its sensitivity was 81% and its specificity 100% (Lyder et al., 1999).

Many gaps exist in the literature related to the variables that place elders at risk for pressure ulcers. The identification of optimal cutoff scores for various instruments in different populations at risk for pressure ulcers is greatly needed.

What Is Known About Skin Care and Pressure Ulcer Prevention?

There continues to be a dearth of research that explores the relationship between skin care and pressure ulcer prevention. Most skin care recommendations are based on expert opinions (Bergstrom et al., 1992) with little scientific research. Most experts would agree that the goal of proper skin care is to identify elders at risk for pressure ulcers and to maintain and improve tissue tolerance to prevent injury.

All elders at risk for pressure ulcers should have a systematic skin inspection at least daily, paying particular attention to the bony prominences. Their skin should be cleansed at the time of soiling—avoiding hot water, and using mild cleansing agents that minimize irritation and dryness of the skin (Bergstrom, Allman, et al., 1992; Rodeheaver, 1999). The avoidance of low humidity during skin cleansing should be promoted since low humidity promotes scaling and dryness, which have been associated with pressure ulcer development (Guralnik et al., 1988). Avoidance of massage over bony prominences is warranted because of evidence that this procedure leads to deep tissue trauma (Dyson, 1978; Ek, Gustavsson, & Lewis, 1985). Skin care should focus on minimizing moisture from incontinence, perspiration, or wound drainage. Skin injury due to friction and shear forces should also be minimized through proper positioning, transferring, and turning techniques. Friction injuries may be relieved by use of lubricants, protective films (i.e., transparent dressings and skin sealants), protective dressings (i.e., hydrocolloids), and protective padding. More research is needed to determine the association between skin care and pressure ulcer prevention.

What Is Known About Mechanical Loading and Pressure Ulcer Prevention?

There continues to be a dearth of research regarding the optimal frequency of turning elders at risk for pressure ulcers. The first study published on frequency of turning (Norton, McLaren, & Exton-Smith, 1975) was an observational nursing study which divided groups of elders into three turning treatment groups (every 2 to 3 hours [$n = 32$], every 4 hours [$n = 27$], or turned 2 to 4 times/day [$n = 41$]). These researchers found that elders turned every 2 to 3 hours had fewer ulcers. This landmark nursing study created the nursing practice standard of turning patients every 2 hours.

A more recent study investigated the length of turning intervals and body position on interface pressure in healthy elders (Knox, Anderson, & Anderson, 1994). These investigators, using a Latin-Square design with 48 subjects, found a significant ($p = .004$) increase in skin surface temperature at the completion of 2-hour turning durations. Thus, a 2-hour minimum turning regimen appears adequate in healthy elders. The effects of blood flows and interface pressure small shifts in position in 50 nursing home residents were examined by Oertwich, Kindschuh, and Bergstrom (1995) using a within-subjects, repeated-measures design. They found a significant decrease in interface pressure under the trochanter and an increase in blood flow ($p \leq .05$). The results of this study suggest that small shifts do relieve pressure and increase blood flow. The researchers noted, however, that the findings reflect only intermediate outcomes. Further studies are needed to test the clinical association between implementing small shifts and the reduction of pressure ulcers.

Studies using multiple turning frequencies that are stratified by level of pressure ulcer risk are needed. The literature suggests that a written schedule for systematic turning and repositioning should be used (Bergstrom et al., 1992). For patients in bed, positioning devices such as pillows or foam wedges should be used to keep bony prominences from direct contact with one another. The head of the bed should be at the lowest elevation possible consistent with medical condition to decrease friction and shear forces. Seller, Allen, and Srahelin (1986) found that lying directly on the trochanters (90-degree angle) produced high interface pressures and low transcutaneous oxygen tension as compared with being positioned on a 30-degree, side-lying angle in which the transcutaneous oxygen tension in the body was normal and interface pressure reduced.

WHAT IS KNOWN ABOUT SUPPORT SURFACES AND PRESSURE ULCER PREVENTION?

The use of support surfaces to assist in offloading pressure has been found to be an important component to pressure ulcer care. Two types of support surfaces exist: static (foam, static air, gel, water, or combination gel/water) and dynamic (alternating air, low air loss, or air fluidized). Both types of support surfaces have been found effective in offloading pressure as compared with standard mattresses. Colin, Loyant, Abraham, and Saumet (1996) studied transcutaneous oxygen tension on the sacrum of 20 healthy adults positioned on five different mattress types. Prior to beginning the intervention, mean transcutaneous oxygen on the sacrum was 68.2 mmHg ($SD = 9.4$). After the intervention, mean transcutaneous oxygen differed depending on the support surface. Mean values were 17.9 mmHg ($SD = 27.9$) for standard hospital mattress, 30.15 mmHg ($SD = 29.5$) for first foam mattress, 30.25 mmHg ($SD = 28.5$) for the second foam mattress, 50.5 mmHg ($SD = 23.1$) for the air mattress, and 50.95 mmHg ($SD = 21.6$) for the water-filled mattress. Clearly the standard mattress exerted the most pressure to the sacral area of these healthy volunteers. However, what is still unknown is the amount of pressure required to cause pressure ulcer development for an individual elder.

To date there are few studies that demonstrate significant differences in the prevention of pressure ulcers across categories of support surfaces within each type (Cullum, Deeks, Sheldon, Song, & Fletcher, 2001; Lazzara & Buschmann, 1991; Fontaine, 2000). A few nursing studies have noted little differences between the classifications. One such study (Ooka, Kemp, McMyn, & Shott, 1995) investigated three types of support surfaces (two dynamic mattress replacements and one static foam mattress) and their ability to prevent pressure ulcers in 110 at-risk patients admitted to a surgical intensive care unit in an urban medical center. These researchers found that 8% of the patients developed a pressure ulcer. However, 9 patients developed pressure ulcers (3 on each support surface) with no statistically significant difference between the support surfaces and risk of pressure ulcer development. It was noted that the average cost to purchase the dynamic surface was $2000 compared with $240 for the static surface. Thus, the cost in selecting a support surface must be considered given the lack of variance in the surface's ability to prevent pressure ulcers. Additional research is needed to investigate the use of support surfaces and their ability to prevent pressure ulcers in a variety of patient care settings.

WHAT IS KNOWN ABOUT THE IMPLEMENTATION OF COMPREHENSIVE PREVENTION PROGRAMS AND DECREASING THE INCIDENCE OF PRESSURE ULCERS?

Because the causes of pressure ulcers are multivariate, effective prevention of all ulcers remains elusive. Comprehensive protocols of care to prevent pressure ulcers have been evaluated in both long-term care and hospital settings. It remains a challenge, however, to prevent all ulcer development (Bergstrom, Braden, Kemp, Champayne, & Rubin, 1996; Xakellis, Frantz, Lewis, & Harvey, 1998). Xakellis and colleagues (1998) evaluated the efficacy of an intensive pressure ulcer prevention protocol for reducing the incidence of ulcers in a 77-bed, long-term care facility. The intensive pressure ulcer prevention protocol consisted of institution-specific risk assessment (Braden Scale), preventive interventions stratified on risk level, with implementation of support surfaces and turning/repositioning residents. The sample included 132 residents, 69 prior to prevention intervention and 63 postprevention intervention. The 6-month incidence rate of pressure ulcers prior to the intensive prevention intervention was 23%. For the 6-month postintensive prevention intervention, the pressure ulcer incidence rate was 5%. This study demonstrated that significant reductions in the incidence of pressure ulcers are possible to achieve within a rather short period of time (6 months) when facility specific intensive prevention interventions are used.

A more recent study examined the effects of implementing the SOLU-TIONS program, which focuses pressure ulcer prevention measures on alleviating risk factors identified by the Braden Scale in two long-term care facilities (Lyder, Shannon, Empleo-Frazier, McGehee, & White, in press). The quasi-experimental study found that after 5 months of implementing the SOLUTIONS program, Facility A (150 beds) experienced an 87% (13.2% to 1.7%) reduction in pressure ulcer incidence ($p = .02$). Facility B (110 beds) experienced a corresponding 76% (15% to 3.5%) reduction ($p = .02$). Thus, the use of comprehensive prevention programs can significantly reduce the incidence of pressure ulcers in long-term care.

Several studies have attempted to demonstrate that comprehensive pressure ulcer prevention programs can decrease the incidence of pressure sores in acute settings. However, no studies could be found that decreased and maintained a zero percent incidence rate. One large study evaluated the processes of care for Medicare patients hospitalized at risk for pressure ulcer development (Lyder et al., 2001). This multicenter, retrospective cohort study used medical record data to identify 2,425 patients age 65 and older discharged from acute care hospitals following treatment for pneumonia, cerebral vascular disease, or congestive heart failure. Charts were evaluated for the presence of six recommended pressure ulcer prevention processes of care—use of daily skin assessment, use of pressure reducing device, documentation of being at risk, repositioning a minimum of every 2 hours, nutritional consultation initiated for patients with nutritional risk factors, and pressure ulcer staged within 48 hours. Researchers found the percentage of charts indicating compliance with process-of-care were: use of daily skin assessment, 94%; use of pressure reducing device, 7.5%; documented at risk, 22.6%; repositioned a minimum of every two hours, 66.2%; received nutritional consultation, 34.3%; Stage I pressure ulcer staged, 20.2%; and Stage II or later-stage ulcer staged, 30.9%. More interesting, this study found that patients who used pressure reducing devices, were documented at pressure ulcer risk, were repositioned every 2 hours, and received nutritional consultations were more likely to develop pressure ulcers than those patients that did not receive the preventive interventions. One explanation for these findings may be derived from the time period (48 hours) used to implement the preventive measures. Given the acuity of patients entering hospitals, waiting 48 hours may be too late to begin pressure ulcer prevention interventions.

Management of Pressure Ulcers

WHAT IS KNOWN ABOUT STAGING OF PRESSURE ULCERS?

There is no agreement on a single system for pressure ulcer classification. Most experts do agree, however, that the correct staging of an ulcer aids in determining the appropriate management plan. Until recently, the most common classification system for pressure ulcers was Shea's (1975). This system used four grades with Grade 1 representing superficial breakdown of the epidermis and Grade 4 representing damage in fascia to bone. Shea's grading system has been criticized by pressure ulcer experts because it did not capture some changes observed within the ulcer. Thus, a new staging system has become standard for classifying pressure ulcers (National Pressure Ulcer Advisory Panel, 1995).

There is more variability in research that attempts to classify the Stage I pressure ulcer than any other stage (Lyder, 1991). In the U.S., initial classification of "wounding" or depth of tissue destroyed in a pressure ulcer is described by several different and not necessarily equivalent staging systems (Ayello et al., 1997; Bergstrom et al., 1994; International Association for Enterstomal Therapy, 1987; National Pressure Ulcer Advisory Panel, 1995; Shea, 1975).

In 1998, the National Pressure Ulcer Advisory Panel (NPUAP) revised its definition of a Stage I pressure ulcer to encompass the skin alterations that might be seen in Stage I pressure ulcers regardless of skin pigmentation (Henderson et al., 1997). This definition notes that a Stage I pressure ulcer is an observable, pressure-related alteration of intact skin whose indicators as compared with an adjacent or opposite area on the body may include changes in one or more of the following: skin temperature (warmth or coolness), tissue consistency (firm or boggy feel), or sensation (pain, itching). The NPUAP definition further states that the pressure ulcer appears as a defined area of persistent redness in lightly pigmented skin, whereas in darker skin tones, the pressure ulcer may appear with persistent erythema, and blue or purple hues. This classification of the Stage I pressure ulcer is the only classification that includes nonwhite skin and is based on clinical expertise. Hence, it has face validity but has never been empirically validated. Given the increasing numbers of elders with darkly pigmented skin, research to validate this classification is warranted.

WHAT INSTRUMENTS ARE AVAILABLE TO MONITOR THE HEALING OF PRESSURE ULCERS?

In the past 8 years two instruments have been developed to measure healing of pressure ulcers. The Pressure Sore Status Tool (PSST) was developed in 1992 (Bates-Jensen, 1997); it is a pencil and paper instrument comprising 15 items. The first 2 items are related to the location and shape of the ulcer; the remaining 13 items are scored and appear with descriptors of each item on a modified Likert scale (1 being the healthiest attribute of the characteristic and 5 being the least healthy attribute of the characteristic). The 13 items are summed to provide a numerical indicator of wound health or degeneration. The content validity of the PSST has been established by a panel of 20 experts (Bates-Jensen, Vredevoe, & Brecht, 1992). Evidence supporting interrater reliability was obtained by the use of two wound, ostomy, and continence nurses who independently rated 20 pressure ulcers on ten patients. Interrater reliability was established at $r = .91$ for the first observation and $r = .92$ for the second observation ($p = .001$) (Bates-Jensen et al., 1992).

The Pressure Ulcer Scale for Healing (PUSH) was developed by the NPUAP in 1997 (Bartolucci & Thomas, 1997). The PUSH tool is a pencil and paper instrument comprising measurements of pressure ulcer surface area, exudate amount, and surface appearance (Thomas et al., 1997). It uses a Likert scale with 1 being the healthiest attribute of the characteristic and 4 or 5 (dependent on the item) being the least healing attribute of the characteristic. A research database of 37 subjects with pressure ulcers was used to test hypothetical models of healing. The model revealed that the PUSH tool had both content validity ($p = .01$) and correlational validity ($p = .05$) to monitor the changing pressure ulcer status.

Several additional measure of healing have not been as thoroughly studied as the PSST and PUSH. These instruments include the Sussman Wound Healing Tool (Sussman & Swanson, 1997), Sessing Scale (Ferrel, 1997), and Wound Healing Scale (Krasner, 1997). However, no data could be found that validated these instruments. Further research is needed to examine the validity and reliability of these instruments.

What Is Known About the Comprehensive Management of Pressure Ulcers?

The comprehensive management of pressure ulcers includes cleansing, controlling infections, debridement, dressings that promote a moist wound environment, nutritional support, and offloading (turning and use of support surfaces). Moreover, the use of adjunctive therapies to heal pressure ulcers should be considered for recalcitrant pressure ulcers.

The first step in the management of pressure ulcers is cleansing the wound to remove devitalized tissue and decrease bacterial burden. Pressure ulcers exhibit delayed healing in the presence of high levels of bacteria (Robson & Heggers, 1969). No randomized control studies could be found that demonstrated the optimal frequency of, or agent for, cleansing the pressure ulcer. Cleansers that do not disrupt or cause trauma to the ulcer should be used (Barr, 1995). Normal saline (0.9%) is usually recommended because it is not cytotoxic to healthy tissue (Bergstrom et al., 1994). Although the active ingredients in newer wound cleansers may be noncytotoxic (surfactants), the inert carrier may be cytotoxic to healthy granulation tissue (Rodeheaver, 1988). Thus, a careful review of all ingredients is warranted. Hellewell, Major, Foresman, and Rodeheaver (1997) found that the antiseptic cleansers were most cytotoxic to granulation tissue. Most research investigating cleansers has been conducted in vitro, with findings extrapolated to the human population. Thus, studies investigating the efficacy of cleansers in the wound environment must be undertaken.

The mechanical method used to deliver the cleanser must provide enough pressure to remove debris, yet not cause trauma to the wound bed. Studies have shown that optimal pressure to cleanse a wound is between 4 to 15 psi (pounds per square inch) (Rodeheaver et al., 1975). Use of a 35 ml syringe with 19-gauge needle to create an 8-psi irrigation pressure stream (Bergstrom et al., 1994) was found to be significantly more effective in removing bacteria than other irrigation pressures (Stevenson et al., 1976). Irrigation pressures exceeding 15 psi causes trauma to the wound bed and may drive bacteria into the tissue (Bhasker, Cutright, & Gross, 1969; Wheeler, Rodeheaver, Thacker, & Edgerton, 1976). New technology such as the battery powered, disposable irrigation devices can provide an alternative to loosen wound debris (Rodeheaver, 1999). Research that investigates multiple methods for cleaning wounds, frequency and evaluating the best methods for cleaning wounds is still needed.

The presence of necrotic, devitalized tissue promotes the growth of pathologic organisms and prevents wounds from healing (Witkowski & Parish, 1992; Yarkoney, 1994). Thus debridement is an important step in the overall management of pressure ulcers. Four types of debridement exist: sharp, autolytic, enzymatic, and mechanical. Sharp (or surgical) debridement is considered the most effective type of debridement because it involves the cutting away (with a scalpel) of necrotic tissue (Dolynchuk, 2001). This form of debridement is relatively quick. Surgical debridement is essential when cellulitis or sepsis is suspected (Galpin, Chow, Bayer, & Guze, 1976). Autolytic debridement involves the use of a semiocclusive or occlusive dressing (hydrocolloids, hydrogels). This form of debridement uses the body's own natural enzymes to breakdown the necrotic tissue. It is a much slower form of debridement and is relatively painless. Enzymatic debridement uses proteolytic enzymes (i.e., papain/urea, collagenase and trypsin) to remove necrotic tissue. This form of debridement is slow and expensive (Dolynchuk, 2001). Mechanical debridement uses wet-to-dry gauze to adhere to the necrotic tissue which is then removed. Upon removal of the gauze dressing, necrotic tissue and wound debris are removed. However, healthy granulation tissue is also removed and this delays wound healing (Dolynchuk, 2001).

There is no optimal debridement method. Selection of the debridement method is based on the goals of the patient, the absence or presence of infection, the amount of necrotic tissue present, and economic considerations for the patient and institution.

The use of dressings is a major component in the effective management of pressure ulcers. There are over 300 different modern dressings available to manage pressure ulcers (Ovington, 1999). Most dressings can be broken down into seven classifications: transparent films, foam islands, hydrocolloids, petroleum-based nonadherents, alginates, hydrogels, and gauze. Few randomized control studies have been conducted to evaluate the efficacy of dressings within a specific classification. Most dressing studies compare gauze (standard) to modern (nongauze) wound dressings (Fowler, 1986; Gorse & Mesner, 1987; Kim et al., 1996). These studies are inherently flawed since gauze dressings are not classified as modern wound dressing, thus equivalent comparisons cannot be made. Four randomized controlled trials were found that compared saline gauze dressings to modern wound dressings in the management of pressure ulcers (Colwell, Foreman, & Trotter, 1993; Sebern, 1986; Thomas, Goode, LeMaster, & Tennyson, 1998; Xakellis & Chrischilles, 1992). In three of the four studies, no significant differences were noted in the number of pressure ulcers healed for the control and experimental groups (Colwell et al., 1993; Thomas et al., 1998; Xakellis & Chriscilles, 1992). In one study, a significant difference ($p \leq .01$) in median decrease in ulcer size was found in a subgroup of subjects with Stage II pressure ulcers using film compared with saline gauze (Sebern, 1986).

Although few studies have been able to demonstrate differences in healing rates using modern wound dressing compared with traditional gauze, there do appear to be significant differences in the time to heal. Several studies have found that compared with traditional gauze, modern wound dressings heal wounds faster, are more economical, and save caregiver time (Bolton, van Rijswijk, & Shaffer, 1997; Kim et al., 1996; Phillips & Davey, 1997; Saydak, 1990). A recent nursing study examined the use of traditional gauze dressing versus a hydrocolloid dressing in healing Stage II pressure ulcers in two groups of elders in two long-term facilities (Lyder, Shannon, Empleo-Frazier, McGehee, & White, under review). This study found that the hydrocolloid dressings significantly healed 40 Stage II pressure ulcers faster (3.44 weeks, $p \leq 0.01$) than the traditional gauze group (32 pressure ulcers, 7.12 weeks). Additional randomized controlled trials are needed comparing modern wound dressings with traditional gauze dressings, and comparing modern wound dressings within specific categories (hydrocolloids or alginates) with each other to determine differences in healing rates and cost.

Optimal nutrition is believed to be critical both to the prevention and healing of pressure ulcers (Thomas, 2001). Good nutritional status has been associated with wound healing (Breslow, Hallfrisch, Guy, Carwley, & Goldberg, 1993; Strauss & Margolis, 1996). Several studies have correlated wound severity with severity of nutritional deficit (Allman, 1989; Berlowitz & Wilking, 1989; Breslow, Hallfrisch, & Goldberg, 1991; Salzberg, Cooper-Vastola, Perez, Viehbeck, & Byrne, 1996). However, there is disagreement regarding which nutritional parameters or interventions consistently improve wound healing, since nutritional status as measured by serum albumin has also not been associated with pressure ulcer healing (Day & Leonard, 1993).

The literature suggests that administering high protein diets for those patients with protein deficiency is essential to wound healing. One small study ($N = 12$) has suggested that 1.25 g protein/L/kg/day to 1.50 g protein/L/kg/day is needed to promote wound healing (Chernoff, Milton, & Lipschitz, 1990). However, Mulholland, Tui, Wright, Vinci, and Shafiroff (1943) suggest that as much as 2.0 g protein/L/kg/day is essential for wound healing. Breslow and colleagues (1993) investigated the importance of dietary protein in healing pressure ulcers. They studied 28 malnourished patients with a total of 33 truncal pressure ulcers. The patients received liquid nutritional formulas as tube feedings or meal supplements containing either 24% (61 g protein/L; $n = 15$) protein or 14% (37 g protein/L; $n = 13$) protein for 8 weeks. They found that patients who received the 24% protein intake had significant decrease ($p = .02$) in truncal pressure ulcer surface area compared with the group on 14% protein intake. Clearly, increasing protein stores for patients with pressure ulcers who are malnourished is essential. It is unclear, however, from the literature what the optimum protein intake requirements are for patients with pressure ulcers (Thomas, 2001).

Vitamin and mineral deficiencies (vitamins A, C, E and zinc) have been found in a majority of elders residing in nursing homes (Bergstrom &

Braden, 1992; Pinchcosky-Devin & Kaminski, 1986). Supplementation of zinc and vitamin C may assist wound healing if deficiencies in these substances are present (Burr, 1973; Taylor, Rimmer, Day, Butcher, & Dymock, 1974; Williams, Lines, & McKay, 1988). However, there is very little evidence that supplementation with these vitamins and minerals aids in wound healing without the presence of the specific deficiency (Ehrlich & Hunt, 1968; Rackett, Rothe, & Grant-Kels, 1993; ter Riet, Kessels, & Knipschild, 1995; Waldorf & Fewkes, 1995). Although many experts believe that overall nutrition is important to good wound healing, beyond increasing protein (for those patients that are protein depleted), there is a lack of literature to support the use of supplemental vitamins and minerals.

WHAT IS THE ROLE OF ADJUNCTIVE THERAPIES IN HEALING PRESSURE ULCERS?

The use of adjunctive therapies is the fastest growing area in pressure ulcer management. Adjunctive therapies include: electrical stimulation, hyperbaric oxygen, low-energy laser radiation, therapeutic ultrasound, radiant heat, growth factors, and skin equivalents. Except for electrical stimulation, there is little research to substantiate the effectiveness of adjunctive therapies in healing pressure ulcers.

Electrical stimulation is the use of electrical current to stimulate a number of cellular processes important to pressure ulcer healing, including increasing fibroblasts, neutrophil macrophage collagen, DNA synthesis and increasing the number of receptor sites for specific growth factors (Kloth et al., 1996). Clinical research in support of electrical stimulation has been well documented (Baker, Chambers, DeMuth, & Villar, 1997; Griffin et al., 1991; Kloth & Feeder, 1988). Eight randomized controlled studies were found in the literature. Electrical stimulation appears to be most effective on Stage III and Stage IV pressure ulcers that have been unresponsive to traditional methods of healing. In a meta-analysis (Gardner, Frantz, & Schmidt, 1999) of 15 studies evaluating the effects of electrical stimulation on the healing of chronic ulcers, researchers found that the rate of healing per week was 22% for the electrical stimulation group compared with 9% for the control group.

Although there is much data to suggest that electrical stimulation is effective in healing pressure ulcers, the optimal electrical charge needed to stimulate pressure ulcer healing remains unclear. The literature suggests that an optimal electrical charge of 300–500 uC/sec produces positive effects on the pressure ulcer (Kloth et al., 1996). However, research is still needed to determine the optimal electrical charge based on the characteristics of pressure ulcers (e.g., stage, depth, drainage).

Hyperbaric oxygen is believed to promote wound healing by stimulating fibroblast, collagen synthesis, epithelialization, and control of infection (Courville, 1998). However, controlled clinical studies of the effects of hyperbaric oxygen and the healing of pressure ulcers could not be found. The literature that does exist suggests that topical hyperbaric oxygen does not increase tissue oxygenation beyond the superficial dermis (Gruber, Heitkamp, Billy, Amato, & Arsenal, 1970).

There is a dearth of research regarding the use of therapeutic ultrasound and ultraviolet light therapy in healing pressure ulcers. Only one controlled study could be found that evaluated the use of therapeutic ultrasound and healing of pressure ulcers (McDiarmid, Burns, Lewith, & Machin, 1985). This study found that there was some improvement in healing rates of the infected ulcers, however no differences in healing rates were noted for the clean ulcers. Several studies have used ultraviolet light in wounds (Nussbaum, Biemann, & Mustard, 1994; ter Riet, Kessels, & Knipschild, 1996). However, no studies were found that demonstrated beneficial effects from the use of ultraviolet light in the healing of pressure ulcers.

Research on the efficacy of radiant heat (normothermia) to heal pressure ulcers is being conducted. It is believed that increasing the thermal wound environment not only increases blood flow, but promotes fibroblasts and other factors associated with pressure ulcer healing (Xia, Sato, Hughes, & Cherry, 2000). Results of three studies (Kloth et al., 2000; Robinson, & Santilli, 1998; Santelli, Valusek, & Robinson, 1999) suggest that radiant heat is beneficial to pressure ulcer healing. The most convincing study was published by Kloth and colleagues (2000). These researchers enrolled 20 patients with 21 Stage III and Stage IV pressure ulcers. The only difference between the experimental group compared with the control group was the addition of radiant heat applied through a semiocclusive dressing (Monday through Friday, 4.5 hours/treatment) for 4 weeks. The results revealed that the experimental group had a mean pressure ulcer surface area reduction of 60.73% compared with the control group's 19.24% reduction. Additional research with larger sample sizes is needed to increase the knowledge of radiant heat and pressure ulcer healing. Studies evaluating the optimal duration of radiant heat treatment on specific stages of ulcers are needed.

The use of growth factors and skin equivalents in healing pressure ulcers is relatively new. The use of cytokine growth factors (e.g., recombinant, platelet-derived growth factor-BB {rhPDGF-BB}) and fibroblast growth factors (bFGF) and skin equivalents are currently being studied. Only one multicenter, randomized double-blind study was found (Mustoe, Cutler, Allman, Goode, & Deuel, 1994). This study enrolled 45 patients with Stage III or Stage IV pressure ulcers who were randomized to either treatment Group 1 (300 ug/ml of rhPDGF), treatment Group 2 (100 ug/ml rhPDGF), or treatment Group 3 (placebo). After 4 weeks of treatment, patients in Group 1 had a 40% reduction in ulcer area, Group 2 had a 71% reduction in ulcer area, and Group 3 had a 17% reduction in pressure ulcer area. This area of research is most promising.

CONCLUSIONS

The review of the literature identified numerous gaps in our understanding of effective pressure ulcer prevention and management. It is evident that pressure ulcer prevention and management is complex. Moreover, much of the current practice is derived from expert opinion rather than empirical evidence. Researchers have made progress in identifying risk factors for pressure ulcer prevention. However, major gaps exist in our understanding of variables that place elders at risk for pressure ulcers. Causal links to pressure ulcer development have not been established. There is a paucity of studies that have included racial minorities. The role of gerontological nurse researchers in conducting pressure ulcer research in vast. To this end, research in the following areas is warranted:

1. Identify major risk factors for pressure ulcer development.
2. Evaluate major risk factors for their cultural sensitivity/appropriateness.
3. Determine optimal cutoff scores for pressure ulcer prediction scales based on various patient populations.
4. Evaluate association of comprehensive skin care and preventing pressure ulcers.
5. Identify optimal turning parameters for various patient populations.
6. Determine efficacy of specific classification of support surfaces to prevent and heal pressure ulcers.
7. Develop universal pressure ulcer classification system.
8. Evaluate the efficacy and cost of implementing comprehensive pressure ulcer prevention programs.

9. Determine optimal methods for pressure ulcer cleansing.
10. Determine efficacy of dressings to effectively heal pressure ulcers.
11. Identify the role of nutrition (vitamins, minerals, etc.) in the prevention and healing of pressure ulcers.
12. Evaluate role of various adjunctive therapies with specific parameters for healing pressure ulcers.

REFERENCES

Allman, R. M. (1989). Epidemiology of pressure sores in different populations. *Decubitus, 2*(2), 30–33.

Allman, R. M., Goode, P. S., Patrick, M. M., Burst, N., & Bartolucci, A. A. (1995). Pressure ulcer risk factors among hospitalized patients with activity limitations. *Journal of the American Medical Association, 273*, 865–870.

Allman, R. M., Laprade, C. A., Noel, L. B., Walker, J. M., Moorer, C. A., Dear, M. R., & Smith, C. R. (1986). Pressure sores among hospitalized patients. *Annals of Internal Medicine, 105*, 337–342.

Ayello, E. A., Sussman, C., Leiby, D., Woodruff, L., Sprigle, S., Bennett, M. A., Dungog, E. F., & Henderson, C. (1997). Classification update: Stage I and darkly pigmented skin. Abstract presented at the National Pressure Ulcer Advisory Panel Fifth National Conference–Monitoring Pressure Ulcer Healing: An Alternative to Reverse Staging. Arlington, VA February 7–8, 1997.

Baker, L., Chambers, R., DeMuth, S., & Villar, F. (1997). Effects of electrical stimulation on wound healing of ulcers in human beings with spinal cord injury. *Wound Repair and Regeneration, 4*, 21–28.

Barbenel, J. C., Jordan, M. M., & Nicol, S. M. (1977). Incidence of pressure sores in the greater Glasgow health board area. *Lancet, 2*, 248–550.

Barr, J. E. (1995). Principles of wound cleansing. *Ostomy Wound Management, 41*, 7A.

Bartolucci, A. A., & Thomas, D. R. (1997). Using principal component analysis to describe wound status. *Advances in Wound Care, 10*(5), 93–95.

Basson, M. D., & Burney, R. E. (1982). Defective wound healing in patients with paraplegia and quadriplegia. *Surgery, Gynecology and Obstetrics, 155*(1), 9–12.

Bates-Jensen, B. M. (1997). The pressure sore status tool a few thousand assessments later. *Advances in Wound Care, 10*(5), 65–73.

Bates-Jensen, B. M., Vredevoe, D. L., & Brecht, M. (1992). Validity and reliability of the pressure sore status tool. *Decubitus, 5*(6), 20–28.

Bergstrom, N., Allman, R. M., Alvarez, O. M., Bennet, M. A., Carlson, C. E., Frantz, R. A., Garber, S. L., Jackson, B. S., Kaminski, M. V., Kemp, M. G., Krouskop, T. A., Lewis, V. L., Maklebust, J., Margolis, D. J., Marvel, E. M., Reger, S. I., Rodeheaver, G. T., Salcido, R., Xakellis, G. C., & Yakony, G. M. (1994). Treatment of pressure ulcers in adults. Clinical practice guideline, Number 15.

U.S. Dept. of Health and Human Services; December 1994. Agency for Health Care Policy and Research publication 95-0652. Rockville, MD: Public Health Service.

Bergstrom, N., Allman, R. M., Carlson, C. E., Eaglstein, W., Frantz, R. A., Garber, S. L., Gosnell, D., Jackson, B. S., Kemp, M. G., Krouskop, T. A., Mravel, E. M., Rodeheaver, G. T., & Xakellis, G. C. (1992). Pressure ulcers in adults: Prediction and prevention. Clinical Practice Guideline, Number 3. U.S. Dept. of Health and Human Services; May 1992. Agency for Health Care Policy and Research publication 92-0047. Rockville, MD: Public Health Service.

Bergstrom, N., & Braden, B. (1992). A prospective study of pressure sore risk among institutionalized elderly. *Journal of the American Geriatrics Society, 40*, 747–758.

Bergstrom, N., Braden, B., Kemp, M., Champayne, M., & Ruby, E. (1996). Multisite study of incidence of pressure ulcers and the relationship between risk level, demographic characteristics, diagnoses, and prescription of preventive interventions. *Journal of the American Geriatrics Society, 44*, 22–30.

Bergstrom, N., Braden, B., Kemp, M. Champagne, M., & Ruby, E. (1998). Predicting pressure ulcer risk: A multisite study of the predictive validity of the Braden Scale. *Nursing Research, 47*, 261–269.

Bergstrom, N., Braden, B., Laguzza, A., & Holzman, V. (1987). The Braden Scale for predicting pressure sore risk. *Nursing Research, 38*, 205–210.

Bergstrom, N., Demuth, P., & Braden, B. (1987). A clinical trial of the Braden Scale for predicting pressure sore risk. *Nursing Clinics of North America, 22*, 417–428.

Berlowitz, D. R., & Wilking, S. V. (1989). Risk factors for pressure sores. A comparison of cross-sectional and cohort-derived data. *Journal of the American Geriatrics Society, 37*, 1043–1050.

Bhasker, S. N., Cutright, D. E., & Gross, A. (1969). Effect of water lavage on infected wounds in the rat. *Journal of Periodontology, 40*, 671–672.

Bolton, L. L., van Rijswijk, L., & Shaffer, F. A. (1997). Quality wound care equals cost-effective wound care: A clinical model. *Advances in Wound Care, 10*, 33–38.

Braden, B., & Bergstrom, N. (1987). A conceptual schema for the study of the etiology of pressure sores. *Rehabilitation Nursing, 12*(1), 8–12.

Brandeis, G. H., Morris, J. N., Nash, D. J., & Lipsitz, L. A. (1990). Epidemiology and natural history of pressure ulcers in elderly nursing home residents. *Journal of the American Medical Association, 264*, 2905–2909.

Breslow, R. A., Hallfrisch, J., & Goldberg, A. P. (1991). Malnutrition in tube-fed home patients with pressure sores. *Journal of Parenteral & Enteral Nutrition, 15*, 663–668.

Breslow, R. A., Hallfrisch, J., Guy, D. G., Carwley, B., & Goldberg, A. P. (1993). The importance of dietary protein in healing pressure ulcers. *Journal of the American Geriatrics Society, 41*, 357.

Burr, R. G. (1973). Blood zinc in the spinal patient. *Journal of Clinical Pathology, 26*, 773–775.

Chernoff, R. S., Milton, K. Y., & Lipschitz, D. A. (1990). The effect of a very high-protein liquid formula on decubitus ulcer healing in long-term tube-fed institutionalized patients. *Journal of the American Geriatrics Society, 90*, A–130.

Colin, D., Loyant, R., Abraham, P., & Saumet, J. (1996). Changes in sacral transcutaneous oxygen tension in the evaluation of different mattresses in the prevention of pressure ulcers.*Advances in Wound Care, 9*(1), 25–28.

Colwell, J. C., Foreman, M. D., & Trotter, J. P. (1993). A comparison of the efficacy and cost effectiveness of two methods of managing pressure ulcers. *Decubitus, 6*(4), 28–36.

Courville, S. (1998). Hyperbaric oxygen therapy: Its role in healing problem wounds. *Caet Journal, 17*(4), 7–11.

Cuddigan, J., Ayello, E. A., Sussman, C., & Baranoski, S. (2001). *Pressure ulcers in America: Prevalence, incidence, and implications for the future.* Reston, VA: National Pressure Ulcer Advisory Panel.

Cullum, N., Deeks, J., Sheldon, T. A., Song, F., & Fletcher, A. W. (2001). *Beds, mattresses and cushions for pressure sore prevention and treatment.* Oxford, England: The Cochrane Library.

Day, A., & Leonard, F. (1993). Seeking quality care for patients with pressure ulcers. *Decubitus, 6*, 32–43.

Dyson, R. (1978). Bed sores—the injuries hospital staff inflict on patients. *Nursing Mirror, 146*(24), 30–32.

Dolychuck, K. N. (2001). Debridement. In D. Krasner, G. T. Rodeheaver, & R. G. Sibbald (Eds.), *Chronic wound care: A clinical source book for health care professionals* (3rd ed., pp. 385–390).

Eckman, K. L. (1989). The prevalence of dermal ulcers among persons in the U.S. who have died. *Decubitus*, May 2, 36–40.

Ek, A. C., Gustavsson, G., & Lewis, D. H. (1985). The local skin blood flow in areas at risk for pressure sores treated with massage. *Scandinavian Journal of Rehabilitation and Medicine, 17*(2), 81–86.

Ek, A. C., Lewis, D. H., Zetterqvist, H., & Svensson, P. G. (1984). Skin blood flow in an area at risk for pressure sore. *Scandinavian Journal of Rehabilitation Medicine, 16*(2), 85–89.

Erlich, H. P., & Hunt, T. K. (1968). Effects of cortisone and vitamin A on wound healing. *Annals of Surgery, 167*, 324–328.

Ferrell, B. (1997). The Sessing scale for measurement of pressure ulcer healing. *Advances in Wound Care, 10*(5), 78–81.

Fontaine, R. (2000). Investigating the efficacy of a nonpowered pressure-reducing therapeutic mattress: A retrospective multi-site study. *Ostomy Wound Management, 46*(9), 39–43.

Fowler, E. (1986). Nursing diagnosis: Actual impairment of skin integrity. *Journal of Gerontological Nursing, 12*(10), 36–37.

Fuhrer, M., Garber, S., Rintola, D., Clearman, R., & Hart, K. (1993). Pressure ulcers in community-resident persons with spinal cord injury: Prevalence and risk factors. *Archives of Physical Medicine and Rehabilitation, 74*, 1172–1177.

Galpin, J. E., Chow, A. W., Bayer, A. S., & Guze, L. B. (1976). Sepsis associated with decubitus ulcers. *American Journal of Medicine, 61*, 346–350.

Gardner, S. E., Frantz, R. A., & Schmidt, F. L. (1999). Effect of electrical stimulation on chronic wound healing: A meta-analysis. *Wound Repair Regeneration, 7*, 495–503.

Gorse, G. J., & Messner, R. L. (1987). Improved pressure sore healing with hydrocolloid dressings. *Archives of Dermatology, 123*, 766–771.

Griffin, J., Tooms, R., Mendius, R., Clifft, J., Vander Zwaag, R., & El-Zeky, F. (1991). Efficacy of high voltage pulsed current for healing of pressure ulcers in patients with spinal cord injury. *Physical Therapy, 71*, 433–444.

Gruber, R. P., Heitkamp, D. H., Billy, L. J., Amato, J. J., & Arsenal, E. (1970). Skin permeability of oxygen and hyperbaric oxygen. *Archives of Surgery, 101*, 69–70.

Guralnik, J. M., Harris, T. B., White, L. R., & Coroni-Huntley, J. C. (1988). Occurrence and predictors of pressure ulcers in the National Health and Nutrition Examination Survey Follow-Up. *Journal of the American Geriatrics Society, 36*, 807–812.

Health Care Financing Administration. Investigative Protocol, Guidance to Surveyors–Long Term Care Facilities. Rev. 274. U.S. Dept. of Health and Human Services; June 2000.

Healthy People 2010. (2001). U.S. Department of Health and Human Services [on-line]. [Available: http://www.health.gov/healthypeople]. Accessed January 7, 2001.

Hellewell, T. B., Major, P. A., Foresman, P. A., & Rodeheaver, G. T. (1997). A cytotoxicity evaluation of antimicrobial wound cleansers. *Wounds, 9*(1), 15–20.

Henderson, C. T., Ayello, E. A., Sussman, C., Leiby, D. M., Bennett, M. A., Dungog, E. F., Sprigle, S., & Woodruff, L. (1997). Draft definition of Stage I pressure ulcers: Inclusion of persons with darkly pigmented skin. *Advances in Wound Care, 10*, 16–19.

Houghton, P. E. (1999). Effects of therapeutic modalities on wound healing: A conservative approach to the management of chronic wounds. *Physical Therapy Reviews, 4*(3), 167–182.

International Association for Enterstomal Therapy. (1987). *Standards of care for dermal wounds: Pressure ulcers.* Irvine, CA: Author.

Kelly, L. S., & Mobily, P. R. (1991). Iatrogenesis in the elderly: Impaired skin integrity. *Journal of Gerontological Nursing, 17*(9), 24–29.

Kim, Y. C., Shin, J. C., Park, C. I., Oh, S. H., Choi, S. M., & Kim, Y. S. (1996). Efficacy of hydrocolloid occlusive dressing technique in decubitus ulcer treatment: A comparative study. *Yonsei Medical Journal, 37*, 181–185.

Kloth, L., & Feeder, J. (1988). Acceleration of wound healing with high voltage, monophasic, pulsed current. *Physical Therapy, 68*, 503–508.

Kloth, L. C., Berman, J. E., Dumit-Minkel, S., Sutton, C. H., Papanek, P. E., & Wurzel, J. (2000). Effects of a normothermic dressing on pressure ulcer healing. *Advances in Skin and Wound Care, 13*(2), 69–74.

Kloth, L. C., & McCulloch, J. (1996). Promotion of wound healing with electrical stimulation. *Advances in Wound Care, 9*, 42–45.

Knox, D. M., Anderson, T. M., & Anderson, P. S. (1994). Effects of different turn intervals on skin of healthy older adults. *Advances in Wound Care, 7*, 48–52, 54–56.

Kosiak, M. (1959). Etiology and pathology of ischemic ulcers. *Archives of Physical Medicine and Rehabilitation, 40*(2), 62–69.

Kosiak, M., Kubicek, W. G., Olson, M., Dantz, J. N., & Kottke, F. J. (1958). Evaluation of pressure as a factor in the production of ischial ulcers. *Archives of Physical Medicine and Rehabilitation, 39*, 623–629.

Krasner, D. (1997). Wound healing scale, version 1.0: A proposal. *Advances in Wound Care, 10*(5), 82–85.

Landis, E. M. (1930). Micro-injection studies of capillary blood pressure in human skin. *Heart, 15,* 209.

Langemo, D. K., Olson, B., Hunter, S., Burd, C., Hansen, D., & Cathcart-Silberberg, T. (1989). Incidence of pressure sores in acute care, rehabilitation, extended care, home health, and hospice in one locale. *Decubitus, 2*(2), 42.

Lazzara, D. J., & Buschmann, M. T. (1991). Prevention of pressure ulcers in elderly nursing home residents: Are special support surfaces the answer? *Decubitus, 4*(4), 42–44.

Lewicki, L. J., Mion, L. C., & Secic, M. (2000). Sensitivity and specificity of the Braden Scale in the cardiac surgical population. *Journal of Wound Ostomy and Continence Nursing, 27*(1), 36–41.

Lyder, C. (1991). Conceptualization of the Stage 1 pressure ulcer. *Journal of ET Nursing, 18,* 162–165.

Lyder, C. H., Grady, J., Mathur, D., Patrello, M., & Meehan, T. (in press). Preventing pressure ulcers in Connecticut hospitals using the plan-do-study-act model for quality improvement. *Journal of Quality Improvement.*

Lyder, C. H., Preston, J., Grady, J., Scinto, J., Allman, R. M., Bergstrom, N., et al. (2001). Quality of care for hospitalized medicare patients at risk for pressure ulcers. *Archives of Internal Medicine, 161,* 1549–1554.

Lyder, C., Preston, J., Scinto, J., Grady, J., & Ahearn, D. (1998). *Medicare quality indicator system: Pressure ulcer prediction and prevention module: Final report.* Baltimore, MD: U.S. Health Care Financing Administration.

Lyder, C. H., Shannon, R., Empleo-Frazier, O., McGehee, D., & White, C. (in press). A comprehensive program to prevent pressure ulcers: Exploring cost and outcomes. *Ostomy Wound Management.*

Lyder, C. H., Shannon, R., Empleo-Frazier, O., McGehee, D., & White, C. (under review). Examining the cost-effectiveness of two methods for healing Stage II pressure ulcers in long-term care.

Lyder, C., Yu, C., Emerling, J., Stevenson, D., Empleo-Frazier, O., Mangat, R., & Mckay, J. (1999). The Braden Scale for pressure ulcer risk: Evaluating the predictive validity in Blacks and Hispanic elderly patients. *Applied Nursing Research, 12*(2), 60–68.

Lyder, C., Yu, C., Stevenson, D., Mangat, R., Empleo-Frazier, O., Emerling, J., & McKay, J. (1998). Validating the Braden Scale for the prediction of pressure ulcer risk in Blacks and Latino/Hispanic elders: A pilot study. *Ostomy/Wound Management, 44,* 42–50.

Mawson, A. R., Siddiqui, F. H., & Biundo J. J. (1993). Enhancing host resistance to pressure ulcers: A new approach to prevention. *Preventive Medicine, 22,* 433–450.

McDiarmid, T., Burns, P. N., Lewith, G. T., & Machin, D. (1985). Ultrasound and the treatment of pressure sores. *Physiotherapy, 71,* 66–70.

Morrison, S. (1984). Monitoring decubitus ulcers: A monthly survey method. *Quarterly Review Bulletin, 10,* 112–117.

Mulholland, J. H., Tui, C., Wright, A. M., Vinci, V., & Shafiroff, B. (1943). Protein metabolism and bedsores. *Annals of Surgery, 118*, 1015–1023.

Mustoe, T. A., Cutler, N. R., Allman, R. M., Goode, P. S., Deuel, T. F., Prause, J. A., Bear, M., Serder, C. M., & Pierce, G. F. (1994). A phase II study to evaluate recombinant platelet-derived growth factor-BB in the treatment of stage 3 and 4 pressure ulcers. *Archives of Surgery, 129*, 213–219.

National Pressure Ulcer Advisory Panel. (1999). Position on reverse staging of pressure ulcers. *Advances in Wound Care, 8*, 32–33.

Norton, D. (1989). Calculating the risk: reflections of the Norton Scale. *Decubitus, 2*(3), 24–31.

Norton, D., McLaren, R., & Exton-Smith, A. (1975). *An investigation of geriatric nurse problems in hospitals*. Edinburgh, Scotland: Churchill Livingston.

Nussbaum, E. L., Biemann, I., & Mustard, B. (1994). Comparison of ultrasound/ ultraviolet–C and laser for treatment of pressure ulcers in patients with spinal cord. *Physical Therapy, 74*, 812–825.

Oertwich, P. A., Kindschuh, A. M., & Bergstrom, N. (1995). The effects of small shifts in body weight on blood flow and interface pressure. *Research in Nursing and Health, 18*, 481–488.

Ooka, M., Kemp, M. G., McMyn, R., & Shott, S. (1995). Evaluation of three types of support surfaces for pressure ulcers in patients in a surgical intensive care unit. *Journal of Wound Ostomy and Continence Nursing, 22*, 271–279.

Ovington, L. (1999). Dressings and adjunctive therapies: AHCPR guidelines revisited. *Ostomy Wound Management, 45*, 94S–106S.

Pang, S. M., & Wong, T. K. (1998). Predicting pressure sore risk with the Norton, Braden, and Waterlow Scales in a Hong Kong rehabilitation hospital. *Nursing Research, 47*, 147–153.

Peterson, N. C., & Bittman, S. (1971). The epidemiology of pressure sores. *Scandinavian Journal of Plastic Reconstruction Surgery and Hand Surgery, 5*(4), 62–66.

Phillips, T., & Davey, C. (1997). Wound cleansing versus wound disinfection: A challenging dilemma. *Perspectives, 21*, 15–16.

Pinchofsky-Devin, G. D., & Kaminski, M. V. (1986). Correlation of pressure sores and nutritional status. *Journal of the American Geriatrics Society, 34*, 435–440.

Rackett, S. C., Rothe, M. J., & Grant-Kels, J. M. (1993). The role of dietary manipulation in the prevention and treatment of cutaneous disorders. *Journal of the American Academy of Dermatology, 29*, 447–453.

Robinson, C., & Santilli, S. M. (1998). Warm-up active wound therapy: A novel approach to the management of chronic venous stasis ulcers. *Journal of Vascular Nursing, 16*(2), 38–42.

Robson, M. C., & Heggers, J. P. (1969). Bacterial quantification of open wounds. *Military Medicine, 134*(1), 19–24.

Rodeheaver, G. (1988). Controversies in topical wound management. *Ostomy Wound Management*, 58–68.

Rodeheaver, G. T. (1999). Pressure ulcer debridement and cleansing: A review of the current literature. *Ostomy Wound Management, 45*, 80S–85S.

Rodeheaver, G. T., Pettry, D., Thacker, J. G., Edgerton, M. T., & Edlich, R. F. (1975). Wound cleansing by high pressure irrigation. *Surgery Gynecology and Obstetrics, 141*, 357–362.

Rousseau, P. (1988). Pressure ulcers in the aged: A preventable problem. *Continuing Care, 17*, 35–42.

Salcido, R., Donofrio, J., & Fisher, S. (1994). Histopathology of pressure ulcers as a result of sequential computer-controlled pressure sessions in a fuzzy rat model. *Advances in Wound Care, 7*(5), 23–40.

Salzberg, C., Cooper-Vastola, S., Perez, F., Viehbeck, M. G., & Byrne, D. W. (1995). The effects of nonthermal pulsed electromagnetic energy on wound healing of pressure ulcers in spinal cord-injured patients: A randomized double-blind study. *Ostomy Wound Management, 41*, 42–51.

Shea, J. D. (1975). Pressure sores: Classification and management. *Clinical Orthopedics, 112*, 89–100.

Santilli, S. M., Valusek, P. A., & Robinson, C. (1999). Use of noncontact radiant heat bandage for the treatment of chronic venous stasis ulcers. *Advances in Wound Care, 12*(2), 89–93.

Saydak, S. (1990). A pilot of two methods for the treatment of pressure ulcers. *Journal of Enterstomal Therapy, 7*, 139–142.

Sebern, M. (1986). Pressure ulcer management in home health care: Efficacy and cost effectiveness of a moisture vapor permeable dressing. *Archives of Physical Medicine and Rehabilitation, 67*, 726–729.

Seller, W. O., Allen, S., & Stahelin, H. B. (1986). Influence of 30° laterally inclined position and the supersoft 3-piece mattress on skin oxygen tension on areas of maximum pressure: Implications for pressure sore prevention. *Gerontology, 32*, 158–166.

Shea, J. D. (1975). Pressure sores: Classification and management. *Clinical Orthopedics, 112*, 89–100.

Spector, W., Kapp, M., Tucker, R., & Sternberg, J. (1988). Factors associated with presence of decubitus ulcers at admission to nursing homes. *Gerontologist, 28*, 830–834.

Stevenson, T. R., Thacker, J. G., Rodeheaver, G. T., Bacchetta, C., Edgerton, M. T., & Edlich, R. F. (1976). Cleansing the traumatic wound by high pressure syringe irrigation. *JACEP, 5*(1), 17–21.

Strauss, E., & Margolis, D. (1996). Malnutrition in patient with pressure ulcers: Morbidity, mortality, and clinically practical assessments. *Advances in Wound Care, 9*(1), 37–40.

Sussman, C., & Swanson, G. (1997). Utility of the Sussman wound healing tool in predicting wound healing outcomes in physical therapy. *Advances in Wound Care, 10*(5), 74–77.

Taylor, T. V., Rimmer, S., Day, B., Butcher, J., & Dymock, I. W. (1974). Ascorbic acid supplementation in the treatment of pressure sores. *Lancet, 2*, 544–551.

ter Riet, G., Kessels, A., & Knipschild, P. (1995). Randomized clinical trial of ascorbic acid in the treatment of pressure ulcers. *Journal of Clinical Epidemiology, 48*, 1452–1460.

ter Riet, G., Kessels, A., & Knipschild, P. (1996). A randomized clinical trial of ultrasound in the treatment of pressure ulcers. *Physical Therapy, 76*, 1301–1311.

Thomas, D. R. (2001). Improving outcome of pressure ulcer with nutritional interventions: A review of the literature. *Nutrition, 17*, 121–125.

Thomas, D. R., Goode, P. S., LeMaster, K., & Tennyson, T. (1998). Acemannan hydrogel dressing versus saline dressing for pressure ulcers: A randomized controlled trial. *Advances in Wound Care, 11*, 273–276.

Thomas, D. R., Goode, P. S., Tarquine, P. H., & Allman, R. M. (1996). Hospital-acquired pressure ulcers and risk of death. *Journal of the American Geriatrics Society, 44*, 1435–1440.

Waldorf, H., & Fewkes, J. (1995). Wound healing. *Advances in Dermatology, 10*, 77–81.

Wheeler, C. B., Rodeheaver, G. T., Thacker, J. G., & Edgerton, R. F. (1976). Side-effects of high pressure irrigation. *Surgical Gynecology and Obstetrics, 143*, 775–778.

Williams, C. M., Lines, C. M., & McKay, E. C. (1988). Iron and zinc status in multiple sclerosis patients with pressure sores. *European Journal of Clinical Nutrition, 42*, 321–328.

Witkowski, J. A., & Parish, L. C. (1992). Debridement of cutaneous ulcers: Medical and surgical aspects. *Clinical Dermatology, 9*, 558–591.

Xakellis, G. C., & Chriscilles, E. A. (1992). Hydrocolloids versus saline gauze dressings in treating pressure ulcers: A cost-effective analysis. *Archives of Physical Medicine and Rehabilitation, 73*, 463–469.

Xakellis, G. C., Frantz, R. A., Lewis, A., & Harvey, P. (1998). Cost-effectiveness of an intensive pressure ulcer prevention protocol in long-term care. *Advances in Wound Care, 11*, 22–29.

Xia, Z., Sato, A., Hughes, M. A., & Cherry, G. W. (2000). Stimulation of fibroblast growth in vitro by intermittent radiant warming. *Wound Repair Regeneration, 8*, 138–144.

Yarkony, G. M. (1994). Pressure ulcers: Medical management. In *Spinal cord injury medical management and rehabilitation* (1st ed., pp. 77–83). Gaithersberg, MD: Aspen.

Chapter 3

Pain in Older Adults

LOIS L. MILLER AND KAREN AMANN TALERICO

ABSTRACT

This chapter reviews 80 published research reports of pain and pain problems in older adults by nurse researchers and researchers from other disciplines. Reports were identified through searches of MEDLINE and the Cumulative Index to Nursing and Allied Health Literature (CINAHL) using the search terms pain, older adult, aged and pain, and dementia. Reports were included if published between 1985 to 2001, if conducted on samples age 60 or older, if conducted by nurses or relevant to nursing research, and if published in English. Descriptive, qualitative, correlational, longitudinal, and intervention studies were included. Key findings include the following: pain is widely prevalent in older adult populations; few studies have included minority groups; underidentification and undertreatment of pain in older adults is a consistent interpretation of research findings; pain intensity rating scales are as valid and reliable in older populations as in younger populations; current observational methods of assessing pain in cognitively impaired older adults must be used with caution; nursing intervention studies demonstrate the beneficial effects of education and interventions aimed at improved pain assessment. The main recommendations are: careful attention should be given to the conceptualization and definition of pain; examination of pain should include physiological, motivational, cognitive, and affective factors; studies evaluating undertreatment of pain should include measures of pain self-report; standardized pain measures should be used; studies of persons over the age of 85 and studies of ethnic minorities are needed; more attention should be given to nursing intervention studies and should include both pharmacological and nonpharmacological, psychosocial interventions.

Keywords: pain, older adults, measurement of pain, nursing interventions

The special issues of pain in older adults have only recently begun to receive serious scientific consideration (AGS Panel on Chronic Pain in Older Persons, 1998). Epidemiological evidence demonstrates that large numbers of older adults experience pain, yet the underidentification and undertreatment of pain is one of the most consistent interpretations of research on pain in older adults. Older adults over the age of 85, the fastest growing age group in the country, have been studied least of all in regard to pain and pain problems. Given what we now know about pain and pain management in older adults, there is a consensus that this is a significant area for future research and improved nursing care (AGS, 1998; NIH Consensus Panel, 1986; NINR, 2001).

Nurses are in a unique position to have a positive impact on pain management because of their interface with older adults in community, acute, and long-term care settings. Institutionalized older adults, whether in acute-care or long-term care settings, rely on nurses to appropriately assess pain, administer treatments for pain, and evaluate the person's response to pain. Additionally, community-based nurses, through educational efforts targeted at the appropriate assessment, overcoming attitudinal barriers, aggressive treatment of pain, and management of medication side effects, can do much to improve the care of older adults who dwell in the community.

This review will evaluate the current state of knowledge and identify ways that nurses can best contribute to the improvement of older adult care in the area of pain management. The review is organized around the following set of questions:

1. How does pain vary across population groups of older adults?
2. How has pain in older adults been measured?
3. What are the attitudes and beliefs of older adults about pain, and what are their experiences with pain and pain treatments?
4. How adequately is pain treated in older adults?
5. What treatments for pain do older adults use and has the full range of interventions been tested?

METHOD

This review focused on research on pain and pain problems in older adults over the age of 60, published between 1985 and 2001. The literature search for the review was conducted using a variety of data collection techniques. Online computer searches of MEDLINE and the Cumulative Index to Nursing and Allied Health Literature (CINAHL) databases yielded most of the studies reviewed. Relevant citations were pulled from key articles and some citations were obtained through informal sharing among faculty and student colleagues. The search included all relevant studies published in English. Because of the potentially large number of studies on pain in the specified time period, the search was limited by searching for the words *pain*, *older adult*, and *aged* in the title or abstract, and a specialized literature search on the key words *pain* and *dementia* was conducted. Studies were reviewed for type of pain, subject source, measurement and design. Studies of both acute and chronic pain were included because authors frequently did not indicate or define the type of pain they were studying. Studies across community and institutional settings were included to give as complete a picture of the state of the science as possible. Because this is a relatively young science, many studies were descriptive and/or correlational, some were qualitative, and few were longitudinal or experimental tests of interventions.

We highlight nursing's contribution wherever possible, but because pain research is multidisciplinary in nature, we included nonnurse-authored research for a complete picture of the state of the science (NIH Consensus Panel, 1986). For each of the key questions, we have presented what is known in general about older adult populations, followed by evidence specific to pain in persons with Alzheimer's disease and related dementias. Because this population represents a vulnerable group with complex nursing needs and presents many challenges for care providers in terms of pain assessment and management, we believe it is worthy of close examination.

RESULTS AND DISCUSSION

How Does Pain Vary Across Population Groups of Older Adults?

Prevalence studies of pain in older adults have increased in recent years, providing much needed information on the size and nature of the problem. Table 3.1 summarizes selected studies that examined prevalence and incidence of pain in older adults across settings. The prevalence of pain in community-dwelling older adults ranges from approximately 36–86% for

TABLE 3.1   Prevalence and Incidence of Pain in Older Adult Populations: Selected Studies 1985–2000

Study	Methods	Pain prevalence findings
The Prevalence of Pain in a General Population: The Results of a Postal Survey in a County in Sweden (Brattberg, Thorsland, & Wikman, 1989)	Design: Mail & telephone survey with 82% response rate. Type/Measure of Pain: Persistent pain. Pain sensation intensity, how much affected, troubled by pain? Sample: Sweden 183 community-dwelling older adults age 18–84 (Gender, ethnicity not reported).	Prevalence rate of 36.1% in 65–84 age group. Prevalence rate in 65–84 age group higher than 18–44 age group (34.2%) and lower than 45–64 age group (50%).
Population-based Study of Pain in Elderly People: A Descriptive Study (Brochet, Michel, Barberger-Gateau, & Dartigues, 1998)	Design: Descriptive, face-to-face interview. Type/Measure of Pain: Pain within last year, location, temporal pattern, severity (by authors). Sample: France 741 general population older adults mean age 74.2 (range not reported). 60.2% women (ethnicity not reported).	Prevalence rate of 71.5% for pain in any body location in last year. Women significantly more likely to report any pain and persistent pain, men reported significantly more episodic pain. No significant gender differences in pain severity.

TABLE 3.1 *(continued)*

Study	Methods	Pain prevalence findings
Pain and Suffering in Seriously Ill Hospitalized Patients (Desbiens & Wu, 2000)	Design: Integration of findings related to pain from the SUPPORT and HELP longitudinal intervention studies. Type/Measure of Pain: Self-reported frequency and severity of pain. Sample: 5176 seriously ill hospitalized patients, median age 52.5 with interquartile range 64.4–73 HELP subsample selected patients > 80 years of age	Prevalence ranged 43–60% of participants, which varied by diagnostic category (colon cancer highest). Pain varied widely by hospital site. Pain prevalence and treatment did NOT improve over a 5-year period, even with complex cognitive and psychological intervention.
Pain in the Nursing Home (Ferrell, Ferrell,* & Osterweil, 1990)	Design: Descriptive, face-to-face interview. Type/Measure of Pain: McGill Present Pain Intensity Scale, Pain Experience Measure (by authors). Sample: US 92 residents of SNF, ICF, Board and Care aged 76–106. 83% female (ethnicity not reported).	Prevalence rate of 71% for at least one pain complaint, which varied by type of pain which was highest for low back pain (40%) and lowest for neuropathies (11%). Constant pain was reported by 24%. Only 15% of those in pain had received analgesics in previous 24 hours.

(continued)

TABLE 3.1 *(continued)*

Study	Methods	Pain prevalence findings
Chronic Musculoskeletal Pain and Depressive Symptoms in the National Health and Nutrition Examination I. Epidemiologic Follow Up Study (Magni, Marchetti, Moreschi, Merskey, & Luchini, 1993)	Design: Descriptive, mail survey. Type/Measure of Pain: Chronic pain, persistent pain. Presence, location of pain in previous 12 months (by authors). Sample: US 2341 general population, 386 (16.5%) age 65–86. Total sample—54% female, 8% African American, 1.5% other race.	Prevalence rate of 37.1% for 65–74 age group. Prevalence rate of 38.2% for 75–86 age group. Increasing prevalence with increasing age in five age groups from age 33 to 86.
An Epidemiologic Analysis of Pain in the Elderly: The Iowa 65+ Rural Health Study, 1994 (Mobily,* Herr,* Clark, & Wallace, 1994)	Design: Descriptive, in-home interview. Type/Measure of Pain: Pain, multiple pain complaints, site(s) of pain. Measure not described. Sample: US 3,097 general population in 2 Iowa counties over age 65 (age range, mean, ethnicity not reported).	Prevalence rate of 86.3% for any pain. Prevalence rate of 59% for multiple pain complaints. Prevalence rate for 85+ age group significantly lower than other age groups. Higher prevalence in women than men.
Musculoskeletal Complaints and Associated Consequences in Elderly Chinese Age 70 Years and Over (Woo, Ho, Lau, & Leung, 1994)	Design: Descriptive, face-to-face interview. Type/Measure of Pain: Not reported. Sample: Hong Kong 2,032 general population age 70–90+. 51% Chinese women.	Prevalence rate of 57%. Slight decreasing prevalence with increasing age. Women consistently reported higher rates than men.

*Nurse Researcher.

some type of pain, usually chronic in nature. A clear pattern of women reporting pain more frequently appeared, but no gender differences were found for reports of pain severity, which was examined inconsistently across studies. Pain prevalence was 75.7% in a home health population (Ross & Crook, 1998) and 80.4% in a disabled, community-dwelling sample (Pahor et al., 1999). No clear ethnic differences were evident, but few studies explicitly included African-American, Native American, or other ethnic minority participants. These studies demonstrate the high prevalence of pain in older adults across settings.

Prevalence of pain in older adults living in institutional settings has been reported at 62%–79% (Ferrell, Ferrell, & Rivera, 1995; Parmelee, Smith, & Katz, 1993). Between 30% and 70% of nursing home residents with dementia have diagnoses of arthritis or musculoskeletal disorders, the most frequent cause of pain in older adults (Feldt, Warne, & Ryden, 1998; Ferrell et al., 1995; Horgas & Tsai, 1998; Marzinski, 1991; Weiner, Peterson, & Keefe, 1999). Those who examined pain in persons with dementia have found similarly high prevalence rates for both those who are institutionalized (62%) (Ferrell et al., 1995) as well as those who live in the community (64%) (McCarthy, Addington-Hall, & Altmann, 1997), demonstrating a significant need for nursing intervention in this population.

The question, "How does pain vary across population groups of older adults?" is difficult to answer definitively with available evidence. There is a real need for researchers explicitly to analyze and report ethnic minority differences, although international studies lead us to believe that pain is a consistent problem across groups of older adults. Women, who disproportionately make up the older population, seem to suffer more from chronic pain than men. Whether the higher prevalence noted in rural versus urban older adults (see Mobily, Herr, Clark, & Wallace, 1994, Table 3.1) truly exists or is an artifact of question construction is unclear, but has implications for health policy planning if indeed pain is more prevalent in rural older adults. Given the differences in how pain has been defined across studies and the fluctuating nature of chronic pain, we recommend that researchers examine not only current pain but also chronic/daily pain complaints for a period of time that would detect ongoing pain issues. Finally, we suggest that prospective epidemiological studies on pain presence, intensity, and impact on function be conducted to understand fully the impact of pain on older adults. These studies are needed across care settings, should explicitly target persons with dementia, and should focus on ethnic minority and rural differences.

How Has Pain in Older Adults Been Measured?

A critical first step in providing optimal pain control is pain assessment. Verbal self-report is widely accepted as the most reliable measure of pain (AGS, 1998; Jacox, Carr, Payne, & the Cancer Pain Management Panel, 1994; McCaffery & Pasero, 1999; Turk & Melzack, 1992). Yet, use of self-report pain measures has been infrequently studied in older populations. Assumptions are often made that existing instruments (e.g., the McGill Pain Questionnaire) are too difficult for older adults to use (Herr & Mobily, 1991), when the instruments have not been fully evaluated.

Subjective intensity is the dimension of pain most often measured in both clinical settings and in research on pain. Nurse researchers Herr and Mobily (1993) have conducted important pioneering research on the psychometric properties of selected pain intensity rating scales with samples of older adults. In their 1993 study, Herr and Mobily compared scores on five pain intensity rating scales in a sample of community-dwelling older adults with leg pain using a horizontal 100 millimeter Visual Analog Scale, a Vertical Visual Analog Scale, a Numeric Rating Scale (0–20), a Verbal Descriptor Scale (*no pain* to *pain as bad as it could be*), and a Pain Thermometer (picture of thermometer with word descriptors—*no pain* to *pain as bad as it can be*). Significant correlations ($r = .84$ to 1.00) existed among all five scales. Failure rates were comparable to rates in younger samples, suggesting that both visual analog scales and verbal descriptor scales can be used with an older population. Most important, participants had a clear preference for using the two scales that included word descriptors—the Verbal Descriptor Scale and the Pain Thermometer.

In a second study, Herr and colleagues (1998) conducted psychometric testing on a Faces Pain Scale (FPS), which they modified from one developed for children. The FPS was tested with 168 community-dwelling older adults, who were asked to rate the intensity of a vividly remembered painful experience. Initial support for content validity was obtained; most subjects agreed that the faces represented pain. However, they also agreed that the faces could represent other constructs as well (sourness, sleepiness, sadness, boredom), and four subjects said they could not use the FPS to communicate pain. There was strong agreement on the rank ordering of the faces as a measure of pain intensity, but there were wide gaps between some of the faces, suggesting that the intervals are not equal, which has implications for quantitative analyses.

Although these studies are important and provide valuable information about the use of pain intensity rating scales with older populations, they do not address other dimensions of pain. In an attempt to tackle this issue, Ferrell, Stein, and Beck (2000) developed and tested a multidimensional pain assessment instrument specifically for use with an older adult population. The Geriatric Pain Measure (GPM) is a 24-item instrument, which was pilot-tested on ambulatory geriatric clinic patients ($N = 176$) with multiple health problems. Initial psychometric testing yielded a Cronbach's alpha of .94, average interitem correlation of .42 (range .17 to .83), and test-retest reliability of .90. Factor analysis identified five subscales: Disengagement because of Pain; Pain Intensity; Pain with Ambulation; Pain with Strenuous Activities; and Pain with Other Activities. The scale consistently demonstrated moderate to strong, highly significant correlations with the McGill Pain Questionnaire (Melzack, 1975), a widely used multidimensional pain assessment instrument with established validity and reliability. The GPM's developers found the instrument easy to administer in the population tested. The GPM holds excellent promise but needs further testing in other older populations.

Although some evidence indicates that self-reports of pain decline as dementia progresses, a growing body of literature indicates that, when asked, sizable proportions of persons with dementia are able to communicate that they have pain (Ferrell et al., 1995; Herr & Mobily, 1993; Parmelee, 1996; Parmelee et al., 1993). Yet, it is clear that the ability to communicate pain declines as dementia progresses and varies widely among individuals. Measures such as the GPM or the Faces Pain Scale often place significant demands on verbal and working memory, which decline in both normal aging and dementia, and thus may not be appropriate for this group. In particular the GPM uses compound sentences with left-branching clauses, placing a burden on grammatical communication skills, which are impaired in many dementias. To overcome these problems with standard self-report measures, research on pain assessment in persons with dementia has focused on observational measures of pain and whether behavioral symptoms are pain indicators in persons with late stage dementia.

Several researchers have attempted to identify observable behaviors that can be reliably associated with discomfort and/or pain. Among one of the first efforts in this direction, the Discomfort Scale for patients with Dementia of the Alzheimer's Type (DS-DAT) was developed by a nurse-led team (Hurley, Volicer, Hanrahan, Houde, & Volicer, 1992). Items are almost exclusively limited to observations of facial expressions and body postures. The DS-DAT is a 9-item observational measure with reported validity and reliability (α = .86–.89). However, replications have been difficult due to poor interrater agreement for three items: relaxed body language, sad facial expression, and frowns, primarily due to wrinkles around the eyes and mouth (Miller, Moore, Schofield, & Ng'andu, 1996). Swedish nurse researchers used the Facial Action Coding System based on facial muscle group movement to measure the response of four severely impaired dementia patients to well-circumscribed pleasurable and aversive (i.e., painful) stimuli (Asplund, Norberg, Adolfsson, & Waxman, 1991). Complex facial expressions, which could be taken as indicators of emotion and pain, were not clearly seen under either condition. Rather, common responses appeared to be primitive reflexive fragments of expressions, suggesting that facial affect of pain may be altered in late stage dementia. Another nurse has recently published results of psychometric testing of the Checklist of Nonverbal Pain Indicators (CNPI) (Feldt, 2000a). This instrument is a dementia-specific adaptation of the University of Alabama Birmingham Pain Behavior Scale and has face validity and good reliability (interrater = 93% agreement, κ = .63–.82), but may be more sensitive to pain when observations occur during movement such as transfers (Feldt, 2000a). This measure appears to have utility for both clinical and research work, but will require additional psychometric testing, particularly with non-Caucasian populations.

Some have conjectured that behavioral symptoms in dementia may be an objective observable sign of pain (Farrell, Katz, & Helme, 1996; Feldt, 2000b; Feldt, Ryden, & Miles, 1998; Galloway & Turner, 1999; Geda & Rummans, 1999; Talerico & Evans, 2000). Parke (1998) conducted an ethnography of nursing personnel in a long-term care setting to determine how nurses realize the presence of pain in cognitively impaired older adults. These nurses thought that overt behaviors and sounds commonly associated with agitation were manifestations of pain. A weakness of this study, however, was the interpretation that nurses relied on "intuition" rather than an assessment of subtle observable nonverbal behaviors, which had been well articulated by participants. Other researchers validated these findings using focus group methodology with nurses in a Canadian hospital (Galloway & Turner, 1999). Both of these qualitative studies identified that behavioral indicators of pain for persons with dementia were "hollering, swearing, agitation, hitting, and resistance to care." These authors point out that it is easiest to detect pain in persons with dementia when there is a long-term relationship between the patient and nurse and thus the ability to detect change in baseline individual behavior. This important

qualification may explain the difficulties of attaining reliability using observational measures for research purposes, which generally are done outside
of long-term therapeutic relationships.

Other nurse researchers used multivariate techniques to examine the
relationship of pain to a behavioral symptom, aggression (Feldt, Warne,
et al., 1998). Pain was examined in nursing home residents ($N = 38$) who
were known to exhibit aggression on a daily basis, with arthritis and
history of hip fracture as the two pain-related diagnoses most frequently
documented. Aggression scores were considerably higher (though not
significant) in residents with pain-related diagnoses, and significantly
higher in those with arthritis and in those with two or more pain-related
diagnoses. This cross-sectional study provides a foundation for future
prospective studies that will begin to tease out whether there are causal
links between pain and behavioral symptoms. Many anecdotal reports have
suggested that analgesic treatment may lead to improvement in behavior,
and an intervention trial investigating this would allow for testing of
causality and hypotheses regarding pain as the origin of some aggression
in persons with dementia.

The challenge for researchers and clinicians will be to determine if
and when behavioral symptoms common in persons with dementia represent pain, when they represent other unmet needs, or when they are the
sequellae of the disease process itself. Seeing these symptoms as potentially
pain-related opens up avenues for treatment that moves beyond traditional
care. However, anecdotal reports of improved behavior through analgesic
treatment must be verified in rigorous studies that examine the causal
nature of pain in behavioral symptoms. An alternative hypothesis is that
analgesia provides alternate sedation to traditional psychoactive drugs for
the treatment of behavioral symptoms.

The final method for pain measurement in older adults is assessment
by surrogates, especially in cases where the older person is unavailable
(e.g., due to death) or is unable to respond to assessment questions. Surrogates have included family members, nurses, nursing assistants, and other
care providers. Community nurses consistently underestimated intense
levels of persistent pain in older adults and overestimated low levels of
pain (Walker, Akinsanya, Davis, & Marcer, 1990). Similar findings have
been reported for acute pain in hospitalized older adults (Bergh & Sjostrom,
1999) and for older persons with dementia in community and institutional
settings (Krulewitch et al., 2000). In a sample of family caregivers of
persons with dementia, none was able to identify nonverbal behaviors

indicating pain and in all cases caregivers discontinued previously used analgesic medications (Fisher-Morris & Gellatly, 1997). Surrogates, especially family members, can often provide valuable information about an older person's pain, especially historical information about types of chronic pain, usual manner of expressing pain, and the use of analgesic medications. However, in light of evidence that older adults and even many with cognitive impairments can reliably report pain, surrogate information should only be used to augment the individual's report of pain and not be used as the first or only source of assessment data.

In summary, although a variety of pain measures exist, few have been tested on older populations. Initial work indicates that older adults respond to standardized measures in a similar manner to younger adults, but prefer measures that include word descriptors. Psychometric testing, as well as clinical utility of existing instruments (e.g., The McGill Pain Questionnaire) and new instruments (e.g., The Geriatric Pain Measure), including testing in minority populations, should be a high priority. The research and clinical utility of observational measures for studies of pain in persons with dementia remains problematic because they are labor-intensive, require extensive training for administration, and may not be valid in persons with dementia who are not able to produce full facial expressions due to brain damage. Additionally, signs of aging (wrinkles), dystonia, and buccal-oral dyskinesia make reliable observation difficult outside of the context of a long-term relationship. Nevertheless, the evidence to date on our ability to detect distress in this population, beginning evidence of a positive relationship between pain and certain common behavioral symptoms, and the lack of other assessment methods in persons who are nonverbal all support the need for additional work on observational measures.

What Are the Attitudes and Beliefs of Older Adults About Pain and What Are Their Experiences with Pain and Pain Treatments?

McCaffery's (1979) definition of pain as "whatever the patient says it is and occurs whenever the patient says it does" reflects the highly subjective nature of the pain experience. This perspective has been critical to moving both practice and research away from attempts to objectively quantify the pain experience in the absence of an understanding of the unique personal factors that influence an individual's experience of pain. Parmelee (1997) provides a cogent examination of psychological influences on pain experience. She identifies the following primary attitudinal influences that sway pain reports: (a) the individual's self-interpretation of pain; (b) ageist attitudes that pain is a "normal" part of the aging process; (c) fear that pain signals a decline in self-care abilities; and (d) attempts to protect caregivers from worry. These attitudinal influences can affect both the older person as well as professional and family caregivers.

It is frequently stated that many barriers to effective pain management exist for older adults, such as fear of addiction and the undesirable side effects of medications. In a qualitative nursing study of 42 older adults in residential care settings using focus group methodology, Yates and colleagues (1995) identified three themes related to attitudes toward pain relief: resignation to pain, ambivalence about the benefits of action, and reluctance to express pain. In a study of 131 community-dwelling older adults with osteoarthritis or rheumatoid arthritis and with persistent/recurring pain, many expressed reluctance to take regular doses of analgesics for fear of tolerance and side effects (Walker et al., 1990). Weiner and Rudy (2000) in their study of attitudinal barriers to effective pain management in the nursing home identified significant patient barriers, such as beliefs that pain treatment is unnecessary for frail older adults without demonstrated functional and physical impairment, and that there seemed to be a general lack of optimism about pain treatment. What was most noteworthy is that staff generally had positive attitudes about pain treatment, although this finding may have been because of social desirability. These researchers suggested that communication breakdown and staff work overload may contribute to the suboptimal treatment of pain in nursing homes.

In summary, early evidence demonstrates that older adults are fearful of the side effects of analgesic drugs, or of developing tolerance, and are reluctant to express and treat pain. However, the depth and breadth of research is extremely limited. Future studies should focus on development of an in-depth understanding of these processes so that ways to overcome older adult-related barriers to effective pain management can be developed.

How Adequately Is Pain Treated in Older Adults?

Despite high pain prevalence rates, one of the most consistent interpretations of findings in research on pain in older adults is its underidentification and undertreatment (Cariaga, Burgio, Flynn, & Martin, 1991; Ferrell,

Ferrell, & Osterweil, 1990; Morrison & Siu, 2000). Analgesic drug treatment of pain is the accepted and recommended treatment for most pain in all age groups (AGS, 1998; Jacox et al., 1994). Yet most studies have identified an alarming trend towards leaving pain untreated in as many as 13 to 85% of persons with pain (Ferrell et al., 1990; Sengstaken & King, 1993; Simons & Malabar, 1995; Wagner et al., 1997). The World Health Organization (WHO) has developed guidelines for the analgesic treatment of mild, moderate, and severe pain (Jacox et al., 1994). According to these guidelines, which recommend analgesics based on three levels of severity—mild (I), moderate (II), and severe (III)—older adults receive less than adequate analgesic treatment. In a population-based study of disabled older adult women ($N = 1002$) in which 48.2% reported severe pain (Level III), 13.2% took no analgesic medications, 22% took between 1 and 19% of the maximum daily dose of the prescribed medication, and 17.1% took between 20 and 50% of the maximum daily dose (Pahor et al., 1999). Only 1.7% of the entire sample reported taking a Level II analgesic (e.g., codeine) recommended by WHO for moderate pain, and none was taking WHO Level III analgesics (e.g., morphine), which are recommended for severe pain. Most were taking acetaminophen (41%), aspirin (34%), and ibuprofen (11.3%), which may explain why 8.6% took more than 100% of the maximum daily dose, due to insufficient pain relief using low potency drugs which are only recommended for mild pain (Level I) (Jacox et al., 1994).

In the hospital setting, Roberts and Eastwood (1994) found that of 98 older adults admitted to the emergency department for femoral neck fracture, 89 (90.1%) reported severe pain. Yet, one-third received no analgesic medication in the emergency department, and eight received no analgesic medication before surgery, indicating that many were left to suffer for significant periods of time. In a comparison between a younger cohort (mean age 33.9 ± 8 years) and an older cohort (mean age 80.6 ± 8 years) of patients admitted to the emergency department for long-bone fractures, 34% of the older group received no analgesia, compared with 20% of the young group (Jones, Johnson, & McNinch, 1996).

Similar findings of untreated pain are reported for nursing homes as well. Two studies involving large samples examined analgesic medication use in all persons admitted to nursing homes in the early 1990's who experienced daily pain. In the first study, examining a sample of 13,625 nursing home residents admitted with a cancer diagnosis, 26% received no analgesic medication; 32% received a WHO Level II analgesic, and

26% received a WHO Level III analgesic (Bernabei et al., 1998). The second study involved a sample of 49,471 nursing home residents, excluding those with a cancer or terminal diagnosis; 25% received no analgesics; 45% received WHO Level II analgesics, and 5% received WHO Level III analgesics (Won et al., 1999). In both studies, residents over the age of 85 with daily pain were significantly more likely to receive no analgesic medication. These two studies demonstrate the relatively greater acceptance of using WHO Level III medications such as morphine for cancer pain (26%) rather than for pain from noncancer sources (5%). Engle and colleagues (1998), in an ethnographic study, found that African-Americans were more likely to report persistent pain that was inadequately treated than Whites in their sample of Southern terminally ill nursing home residents. These studies provide evidence of a consistent trend for leaving pain undertreated in older adults, which may be worse for the oldest-old and older adults belonging to minority groups.

Persons with dementia are at even greater risk for undertreatment of pain, and nurses have made important contributions in this area, with reports comparing analgesic medication administration between persons with and without dementia. In an acute-care setting, nurse researchers found that cognitively impaired persons received significantly less opioid analgesics than cognitively intact persons in the first and second 48 hours post operatively status post-hip fracture (Feldt, Ryden, et al., 1998). Likewise, in a nursing home setting, persons with a diagnosed cognitive impairment were prescribed and administered significantly less analgesic medication, both in number and in dosage, than their more cognitively intact peers (Horgas & Tsai, 1998; Kaasalainen et al., 1998). In a correlational study, 60% of nursing home residents who had at least one diagnosis known to cause pain (e.g., arthritis, fractured hip) had not received analgesics in the previous month (Feldt, Warne, et al., 1998). Nonnurses have reported similar findings in that persons in acute care with dementia consistently received less analgesic medication than persons without dementia (Morrison & Siu, 2000) and in nursing homes (Bernabei et al., 1998; Won et al., 1999). These findings of lower analgesic drug use have been generally interpreted as evidence of substantial undertreatment of pain for persons with dementia.

Clinicians and researchers have struggled with the question of whether persons with dementia actually perceive less pain due to changes in brain functioning or merely report less pain due to language impairments, and some have suggested that evidence of lower analgesic use in persons with dementia implies that pain is less prevalent in this population (Scherder, 2000). Scherder and colleagues (1999) were the first to propose neurobiological explanations for "reduced pain reporting" in persons with dementia. They suggest that the affective components of pain (pain intensity and pain affect) are altered in Alzheimer's disease because of damage to the spinothalamic tract, the spinoreticular tract, and spinoseptal and spinohypothalamic projections, through which nociceptive information reaches the hypothalamus. They compared pain intensity and pain affect in 19 persons with Alzheimer's disease to 18 control older adults without dementia, matching the groups for chronic painful conditions and found that persons with dementia scored significantly lower on pain intensity, pain affect, energy, sleep, and physical mobility. Other evidence suggests no differences in the perception of pain between persons with dementia and those with normal cognitive functioning. When Benedetti and colleagues (1999) compared painful stimuli in a group of persons with moderate dementia and a nondemented control group, they found that there were no differences in stimulus detection (i.e., first tactile sensation) and pain thresholds (i.e., the smallest intensity that produced pain) between the groups. On the other hand, they also report that pain tolerance, or the smallest pain intensity capable of inducing an unbearably painful sensation, was significantly higher in persons with dementia. Porter and colleagues (1996) found that a physiologic measure (heart rate) of response to a painful stimulus (venipuncture) weakened significantly as cognitive impairment increased.

These results must be interpreted with great caution because of methodological difficulties. Scherder and colleagues (1999) used a measure of pain that required subjects to recall pain experience over the previous week, a task that many persons with dementia have difficulty doing. In addition, visual analog scales (used by Roberts and Eastwood, and by Scherder and colleagues) have been found to be the most difficult for older persons with dementia to use (Ferrell et al., 1995; Miller, Neelon, et al., 1996). Finally, pain that is experimentally induced, the method used by Benedetti and colleagues (1999) and Porter and colleagues (1996), may be an oversimplification of the pain experience and may not apply to pain seen in the clinical setting (Gagliese & Melzack, 1997). Our current methods for assessing perception of pain may be inappropriate for the working memory and expressive language impairments in persons with dementia. It is premature to make conclusions that persons with dementia experience less pain on the basis of these current studies. Future studies that are based on a sound conceptual understanding of the brain physiology of pain and the changes caused by Alzheimer's disease are warranted, but caution is urged in attributing failures of our measurement instruments to decreased pain perception in persons with dementia. There is much we can learn from our previous experience with neonatal pain perception. Not many years ago anesthesia and analgesia were thought unnecessary for procedures on neonates. We have since learned that untreated pain for neonates can add unnecessary stress and suffering and have long-term consequences. We are in danger of committing the same error in persons with dementia as we have made in neonates, based upon assumptions and equivocal evidence. As a clinical discipline, nursing has an obligation to assume that, based on the currently available evidence, pain is as distressing to persons with dementia as to those without and to act accordingly.

The question, "How adequately is pain treated in older adults?" is not answered satisfactorily with existing research. The epidemiological and undertreatment evidence strongly suggests that nurses should have a place in improving the care of the older adult population through both individual and public health efforts. The consistent findings that pain is inadequately treated across settings suggest that African-American older adults may be at particular risk of undertreatment, as well as the oldest old. Future research is recommended in examining reasons for this inadequate treatment and professional attitudes toward treating pain in older adults. The undertreatment of pain has important implications for nursing, in that there is an ethical obligation to relieve suffering and prevent harm when means are available to do so (Greipp, 1992; Miller, Nelson, & Mezey, 2000).

What Treatments for Pain Do Older Adults Use and Has the Full Range of Interventions Been Tested?

A small number of descriptive and qualitative studies have examined the treatments for pain used by older adults and by nurses with older adults. Nonpharmacological strategies used by a community-dwelling sample of older adults with persistent or recurrent pain included exercise, heat, topical ointments, dressings, massage, and physical therapy; these were reported as largely ineffective in this study (Walker et al., 1990). Nurse researchers reported increased use of nonpharmacological pain reducing strategies by cancer patients after a pain education program (Ferrell, Ferrell, Ahn, & Tran, 1994). Weiner et al. (1999) examined chronic pain in a nursing home and found that residents, 25% of whom were African American, reported using supportive devices, medication, position changes, lying down, and talking as ways to cope with pain. Older adults in long-term and assisted living facilities identified that giving pain medication on time was among the most important of nurse caring behaviors in a descriptive study based on Watson's Theory of Transpersonal Care (Marini, 1999). In a phenomenological case analysis, nurse researchers reported that a nurse was able to relieve the severe chronic pain from osteoporosis of an older woman through (a) sensitive interaction, (b) bathing in warm water with lavender, and (c) attention to psychosocial influences on pain coping (Taylor, 1992). Simons and Malabar (1995) found that nurses primarily used medications, but also used nonmedication interventions, including change of position, reassurance, ice packs, and passive exercise as interventions, which they offered to male patients more frequently than to female patients. The authors found that nurses often underreported the use of nonmedication interventions, particularly the use of psychosocial strategies.

Older adults have been underrepresented in pain intervention research. Nurses have tested education interventions and interventions aimed at improved pain assessment. In one study, a structured pain education program for older adult cancer patients and their family caregivers was evaluated (Ferrell et al., 1994). Improvements in pain intensity, pain distress, the amount of analgesic medications taken, and the use of nonmedication interventions (e.g., heat, cold, massage) were reported. Imagery and relaxation were used by few subjects and were found to be the least helpful of nonmedication intervention strategies. Although these results are promising, they are limited by the absence of comparison data from a control group. De Rond and colleagues (2000) demonstrated that an education program that focused on improved pain monitoring by nurses could reduce pain intensity and increase opioid use in the acute care intervention group ($N = 345$). English nurses conducted a pilot study to assess the effects of improved pain assessment in nonverbal older adult patients on the use of interventions (Simons & Malabar, 1995). They demonstrated that pain assessments could be significantly improved (although this varied widely by unit and was best in the rehabilitation unit), and that improved education and reinforcement are needed for optimal practice.

Pain intervention studies by other disciplines have reported beneficial effects of exercise (Ettinger et al., 1997; Kovar et al., 1992), cognitive-behavioral therapy such as cognitive restructuring, relaxation, biofeedback (see Gagliese & Melzack, 1997, and Wisocki & Powers, 1997, for reviews), acupuncture and transcutaneous electrical nerve stimulation (TENS)

(Grant, Bishop-Miller, Winchester, Anderson, & Faulkner, 1999), and patient controlled analgesia (PCA) delivery methods for morphine in acute care (Egbert, Parks, Short, & Burnett, 1990). For a review of exercise interventions to decrease pain in older adults, see Fuchs and Zaichkowsky (1997). These intervention studies have been limited by lack of a clear definition of pain, lack of hypotheses, small sample sizes, mixing of age groups, lack of a control group, and use of nonstandardized measures of pain. In addition, most samples have an average age in the 60s, and thus have likely restricted inclusion of persons in the older age groups (i.e., over age 85). Testing of interventions designed specifically for nurses is an important area for future research, given their frequent contact with this population, but the identified limitations of previous studies must be addressed.

Pain intervention studies with populations of older adults with dementia are extremely limited. The two reported here were either conducted by nurse researchers or teams that included nurse researchers. Volicer and Hurley's group (Volicer, Collard, Hurley, Bishop, et al., 1994) reported decreased discomfort levels (measured by the DS-DAT) in older adults on a dementia care unit who received a palliative care intervention in comparison with a group that received usual nursing home care. The intervention focused on palliation of symptoms and reduced use of antibiotics, tube feedings, and transfer to an acute care setting. Specific pain treatments were not described. Kovach and colleagues (1996) report similar findings in an evaluation of hospice interventions in nursing home residents with end-stage dementia. Discomfort levels were significantly lower in subjects who received the intervention in comparison with the control group. Behavioral symptoms were also lower in the intervention group, although these results were not significant and were measured by a single question. The pain management strategy was limited to giving participants acetaminophen (a weak Level I analgesic) as needed, in contrast to standard hospice practice of giving analgesic medication on a routine schedule. These studies are very promising, but are limited as interventions for the treatment of pain because of the multidimensional nature of the intervention. Thus, it is not possible to determine the relative effectiveness of the various aspects of the interventions in reducing pain.

STRENGTH OF EVIDENCE ON PAIN IN OLDER ADULTS

The evidence demonstrates that pain is widely prevalent in older adult populations. This, in combination with the inferential evidence of the underidentification and undertreatment of pain, makes a strong argument for increased study of pain in this population. The early work on pain measure validation demonstrates that older adults respond similarly to younger adults, though they have a preference for measures with word descriptors. Nurses have made important contributions to this literature, especially in the areas of pain assessment, undertreatment of pain, and pain in persons with dementia. The work on observational pain measures for use in nonverbal persons with dementia is especially promising, and some agreement across measures regarding behaviors that are indicative of pain has been demonstrated. Valid and reliable observational measures of pain, like the Checklist of Nonverbal Pain Indicators (CNPI) (Feldt, 2000a) will assist in moving the knowledge of pain in this population forward.

LIMITATIONS OF EVIDENCE AND RECOMMENDATIONS FOR RESEARCH

Failing to specify or define the type of pain being studied, and inconsistency in the terms used for pain make it difficult to generalize findings across studies. For example, although we may conclude that studies of postsurgical pain examine acute pain, many older adults experience chronic pain at the same time, which could contribute to postsurgical pain experiences. Some investigators included definitions of pain so broad (e.g., any pain in the past year) that they, too, made it difficult to interpret findings. Inconsistency in the terms used for pain is demonstrated by the use of the terms *persistent pain* and *chronic pain* to describe similar pain states. In future studies, more careful attention should be paid to conceptualization and definitions of pain.

Researchers have shown a preference for one-dimensional measurement of pain, with reported pain intensity being the most common measure. This practice results in use of an impoverished construct in pain research and may present a challenge for measurement of pain in older adults (Duggleby & Lander, 1994). A widely accepted conceptualization is that pain is a combination and interaction of physiological, motivational, cognitive, and affective factors (Melzack, Wall, & Ty, 1982), yet these factors have been infrequently addressed. A more comprehensive examination of these factors will add considerably to this literature and ought to be undertaken.

Although the literature on the prevalence of pain and the undertreatment of pain in older adults seems compelling, it is limited by several methodological weaknesses. First, the measures of pain used in the prevalence studies varied widely. Many measures of pain were developed by investigators for a specific study, with no psychometric testing reported. None of the population-based studies screened for cognitive impairment, and it seems likely that these samples contained a mix of cognitively intact and impaired individuals, raising questions about the appropriateness of methods and instruments. Few prevalence studies included minority groups, and future studies are sorely needed in this area. In the studies on undertreatment, often no direct measure of pain was used, and conclusions about undertreatment were based on the amount of analgesic drugs given. For example, reports of undertreatment of pain in nursing home residents in one study was based on the result that 25% of residents with a cancer diagnosis received no analgesic medication (Bernabei et al., 1998). An alternative interpretation of this finding is that the cancer was not active at the time of the study and/or did not actually cause pain. Future studies must endeavor to obtain the self-report of pain from the individuals being studied and compare these to the type and amount of analgesic drug given.

In view of the inadequate management of pain in older adults, there is a need for research in many areas. Studies of pain in persons over the age of 85 and studies of ethnic minorities are seriously underrepresented in this literature. Self-medication practices with analgesic drugs, specifically examination of the type and amount of analgesic drug used, dosing schedules, effectiveness of drug regimens and management of drug side effects are needed. Collaborative studies with physicians using analgesic medications as well as studies of psychosocial interventions are needed. Studies using opioid analgesics are especially needed to determine whether the fears surrounding these drugs are warranted, whether they are effective in reducing pain, improving function and reducing depression, and how side effects can be effectively managed. Nursing has much to contribute in terms of nonmedication treatments. Such psychosocial treatments would benefit from exploration using techniques that promote measurement of their dose and comparison of their efficacy with that of analgesic drugs. In persons with dementia, assessment and treatment of pain remains problematic, and research in this area is desperately needed, even though such studies are difficult to design.

ACKNOWLEDGMENTS

The authors gratefully acknowledge Una Beth Westfall and members of the Oregon Health & Science University School of Nursing, Gerontological Nursing Research Group who offered helpful comments on earlier drafts of this chapter.

REFERENCES

AGS Panel on Chronic Pain in Older Persons. (1998). The management of chronic pain in older persons: AGS Panel on Chronic Pain in Older Persons. *Journal of the American Geriatrics Society, 46,* 635–651.

Asplund, K., Norberg, A., Adolfsson, R., & Waxman, H. (1991). Facial expressions in severely demented patients—a stimulus response study of four patients with dementia of the Alzheimer type. *International Journal of Geriatric Psychiatry, 6,* 599–606.

Benedetti, F., Vighetti, S., Ricco, C., Lagna, E., Bergamasco, B., Pinessi, L., & Rainero, I. (1999). Pain threshold and tolerance in Alzheimer's disease. *Pain, 80,* 377–382.

Bergh, I., & Sjostrom, B. (1999). A comparative study of nurses' and elderly patients' ratings of pain and pain tolerance. *Journal of Gerontological Nursing, 25*(5), 30–36.

Bernabei, R., Gambassi, G., Lapane, K., Landi, F., Gatsonis, C., Dunlop, R., Lipsitz, L., Steel, K., & Mor, V. (1998). Management of pain in elderly patients with cancer. SAGE Study Group. Systematic Assessment of Geriatric Drug Use via Epidemiology. *Journal of the American Medical Association, 279,* 1877–1882.

Brattberg, G., Thorslund, M., & Wikman, A. (1989). The prevalence of pain in a general population. The results of a postal survey in a county of Sweden. *Pain, 37,* 215–222.

Brochet, B., Michel, P., Barberger-Gateau, P., & Dartigues, J. (1998). Population-based study of pain in elderly people: A descriptive survey. *Age & Ageing, 27,* 279–284.

Cariaga, J., Burgio, L., Flynn, W., & Martin, D. (1991). A controlled study of disruptive vocalizations among geriatric residents in nursing homes. *Journal of the American Geriatrics Society, 39,* 501–507.

de Rond, M. E., de Wit, R., van Dam, F. S., & Muller, M. J. (2000). A pain monitoring program for nurses: Effect on the administration of analgesics. *Pain, 89,* 25–38.

Desbiens, N. A., & Wu, A. W. (2000). Pain and suffering in seriously ill hospitalized patients. *Journal of the American Geriatrics Society, 48*(5 Suppl.), S183–S186.

Duggleby, W., & Lander, J. (1994). Cognitive status and postoperative pain: Older adults. *Journal of Pain Symptom Management, 9*(1), 19–27.

Egbert, A. M., Parks, L. H., Short, L. M., & Burnett, M. L. (1990). Randomized trial of postoperative patient-controlled analgesia vs. intramuscular narcotics in frail elderly men. *Archives of Internal Medicine, 150,* 1897–1903.

Engle, V. F., Fox-Hill, E., & Graney, M. J. (1998). The experience of living and dying in a nursing home: Self-reports of Black and White older adults. *Journal of the American Geriatrics Society, 46,* 1091–1096.

Ettinger, W. H., Jr., Burns, R., Messier, S. P., Applegate, W., Rejeski, W. J., Morgan, T., Shumaker, S., Berry, M. J., O'Toole, M., Monu, J., & Craven, T. (1997). A randomized trial comparing aerobic exercise and resistance exercise with a health education program in older adults with knee osteoarthritis. *Journal of the American Medical Association, 277*(1), 25–31.

Farrell, M. J., Katz, B., & Helme, R. D. (1996). The impact of dementia on the pain experience. *Pain, 67*(1), 7–15.

Feldt, K. S. (2000a). The Checklist of Nonverbal Pain Indicators (CNPI). *Pain Management Nursing, 1*(1), 13–21.

Feldt, K. S. (2000b). Improving assessment and treatment of pain in cognitively impaired nursing home residents. *Annals of Long-Term Care, 8*(9), 36–42.

Feldt, K. S., Ryden, M. B., & Miles, S. (1998). Treatment of pain in cognitively impaired compared with cognitively intact older patients with hip fracture. *Journal of the American Geriatrics Society, 46*, 1079–1085.

Feldt, K. S., Warne, M. A., & Ryden, M. B. (1998). Examining pain in aggressive cognitively impaired older adults. *Journal of Gerontological Nursing, 24*(11), 14–22.

Ferrell, B. A., Ferrell, B. R., & Osterweil, D. (1990). Pain in the nursing home. *Journal of the American Geriatrics Society, 38*, 409–414.

Ferrell, B. A., Ferrell, B. R., & Rivera, L. (1995). Pain in cognitively impaired nursing home patients. *Journal of Pain Symptom Management, 10*, 591–598.

Ferrell, B. A., Stein, W. M., & Beck, J. C. (2000). The Geriatric Pain Measure: Validity, reliability and factor analysis. *Journal of the American Geriatrics Society, 48*, 1669–1673.

Ferrell, B. R., Ferrell, B. A., Ahn, C., & Tran, K. (1994). Pain management for elderly patients with cancer at home. *Cancer, 74*(7 Suppl.), 2139–2146.

Fisher-Morris, M., & Gellatly, A. (1997). The experience and expression of pain in Alzheimer patients. *Age & Ageing, 26*, 497–500.

Fuchs, C. Z., & Zaichkowsky, L. D. (1997). Exercise in aging and pain control. In D. I. Mostofsky & J. Lomranz (Eds.), *Handbook of pain and aging* (pp. 347–365). New York: Plenum Press.

Gagliese, L., & Melzack, R. (1997). Chronic pain in elderly people. *Pain, 70*(1), 3–14.

Galloway, S., & Turner, L. (1999). Pain assessment in older adults who are cognitively impaired. *Journal of Gerontological Nursing, 25*(7), 34–39.

Geda, Y. E., & Rummans, T. A. (1999). Pain: Cause of agitation in elderly individuals with dementia [letter]. *American Journal of Psychiatry, 156*, 1662–1663.

Grant, D. J., Bishop-Miller, J., Winchester, D. M., Anderson, M., & Faulkner, S. (1999). A randomized comparative trial of acupuncture versus transcutaneous electrical nerve stimulation for chronic back pain in the elderly. *Pain, 82*(1), 9–13.

Greipp, M. E. (1992). Undermedication for pain: An ethical model. *Advances in Nursing Science, 15*(1), 44–53.

Herr, K. A., & Mobily, P. R. (1991). Complexities of pain assessment in the elderly. Clinical considerations. *Journal of Gerontological Nursing, 17*(4), 12–19.

Herr, K. A., & Mobily, P. R. (1993). Comparison of selected pain assessment tools for use with the elderly. *Applied Nursing Research, 6*(1), 39–46.

Herr, K. A., Mobily, P. R., Kohout, F. J., & Wagenaar, D. (1998). Evaluation of the Faces Pain Scale for use with the elderly. *Clinical Journal of Pain, 14*(1), 29–38.

Horgas, A. L., & Tsai, P. (1998). Analgesic drug prescription and use in cognitively impaired nursing home residents. *Nursing Research, 47,* 235–242.

Hurley, A. C., Volicer, B. J., Hanrahan, P. A., Houde, S., & Volicer, L. (1992). Assessment of discomfort in advanced Alzheimer patients. *Research in Nursing & Health, 155,* 369–377.

Jacox, A., Carr, D. B., Payne, R., & the Cancer Pain Management Panel. (1994). *Management of cancer pain: Clinical practice guideline.* No. 9 (AHCPR Publication 94-0592). Rockville, MD: Agency for Health Care Policy and Research, U.S. Department of Health and Human Services, Public Health Service.

Jones, J. S., Johnson, K., & McNinch, M. (1996). Age as a risk factor for inadequate emergency department analgesia. *American Journal of Emergency Medicine, 14*(2), 157–160.

Kaasalainen, S., Middleton, J., Knezacek, S., Hartley, T., Stewart, N., Ife, C., & Robinson, L. (1998). Pain and cognitive status in the institutionalized elderly: Perceptions and interventions. *Journal of Gerontological Nursing, 24*(8), 24–31.

Kovach, C. R., Wilson, S. A., & Noonan, P. E. (1996). The effects of hospice interventions on behaviors, discomfort, and physical complications of end-stage dementia nursing home residents. *American Journal of Alzheimer's Disease, 11*(4), 7–10.

Kovar, P. A., Allegrante, J. P., MacKenzie, C. R., Peterson, M. G., Gutin, B., & Charlson, M. E. (1992). Supervised fitness walking in patients with osteoarthritis of the knee. A randomized, controlled trial. *Annals of Internal Medicine, 116,* 529–534.

Krulewitch, H., London, M. R., Skakel, V. J., Lundstedt, G. J., Thomason, H., & Brummel-Smith, K. (2000). Assessment of pain in cognitively impaired older adults: A comparison of pain assessment tools and their use by nonprofessional caregivers. *Journal of the American Geriatrics Society, 48,* 1607–1611.

Magni, G., Marchetti, M., Moreschi, C., Merskey, H., & Luchini, S. R. (1993). Chronic musculoskeletal pain and depressive symptoms in the National Health and Nutrition Examination. I. Epidemiologic follow-up study. *Pain, 53*(2), 163–168.

Marini, B. (1999). Institutionalized older adults' perceptions of nurse caring behaviors. A pilot study. *Journal of Gerontological Nursing, 25*(5), 10–16.

Marzinski, L. R. (1991). The tragedy of dementia: Clinically assessing pain in the confused nonverbal elderly. *Journal of Gerontological Nursing, 17*(6), 25–28.

McCaffery, M. (1979). *Nursing management of the patient with pain* (2nd ed.). Philadelphia: Lippincott.

McCaffery, M., & Pasero, C. (1999). *Pain clinical manual.* St. Louis: Mosby.

McCarthy, M., Addington-Hall, J., & Altmann, D. (1997). The experience of dying with dementia: A retrospective study. *International Journal of Geriatric Psychiatry, 12,* 404–409.

Melzack, R. (1975). The McGill pain questionnaire: Major properties and scoring methods. *Pain, 1,* 277–299.

Melzack, R., Wall, P. D., & Ty, T. C. (1982). Acute pain in an emergency clinic: Latency of onset and descriptor patterns related to different injuries. *Pain, 14*(1), 33–43.

Miller, J., Moore, K., Schofield, A., & Ng'andu, N. (1996). A study of discomfort and confusion among elderly surgical patients. *Orthopaedic Nursing, 15*(6), 27–34.

Miller, J., Neelon, V., Dalton, J., Ng'andu, N., Bailey, D., Layman, E., & Hosfeld, A. (1996). The assessment of discomfort in elderly confused patients: A preliminary study. *Journal of Neuroscience Nursing, 28,* 175–182.

Miller, L. L., Nelson, L. L., & Mezey, M. (2000). Comfort and pain relief in dementia: Awakening a new beneficence. *Journal of Gerontological Nursing, 26*(9), 32–40.

Mobily, P. R., Herr, K. A., Clark, M. K., & Wallace, R. B. (1994). An epidemiologic analysis of pain in the elderly: The Iowa 65+ Rural Health Study. *Journal of Aging & Health, 6* 139–154.

Morrison, R. S., & Siu, A. L. (2000). A comparison of pain and its treatment in advanced dementia and cognitively intact patients with hip fracture. *Journal of Pain & Symptom Management, 19*, 240–248.

NIH Consensus Panel. (1986). *The integrated approach to the management of pain.* NIH Consensus Panel Statement Online (6(3):1–8), [Web site]. Available: http://odp.od.nih.gov/consensus/cons/055/055_statement.htm#6_Conclus [2001, August 17].

NINR. (July 2, 2001). *The management of chronic pain—Program announcement* (PA-01-115). NINR. Available: http://grants.nih.gov/grants/guide/pa-files/PA-01-115.html [2001, August 17].

Pahor, M., Guralnik, J. M., Wan, J. Y., Ferrucci, L., Penninx, B. W., Lyles, A., Ling, S., & Fried, L. P. (1999). Lower body osteoarticular pain and dose of analgesic medications in older disabled women: The Women's Health and Aging Study. *American Journal of Public Health, 89*(6), 930–934.

Parke, B. (1998). Gerontological nurses' ways of knowing: Realizing the presence of pain in cognitively impaired older adults. *Journal of Gerontological Nursing, 24*(6), 21–28.

Parmelee, P. A. (1996). Pain in cognitively impaired older persons. *Clinics in Geriatric Medicine, 12*(3), 473–487.

Parmelee, P. A. (1997). Pain and psychological function in late life. In D. I. Mostofsky & J. Lomranz (Eds.), *Handbook of pain and aging* (pp. 207–226). New York: Plenum Press.

Parmelee, P. A., Smith, B., & Katz, I. R. (1993). Pain complaints and cognitive status among elderly institution residents. *Journal of the American Geriatrics Society, 41*(5), 517–522.

Porter, F. L., Malhotra, K. M., Wolf, C. M., Morris, J. C., Miller, J. P., & Smith, M. C. (1996). Dementia and response to pain in the elderly. *Pain, 68*(2–3), 413–421.

Roberts, H. C., & Eastwood, H. (1994). Pain and its control in patients with fractures of the femoral neck while awaiting surgery. *Injury, 25*(4), 237–239.

Ross, M. M., & Crook, J. (1998). Elderly recipients of home nursing services: Pain, disability and functional competence. *Journal of Advanced Nursing, 27*(6), 1117–1126.

Scherder, E., Bouma, A., Borkent, M., & Rahman, O. (1999). Alzheimer patients report less pain intensity and pain affect than non-demented elderly. *Psychiatry: Interpersonal & Biological Processes, 62*, 265–272.

Scherder, E. J. A. (2000). Low use of analgesics in Alzheimer's disease: Possible mechanisms. *Psychiatry, 63*(1), 1–12.

Sengstaken, E. A., & King, S. A. (1993). The problems of pain and its detection among geriatric nursing home residents. *Journal of the American Geriatrics Society, 41*, 541–544.

Simons, W., & Malabar, R. (1995). Assessing pain in elderly patients who cannot respond verbally. *Journal of Advanced Nursing, 22*, 663–669.

Talerico, K. A., & Evans, L. K. (2000). Making sense of aggressive/protective behaviors in persons with dementia. *Alzheimer's Care Quarterly, 1*(4), 77–88.

Taylor, B. J. (1992). Relieving pain through ordinariness in nursing: A phenomenologic account of a comforting nurse-patient encounter. *ANS—Advances in Nursing Science, 15*(1), 33–43.

Turk, D. C., & Melzack, R. (1992). The measurement of pain and the assessment of people experiencing pain. In D. C. Turk & R. Melzack (Eds.), *Handbook of pain assessment*. New York: Guilford Press.

Volicer, L., Collard, A., Hurley, A., Bishop, C., Kern, D., & Karon, S. (1994). Impact of special care unit for patients with advanced Alzheimer's disease on patients' discomfort and costs. *Journal of the American Geriatrics Society, 42*, 597–603.

Wagner, A. M., Goodwin, M., Campbell, B., Eskro, S., French, S. A., Shepherd, P. A., & Wade, M. (1997). Pain prevalence and pain treatments for residents in Oregon nursing homes. *Geriatric Nursing, 18*, 268–272.

Walker, J. M., Akinsanya, J. A., Davis, B. D., & Marcer, D. (1990). The nursing management of elderly patients with pain in the community: Study and recommendations. *Journal of Advanced Nursing, 15*, 1154–1161.

Weiner, D., Peterson, B., & Keefe, F. (1999). Chronic pain-associated behaviors in the nursing home: Resident versus caregiver perceptions. *Pain, 80*, 577–588.

Weiner, D. K., & Rudy, T. E. (2000). Attitudinal barriers to effective pain management in the nursing home. In M. Devor, M. C. Rowbotham, & Z. Wiesenfeld-Hallin (Eds.), *Proceedings of the 9th World Congress on Pain, Progress in pain research and management (Vol. 16)*. Seattle, WA: IASP Press.

Wisocki, P. A., & Powers, C. B. (1997). Behavioral treatments for pain experienced by older adults. In D. I. Mostofsky & J. Lomranz (Eds.), *Handbook of pain and aging* (pp. 365–382). New York: Plenum Press.

Won, A., Lapane, K., Gambassi, G., Bernabei, R., Mor, V., & Lipsitz, L. A. (1999). Correlates and management of nonmalignant pain in the nursing home. SAGE Study Group. Systematic Assessment of Geriatric drug use via Epidemiology. *Journal of the American Geriatrics Society, 47*, 936–942.

Woo, J., Ho, S. C., Lau, J., & Leung, P. C. (1994). Musculoskeletal complaints and associated consequences in elderly Chinese aged 70 years and over. *Journal of Rheumatology, 21*, 1927–1931.

Yates, P., Dewar, A., & Fentiman, B. (1995). Pain: The views of elderly people living in long-term residential care settings. *Journal of Advanced Nursing, 21*, 667–674.

Chapter 4

Interventions for Persons
with Irreversible Dementia

SANDY C. BURGENER AND PRUDENCE TWIGG

ABSTRACT

This chapter provides an overview and critique of the theoretical and research literature by nurse researchers and researchers in other disciplines regarding interventions for persons with dementia (PWD). Reports were included if published in English between 1990 and 2000 and if a descriptive, correlational, longitudinal, or intervention design was used. Case studies and narrative descriptions were not included. No specific age criteria for study participants were applied; however, PWD are generally over age 55. The theoretical literature and various disease stages were reviewed, including clinical and behavioral indicators for disease progression. Using a variety of approaches to survey the extant literature (review of computer databases, contacts with experts in the field, ancestry method, and manual searches of key gerontology journals), over 1,200 citations were initially reviewed, allowing for approximately 375 publications undergoing thorough analysis with 157 research publications being included in this synthesis. Key findings include the identification of well-supported cognitive-behavioral interventions to enhance cognitive functioning and memory, and to relieve depression in the early disease stages; multiple environmental and behavioral approaches for improvement in functioning, maintenance of activities, and alleviation of behavioral symptoms in the middle disease stages; and behavioral, interactive, and staff support and education interventions for adequate nutritional intake, urinary incontinence, and management of problematic vocalizations and other behavioral symptoms in the later disease stages. Recommendations for future studies include the need for development of operational definitions of behavioral symptoms, inclusion of the perspective of PWD, evaluation of long-term outcomes, adequate sample size, community rather than institutional-based studies, and increased intervention testing at various stages of the disease.

Keywords: dementia research, care interventions, critical review, stages of dementia, management strategies

The need for understanding appropriate care and interventions to facilitate positive outcomes in persons with dementia (PWD) is evident when reviewing current knowledge and statistics regarding the impact of dementing disorders on afflicted persons and caregivers. With an estimated 50% of individuals 85 years of age or older suffering from dementia, the total number of PWD will increase dramatically over the next two decades (American Psychiatric Association, 1997; Dashiell & Kirk, 1989; Evans et al., 1989). Thus, in the absence of effective prevention and treatment strategies, by 2030 the number of persons with irreversible dementia such as Alzheimer disease (AD) will double from 4.5 million to 9 million. Currently, AD is the fourth leading cause of death in the United States and the third most expensive disease to treat, with estimated costs to patients and their families of over $200,000 during the course of the disease (Duncan & Siegal, 1998). The course of a dementing disease causes anguish to millions more family members and caregivers who attempt to manage and accept the steady and irreversible losses in their loved ones. Although no current therapy can stop or reverse the cognitive decline, a variety of psychosocial and pharmacological approaches have provided some relief from the accompanying psychological, cognitive, and behavioral symptoms associated with dementia, providing a basis for hope and positive interventions (Lawton & Rubinstein, 2000). The central purpose of this chapter is to present a comprehensive review of the empirical literature from nursing and the related health disciplines to identify research-based approaches to interventions for PWD throughout the disease process. To address this central aim, the following two questions will be answered:

1. What theoretical approaches have been used to underpin interventions for PWD?
2. What interventions from nursing and health-related disciplines have been found to be effective at the various stages of the disease process?

Dementia is generally defined as a progressive, nonreversible patho-logical condition in which the decline in memory and other cognitive functions is sufficient to affect the daily life of the person. A number of different forms of dementia have been identified, with Alzheimer disease the most common, accounting for approximately 50% of all cases. Due to recent advances in diagnostic procedures, Lewy body disease, a form of dementia associated with the formation of Lewy inclusion bodies in the cerebral cortex, has been found in approximately 7% to 26% of all persons diagnosed with dementia (American Psychiatric Association, 1997). Although clinically very similar to Alzheimer, Lewy body disease tends to have earlier visual hallucinations and a more rapid evolution, accompanied by Parkinson-like movement disorders. Vascular dementia accounts for another 10% of all dementias, with mixed dementia (con-taining elements of Alzheimer, Lewy body, and vascular dementia) ac-counting for another 10% of dementia types (Small et al., 1997). In addition to these three main categories, other types of pathology are responsible for damage to the central nervous system: degenerative (Pick's disease, frontal lobe pathology), infective processes (Creutzfeld-Jacob disease, neu-rosyphilis, AIDS-related dementia), toxic (alcohol-related brain damage, lead poisoning), and structural damage (head injuries). Dementia can be further broken down into two basic types: cortical, with primary damage in the cerebral cortex, and subcortical, with primary damage in the deeper subcortical regions. While the more common dementias (Alzheimer, Lewy body) are categorized as cortical dementia, subcortical dementias include those associated with Parkinson's disease, Huntington's disease, Wilson's disease, progressive supranuclear palsy, and multiple sclerosis (Kitwood, 1997). As Alzheimer, Lewy body, vascular, and mixed dementia together account for approximately 90% of all dementia cases, progress in much the same manner, and result in similar patterns of care needs, the implica-tions of research for care are congruent within these major diagnostic categories. Research findings are applicable to care for persons within all four diagnostic categories and may be applied to persons with other forms of dementia with similar care needs.

METHOD

The research literature was searched using several modalities, including the CINAHL and MEDLINE databases. Key variables included in the search were *dementia, dementia care, psychological interventions,* and terms representing specific intervention types, such as *reality orientation.* A manual search of 11 key interdisciplinary and nursing gerontological journals was also conducted. An ancestry approach was also used to examine reference lists of relevant articles for identification of related research reports. The same search strategy was used to answer each question guiding the review. Articles self-identified as 'research' were reviewed, both quantitative and qualitative. With over 1,200 research reports undergoing initial examination, 157 were included in this analysis using the following criteria: Research procedures were appropriate to the study design, the study addressed theoretical underpinnings and/or interventions for PWD, PWD were included as research participants, and the study was published between 1990 and 2000. No specific age criteria for study participants were applied, although PWD are generally over age 55. Case studies and narrative descriptions were not accepted for the analysis. Meta-analyses were included as they met the criteria for acceptable conduct of a systematic review of the research literature. Full-text papers presented at research conferences were also included if they met the stated criteria. Studies represent nursing and nonnursing research with all studies being published in English. No attempt was made to separate the research by discipline as much of this research is inherently interdisciplinary. Also, nurse and nonnurse researchers are actively involved in research conducted in many of the interventions discussed, representing a significant overlap in scientific knowledge.

RESULTS AND DISCUSSION

What Theoretical Approaches Have Been Used to Underpin Nursing Interventions for PWD?

Several middle-range nursing theories of dementia care that relate outcomes to person-centered and environmental variables have been developed. The Progressively Lowered Stress Threshold (PLST) model of Hall and Buckwalter (1987) focuses on the interaction between environmental stimuli, stress threshold of the PWD, and dysfunctional behaviors in PWD, identifying common stressors which lead to excess disability: misleading or inappropriate stimuli, excessive external demands, physical stressors, and changes in the environment, routine, or caregiver (Hall, 1994). Fatigue and excessive internal demands are also thought to contribute to dysfunctional behavior, but are internal to the person. Interventions derived from this model focus on reducing, eliminating, or controlling the timing of these stressors.

Meddaugh (1990) suggested using Brehm's (1966, 1981) reactance theory to explain aggressive behaviors in PWD residing in institutions. The theory posits that behavioral restrictions (lack of control) in institutional settings, along with physiological impairments and one's personal history of experiences with constraints, all contribute to aggressive behaviors. Kolanowski, Hurwitz, Taylor, Evans, and Strumpf (1994) also emphasized the role of the environment as an antecedent to disturbing behaviors, using the theoretical framework of Kayser-Jones (1989, 1991). Kayser-Jones used a person–environment framework, derived from Lawton (1983), to describe the relationships between the institutional environment and quality of life (QOL) outcomes.

Dawson, Wells, and Kline (1993) developed an Enablement Model of dementia care which, like Kitwood (1997) and Lyman's (1989), rejects strictly biomedical explanations of declining function and quality of life for PWD, and using Lawton's (1983) concept of environmental press, focuses instead on supporting the remaining abilities of the PWD and avoiding *excess disability*. More recently, the Need-Driven Dementia-Compromised Behavior Model (NDB) has been used to conceptualize behavior difficulties in PWD as the result of background and proximal (including the environment) factors (Algase et al., 1996; Kolanowski, 1999). A variety of terms are used for behavioral symptoms, with *problem behaviors*, *difficult behaviors*, and *dysfunctional behaviors* being common descriptors. In this chapter, we have used the term used by each author and have used *behavioral symptoms* when not referring to a specific author's work consistent with current trends.

All of the middle-range nursing theories of problem behaviors share recognition of the multifaceted nature of the antecedents: person-centered (personality, physical health, life experiences), environmental (social climate, constraints on personal freedom), and dementia-specific (decreased cognition) variables. The PLST and NBD models have been used primarily to investigate specific behavior difficulties in PWD, that is, identifying antecedents to behaviors and developing nursing interventions to affect outcomes. Although the models are effective for that purpose, a focus on problem behaviors may limit the ability of nurse researchers to improve overall QOL for PWD. Some interventions were developed from larger theoretical frameworks. For example, validation therapy (Feil, 1993) is based on the lifespan developmental perspective of Erikson (1963) and includes: reminiscing, recognizing unmet human needs, touch, and music. Ryden (1998) proposed the use of Swanson's (1991) caring model for PWD, with nursing interventions being derived from five processes: maintaining belief, knowing, being with, doing for, and enabling.

STAGING OF THE DISEASE

To facilitate the application of research-based interventions, it is useful to differentiate the various disease stages, as behaviors, abilities, and subsequent care needs vary as PWD move through the disease stages. Although several models exist for staging of dementia, the FAST-ACT staging by Reisberg (1986, 1988) and Clinical Dementia Rating Scale (CDR) by Hughes, Berg, Danzinger, Coben, and Martin (1982) provide an easy-to-apply staging that basically falls into three categories, as found in Table 4.1. Many researchers use these staging categories to describe PWD, facilitating the application of stage-appropriate interventions (Mac-Donald-Connolly, Pedlar, MacKnight, Lewis, & Fisher, 2000). Kitwood (1997) suggests a general categorization where PWD are *mild* if they still retain the ability to manage independently, *moderate* if some help is needed in the ordinary tasks of living, and *severe* if continual help and support are required. Although some overlap in care interventions is evident, the losses and resulting care needs of PWD vary by stage and will be described within this three-stage model.

Stage 1: What Interventions Have Been Found to Be Effective for Persons with Mild to Early–Moderate Dementia?

As persons in the early disease stages are often functionally intact, care needs at this early disease stage are centered around optimizing memory and cognitive function, maintaining engagement in activities, minimizing loss and depression, and increasing general functioning and QOL (Kitwood, 1997). Studies were identified as addressing care needs of persons in the mild to moderate disease stage if the majority of the sample was identified as being in the early to early-middle disease stages and had mean Mini-Mental State Exam (MMSE) scores greater than 17. The majority

TABLE 4.1   Stages of Dementia

Stage	Staging scores			Behavioral characteristics
	FAST	CDR	Mental status (MMSE)	
Stage 1: Mild to Moderate Dementia	1–3	.5–1.9	18–25	Mild to moderate memory impairment; mild impairment in functional activities of daily living; abandonment of more difficult tasks and hobbies; intact social behaviors.
Stage 2: Moderate to Severe	4–5	2.0–3.0	9–17	Increased memory loss; speech difficulties; disorientation; impaired ADLs; requires assistance with personal care; increased safety concerns; increased agitation, delusions and/or hallucinations; increased need for supervision.
Stage 3: Advanced to Vegetative	6–7	4.0–5.0	< 9	Pronounced loss of self-care ability; problem vocalizations; requires assistance with eating, toileting; unable to follow simple directions; speech often unintelligible or irrelevant; progresses to totally dependent state requiring support for nutrition, comfort, skin integrity, and continued integration of self.

of studies reviewed utilized a quasi-experimental design (nonequivalent control group or one-group pretest-posttest design) and small sample sizes.

INTERVENTIONS TO IMPROVE COGNITIVE PERFORMANCE

In studies examining general cognitive performance as an outcome, tested interventions include exercise, cognitive-behavioral therapies, dyadic counseling, social interaction using recreational activities, and reality orientation (RO). These studies generally use institutionalized PWD or participants in day programs, although PWD were described as being in the mild to moderate disease stages, with one reported mean MMSE score of 20 (Baldelli et al., 1993) and four studies being conducted with community-residing PWD (Quayhagen & Quayhagen, 1996; Quayhagen et al., 2000; Topp & Burgener, 1994; Zanetti et al., 1995). Sample sizes varied from 10 to 43 per group, with only two studies (Abraham & Reed, 1992; Quayhagen et al., 2000) using a true experimental design. The length of the treatment varied, with cognitive-behavioral interventions lasting from 8 to 24 weeks, an exercise intervention being delivered four times weekly for 8 weeks, and RO treatments varying from 4 weeks to 24 weeks, with most being delivered three times weekly (Ferrario, Cappa, Molaschi, Rocco, & Fabris, 1991; Gerber et al., 1991; Zanetti et al., 1995), with the cognitive stimulation program described by Quayhagen and colleagues being delivered by the family caregiver 1 hour daily/5 days per week.

Positive effects for all interventions have been found, with the outcomes including improved memory and concentration, functional ability, and affective states (Abraham & Reed, 1992; Baldelli et al., 1993; Gerber et al., 1991; Lindemuth & Moose, 1990; Quayhagen & Quayhagen, 1996; Quayhagen et al., 2000; Zanetti et al., 1995), increased engagement (Ferrario et al., 1991), and improved psychomotor skills (Topp & Burgener, 1994), with the Zanetti study indicating a gain of 3.12 points on the MMSE using an 8-month RO program and Quayhagen and colleagues finding gains of 2 to 6 points (total of 25 points) on cognitive performance exams. In a review of six randomized trials testing RO interventions for dementia, Spector, Davies, Woods, and Orrell (2000) report an average 2.1-point benefit on the MMSE for RO participants compared with control group participants, equating the benefits of RO to a 6-month delay in the usual cognitive decline found in dementia, a clinically significant outcome. Outcomes from exercise interventions have been mixed, with low sample sizes possibly contributing to Type II error. Findings support the statistical and clinical significance of cognitive-behavioral interventions on cognitive performance in PWD, with some support for their long-term effectiveness.

INTERVENTIONS TO IMPROVE MEMORY

Six research reports were identified as including memory as the primary dependent variable, with sample sizes ranging from 5 to 29 per group. Studies generally used well-accepted measures of outcomes, such as the MMSE, neuropsychological testing, or performance on specific cognitive learning tasks, such as item retrieval. All studies were conducted in either the home or community setting. Interventions utilizing repetition (i.e., tape recorded messages, quizzes, spaced retrieval techniques, and visual imagery) (Arkin, 1997, 1998; Frey, Leach, Nelson, Priozzola, & Mahurin, 1991), individualized interventions (Moniz-Cook, Agar, Gibson, Win, & Wang, 1998), and cueing techniques (Byrd, 1990) have had positive effects on memory, with some PWD having learning rates approaching those of normal controls (Byrd, 1990). Although most outcomes were assessed immediately following the memory-enhancing intervention, in a small study ($n = 14$), 63% to 100% of learned material was recalled on a 2-week follow-up testing (Arkin, 1998) with an average 15% gain in mental status scores in another study (Frey et al., 1991), supporting the clinical significance of the findings. In an early review of memory training in PWD, Arkin (1991) concluded that studies failed to demonstrate a significant global improvement in cognitive performance as a result of training, although persons scoring between 18 to 24 on the MMSE showed improvement in test scores. Generally, studies have revealed significant gains in memory, although most have been hampered by small sample sizes, nonblinding of raters to experimental condition, and lack of evaluation of long-term outcomes. The clinical significance of the findings would be enhanced by further studies examining the long-term effects of memory improvement.

INTERVENTIONS TO INCREASE ENGAGEMENT

Three studies identified *engagement* of PWD as a primary outcome, with two studies using a Montessori approach to activity participation (Camp et al., 1997; Judge, Camp, & Orsulic-Jeras, 2000) and the third study utilizing participation in familiar and unfamiliar tasks (Namazi & Johnson, 1992b). All studies used a one-group, pretest–posttest design and descriptive statistics only, with sample sizes ranging from 7 to 19, and average MMSE scores between 17 and 18. In the study by Camp and colleagues, PWD were paired with school-age children, with learning in children also being a measured outcome from this study. Generally, positive effects for engagement were found, with 76% to 86% of participants completing a task successfully (Namazi & Johnson) and periods of disengagement decreasing to 0% from 67% (Judge et al., 2000). Limitations to research in this area include small sample sizes, lack of comparison groups, and lack of reliability estimates for observational measures, with only one study reporting adequate rater reliability of 90% (Judge et al., 2000). Also, the intensity of the Montessori intervention raises questions regarding the feasibility of utilizing this intervention in other settings. Generally, experimental studies utilizing adequate sample sizes are needed to demonstrate long-term, clinically significant outcomes to justify the resources required to implement these interventions.

INTERVENTIONS TO REDUCE DEPRESSION

Depression in PWD has been found to be more prevalent in the early dementia stages (Migiorelli et al., 1995) and higher than in age-matched controls, with reported rates ranging from 11.8% (Onega & Abraham, 1997) to 51% (Migiorelli et al., 1995). Additionally, persons presenting with *preclinical dementia* with disease confirmation at 2 and 5 years have reported high rates of depression (60%), although the total sample ($N = 25$) was small (Visser, Verhey, Ponds, Kester, & Jolles, 2000). Depression has been found to be higher in women (Migiorelli et al., 1995), and associated with poorer performance on cognitive tasks (Visser et al., 2000), lack of energy, loss of interest, psychomotor disturbances (Onega & Abraham, 1997), impairment in ADL's, frequent wandering (Lyketsos et al., 1997), and higher risk for abuse and neglect (Dyer, Pavilik, Murphy, & Hyman, 2000). In a descriptive study of 55 PWD in nursing homes (MMSE: 15–23), McDougall (1995) found depression was associated with the capacity ($r = -.31$) and change ($r = -.44$) aspects of metamemory, defined as knowledge, perceptions, and beliefs about one's own memory. Findings indicate that less depression is associated with better perceived memory capacity and stability.

In addition to pharmacotherapy and electronconvulsive treatments (ECT) (Draper, 1999; Huber & Dietrich, 1999; Rao & Lyketsos, 2000), psychosocial strategies utilizing support groups, behavioral therapies, and validation therapy have been tested to treat depression (Small et al., 1997). Studies testing support group interventions have used one-group, pretest–posttest designs, have included small sample sizes (13 to 22), and have failed to demonstrate a quantitative effect on depression (Morhardt & Johnson, 1998; Yale, 1998) although qualitative findings support positive effects for mood, coping, and positive outlook. One study utilizing a family support intervention ($n = 33$) and a quasi-experimental design found no effect on mood, but did demonstrate increased activity (effect size $d = 0.66$) and social behavior ($d = 0.61$) (Droes, Breebaart, Ettema, van Tilburg, & Mellenbergh, 2000). Teri (1994) and Teri, Logsdon, Uomoto, and McCurry (1997) have used an experimental design to test behavior therapy interventions (problem solving and participation in pleasant events) with significant improvements in depression being found in treatment groups compared with controls ($d = 0.4$ to $d = 1.0$), and continued improvement in depression in treatment group participants at a 6-month evaluation. Validation therapy (VT), developed by Feil as a therapy for restoration of self worth, interaction, facilitation of independent living, and resolution of uncompleted tasks, has been utilized with a variety of older adult populations including PWD. In a critical review of validation therapy in PWD, Neal and Briggs (2000) found one controlled trial of validation therapy since 1990, a 1997 study by Toseland and colleagues that failed to reveal statistically significant results, although one study ($N = 5$) found modest gains in interaction in PWD following a 40-week VT intervention (Morton & Bleathman, 1991). Generally, high rates of depression have been consistently found in PWD in the preclinical and early dementia stages, and have been shown to be associated with decreased functioning and poorer outcomes across studies. Positive effects for behavioral therapies have been found, with well-controlled clinical trials supporting the immediate and long-term effectiveness of behavior therapies, while research support for the effectiveness of validation therapy on depression has not been found.

INTERVENTIONS TO IMPROVE GENERAL FUNCTIONING AND QUALITY OF LIFE

General outcomes have also been examined in PWD in the early disease stages, including driving behaviors. Studies have used a variety of designs, with most being cross-sectional, descriptive studies, and sample sizes ranging from 37 to 194. In studies of driving behavior, findings include lower rates of driving (22% to 46% in PWD compared with 78% in controls), tendency to use a *copilot* when driving (10%), lower traffic sign recognition in dementia ($M = 5.95$ of 10) compared with controls ($M = 8.77$), and particular difficulty with *slow moving vehicle* and *stop* sign recognition (Brashear et al., 1998; Foley, Masaki, Ross, & White, 2000).

Reminiscence therapy (RT) has been used widely with cognitively intact older adults, although only two studies were found specific to PWD (Burnside & Haight, 1994). In a critical review of the RT literature, Spector, Orrell, Davies, and Woods (2000) concluded that no firm support could be found for the effectiveness of RT on cognition or behavior, based on randomized trials to date. QOL in PWD has been found to be associated with personality of PWD ($r = -.35$ to $r = -.58$); caregiver behaviors, stress and relationship with the PWD ($r = -.34$ to $-.58$); and maintenance of activities ($r = -.29$ to .35) in one longitudinal study of 96 community-dwelling PWD (Burgener & Dickerson-Putman, 1999). Finally, in a different approach to examining interventions for PWD, persons taking antipsychotic agents were found (cross-sectional design) to have lower MMSE scores and greater impairment in ADLs than persons not taking medications, with an average of 49.5 months of follow-up (Lopez, Wisniewski, Becker, Boller, & DeKosky, 1999). Development of psychosis was associated with functional decline, institutionalization, aggression, and agitation after controlling for demographic and lagged variables. Use of sedatives and hypnotics were also associated with mortality, with findings indicating that use of antipsychotropic agents and sedatives can affect the outcomes and course of dementia.

In summary, descriptive studies to date have begun to identify driving behaviors in PWD, pointing to potential areas of difficulty. The strength of descriptive studies in identifying factors associated with QOL and functional outcomes are adequate sample sizes and longitudinal design, pointing to variables important in the design and testing of interventions to improve outcomes in PWD in the early disease stages. Beginning empirical support has been found for the negative long-term effects of psychotropic and hypnotic drug use in PWD, requiring systematic studies regarding this important aspect of care for PWD. Although support for RT has yielded mixed findings, the practical and humane benefits of including this personalized therapy into care routines may well justify the effort required.

Stage 2: What Interventions Have Been Found to Be Effective for Persons in the Moderate to Severe Disease Stages?

Middle disease stages are often characterized by increasing difficulties in managing self-care, with some social and interaction skills being preserved, as noted in Table 4.1. The goals of care during the middle disease stages are to promote independence in self care to the fullest extent possible, prevent harm, manage mood and behavioral symptoms to optimize mental comfort, and promote retention of mental abilities.

INTERVENTIONS TO MANAGE BEHAVIORAL SYMPTOMS

The largest number of intervention studies for the middle disease stages are focused on preventing and/or decreasing the occurrence and intensity of behavioral symptoms. The difficulties with conceptualizing, operationalizing, and measuring behavioral symptoms in dementia are well documented (Beck, Cronin-Stubbs, Buckwalter, & Rapp, 1999; Buckwalter, Stolley, & Farran, 1999; Davis, Buckwalter, & Burgio, 1997; Gerdner & Buckwalter, 1994; Kolanowski, 1995a,b; Taft & Cronin-Stubbs, 1995; Weinrich, Egbert, Eleazer, & Haddock, 1995). Environmental and caregiver variables have been related to behavioral symptoms of PWD in institutions (Burgener, Jirovec, Murrell, & Barton, 1992; Kolanowski, Hurwitz, Taylor, Evans, & Strumpf, 1994). The extensive literature on environmental interventions for PWD has been recently and comprehensively reviewed (Day, Carreon, & Stump, 2000; Phillips & Ayres, 1999). Beck and Shue (1994) reviewed interventions for managing behavioral symptoms in PWD and noted the lack of conceptual frameworks for the causes of the behaviors and the development of interventions to decrease behavioral symptoms.

Most studies have focused on active behavioral symptoms, often grouped together as *agitation*. The work of Cohen-Mansfield, Marx, and Rosenthal (1989) has been particularly influential as evidenced by the use of the Cohen-Mansfield Agitation Inventory (CMAI) as the most frequent dependent variable measure in intervention studies for agitation. Only recently have researchers begun to conceptualize passivity as a type of behavioral symptom in dementia (Colling, 1999a, 1999b). Bair, Toth, Johnson, Rosenberg, and Hurdle (1999) found that even acute-care nursing staff with specialized geriatric training failed to identify disruptive behaviors about 50% of the time when compared with direct observations by the researchers. Behaviors disruptive to care were more often identified and interventions instituted when they were "hyperactive," and perceived as interfering with the time and tasks of the nursing staff. Similarly, Whall, Gillis, Yankou, Booth, and Beel-Bates (1992), in a survey of nursing home staff, found that mostly excessive behaviors, not behavioral deficits, were reported as disruptive. Some of the behaviors described as disruptive by the staff may not be harmful to the well being of the residents themselves (e.g., wandering, repetitive verbal remarks, making noises, handling things, requests for attention), a conceptual problem discussed by Burgener and Chiverton (1992). Fopma-Loy and Austin (1993), in a study that presented a vignette of a resident with dementia, found that nursing home staff attributed agitation to the disease process, and considered agitation to be unpreventable and irreversible

Several areas of weakness in the intervention studies for behavioral symptoms emerged during the review. Many studies of specific behavioral symptoms failed to select participants with clinically significant baseline scores on the target behaviors (Buettner, 1999; Camberg et al., 1999; Goddaer & Abraham, 1994; Holmberg, 1997). Although reaching statistical significance, the clinical significance of the interventions to reduce these behaviors is placed in doubt. Outcome variables in the studies were often poorly operationalized, for example, anxiety measured by pulse rate (Kim & Buschman, 1999), relied on researcher-developed scales without information on content and construct validity (Clark, Lipe, & Bilbrey, 1998; Judge et al., 2000), or used published instruments lacking validity for PWD, for example, agitation after traumatic brain injury scale (Tabloski, McKinnon-Howe, & Remington, 1995). With a few exceptions, sample sizes tended to be small and were often obtained from multiple settings without comparison of the environments (Whall et al., 1997; Witucki & Twibell, 1997). A few studies used direct participant observation but most relied instead on caregiver reports; and in many studies the raters were not blinded to the treatment conditions (Clark et al., 1998; Watson, Wells, & Cox, 1998). The choice of outcome measures is not always clearly related to the intervention, for example, a walking intervention for wanderers with total aggressive episodes on the unit as the outcome (Holmberg, 1997). When a specific theory base was identified for the intervention, the Progressively Lowered Stress Threshold Model (Hall & Buckwalter, 1987) was most commonly cited.

The major dementia care theories identify elements of the environment as an important variable, potentially amenable to change. Day and colleagues (2000), in an extensive review of therapeutic environments for PWD, have identified several desirable attributes of the environment including noninstitutional design, small unit sizes, moderate levels of sensory stimulation, and higher light levels, among others. Although the institutional environment may be viewed as more static than other variables affecting behavior, a simple intervention to enrich a unit in the nursing home (added visual, auditory, and olfactory stimuli) resulted in decreased pacing and agitated behaviors (Cohen-Mansfield & Werner, 1998).

A variety of specific interventions have been studied to reduce problem behaviors in PWD: bright light therapy (Rheaume, Manning, Harper, & Volicer, 1998; Thorpe, Middleton, Russell, & Stewart, 2000), simulated presence via audiotapes (Camberg et al., 1999), rocking chair therapy (Watson et al., 1998), sensory stimulation (Buettner, 1999; Witucki & Twibell, 1997), use of recreational items (Aronstein, Olsen, & Schulman, 1996), individualized reinforcement interventions delivered in the home setting (Bourgeois, Burgio, Schulz, Beach, & Palmer, 1997), and physical touch (Kim & Buschmann, 1999; Snyder, Egan, & Burns, 1995). Several small studies using music to decrease problem behaviors (Gerdner & Swanson, 1993; Goddaer & Abraham, 1994; Tabloski et al., 1995) and repetitive disruptive vocalizations (Casby & Holm, 1994), and to promote sleep (Lindemuth, Patel, & Chang, 1992) are promising, although larger samples are needed to replicate the results. For a more detailed discussion of music therapy, the reader is referred to the comprehensive review of Brotons, Koger, and Pickett-Cooper (1997). Koger and Brotons (1999), however, found no randomized controlled trials of music therapy for PWD. A multicomponent program consisting of structured day activities for residents, psychotropic medication management by a psychiatrist, and weekly staff education rounds demonstrated significantly less behavioral problems and physical/chemical restraint use in the treatment group (Rovner, Steele, Shmuely, & Folstein, 1996). Although these studies suffer from some of the methodological weaknesses previously noted, the direction of the findings show enough promise to merit further research.

A particularly fruitful area of dementia care research has centered around decreasing the behavioral symptoms that commonly occur during bathing. Calm, relaxed caregiver behaviors during bathing have been related to decreased disruptive behaviors in PWD (Burgener et al., 1992). In a small pilot study, Hoeffer, Rader, McKenzie, Lavelle, and Stewart (1997) demonstrated improvements in resident behavior and the caregivers' experience using a geriatric clinical nurse specialist for bedside consultation along with an individualized bathing care plan for each resident. In a similar but larger study incorporating staff training and expert consultation, staff knowledge increased and the number of aggressive incidents during bathing decreased after the intervention (Maxfield, Lewis, & Cannon, 1996). Whall and colleagues (1997) used a "natural" environment incorporating visual, auditory, and gustatory stimuli to reduce agitation during bathing with modest results. The addition of music to the bathing experience has also been reported to decrease problem behaviors.

The theoretical basis for interventions for behavioral symptoms in middle-stage dementia is generally strong with a multifaceted approach most frequently advocated. Possible physical causes of the behaviors (e.g., pain—please see the chapter by Miller and Talerico in this volume) should be addressed, as well as environmental factors such as excessive sensory stimuli (e.g., noise, crowding). Behavioral diaries should be used to document the specific behavioral symptom (frequency, severity), precipitating events (e.g., bathing, mealtime), and the response to particular interventions. The major theories support the use of individualized interventions that include a consideration of personal variables such as premorbid personality, social/occupational history, and retained abilities. Pharmacological interventions should generally be reserved for those persons not responding to the above methods and should adhere to established guidelines (International Psychogeriatric Association, 2000). The use of physical restraints is generally not recommended, except in emergency circumstances. Not surprisingly, some of the best studies used intensive time and skill (e.g., evaluations by advanced practice nurses) to plan and implement individualized care and included the caregivers in the process through education, support, and follow-up (Beck, Heithoff, et al., 1997; Bourgeois et al., 1997; Hoeffer et al., 1997). Using a combination of methods and data sources also led to rich and clinically useful findings (Taft, Matthiesen, Farran, McCann, & Knafl, 1997). Additionally, studies that include attention to patient preferences (Clark et al., 1998) and participation/evaluation of family, staff, and/or community members (Beck, Heithoff, et al., 1998; Buettner, 1999; Hoeffer et al., 1999; Taft et al., 1997) are more likely to lead to adoption and acceptance of the interventions.

INTERVENTIONS TO PROMOTE INDEPENDENCE IN FUNCTIONAL ABILITIES

The Enablement Model (Dawson, Wells, & Kline, 1993) provides a strong theoretical basis for rehabilitative interventions for PWD. The general approach is to identify the retained abilities of PWD, provide practice opportunities, and train caregivers to support and improve function through simplification of tasks, adaptation of the environment, and verbal cueing. Existing studies support the benefits of specific skills training for PWD, even into the later disease stages. A common barrier to rehabilitative interventions is the tendency of caregivers, particularly staff, to "care for" the PWD rather than facilitate self-care. Although the maintenance of function in the middle stages of dementia has not been studied as extensively as behavioral symptoms, the benefits of rehabilitation training for activities of daily living (ADLs) have been demonstrated across disease stages and settings for PWD, either directly or indirectly through caregiver education. Persons with mild to mild-moderate dementia attending a day hospital showed a significant improvement in performance of ADLs after 3 weeks of training to stimulate procedural memory (Zanetti et al., 1997). Tappen (1994) demonstrated that even institutionalized PWD with relatively advanced disease (MMSE = 6.4) benefited from graded functional skill training in ADLs. The most successful regimen (skill training), however, was intensive (2.5 hours per day) and depended upon the expertise of a gerontological clinical nurse specialist. Similarly, increased self-care behaviors were exhibited by persons with moderate to severe dementia (mean MMSE = 8.9) after family caregivers received instruction in behavioral approaches to specific activities (Burgener, Bakas, Murray, Dunahee, & Tossey, 1998). Simple modification of closet space, along with caregiver training, increased the level of independence in ADLs in one small intervention study (Namazi & Johnson, 1992a). Beck, Heacock, and colleagues (1997) demonstrated the success of an intervention to improve independent dressing behaviors in nursing home residents ($n = 90$, mean MMSE = 7.35) without significantly increasing care time by the nursing assistants. Rogers and colleagues (1999) studied the effects of skill elicitation and habit training during morning care for institutionalized PWD ($n = 84$, mean MMSE = 6.07), and found functional gains in dressing behaviors, a finding supported in a later study by Wells, Dawson, Sidani, Craig, and Pringle (2000). Collectively, these studies indicate the effectiveness of skill training and environmental modification in improving self-care behaviors in PWD, although some interventions require advanced skills and training.

Most studies reviewed did not report effect sizes in terms of variance accounted for (r-squared), but provided t-scores and F-scores for differences between groups (treatment and control) or pre- and postintervention scores. For some studies, the r-square could be calculated from the published data tables using the method of Cohen (1988), although not all studies provided enough data to do so. For example, the use of a "natural" environment intervention during bathing accounted for up to 70% of the variance in agitation between groups (Whall et al., 1997). Because the intervention combined several different sensory elements, however, the effective treatment element cannot be isolated. Large group differences in the standard deviations for agitated behavior of PWD complicated many of the statistical analyses. This problem may render the pre-post and/or crossover designs, using patients as their own controls, more feasible than treatment/control group designs.

INTERVENTIONS TO MAINTAIN THERAPEUTIC ACTIVITIES

Pulsford (1997) identified numerous goals in the provision of activities for PWD: preserving/enhancing remaining cognitive abilities, reducing behavior problems, improving quality of life, and enhancing caregiver morale. In a study of PWD ($n = 109$) in nine settings, Perrin (1997) used dementia care mapping (DCM), an observational method developed by Kitwood and Bredin (1992), to describe the daytime activity and relative well-being of residents rated as severely impaired. Passive behaviors were documented during 50% of the total observational time, a finding that supports Colling's (1999a, 1999b) concerns. The only significant active behaviors observed were eating/drinking and walking (15% and 10% of the time, respectively).

A variety of approaches to activities have been suggested for PWD including the introduction of stimulus objects (Mayers & Griffin, 1990), activity kits (Hutchinson & Marshall, 2000), Montessori-based activities (Judge et al., 2000), simple recreational items (Aronstein et al., 1996; Buettner, 1999), rocking chair therapy (Watson et al., 1998), and Snoezelen or sensory stimulation therapy (Morrissey & Biela, 1997). Few of these activities, however, have been systematically evaluated in controlled studies. Furthermore, many of the activities studied do not necessarily require active participation by PWD: simulated presence with audiotapes (Camberg et al., 1999), sensory stimulation activities (Witucki & Twibell, 1997), and slow-stroke massage (Rowe & Alfred, 1999), that might be more properly categorized as psychological comfort measures. Interventions that "pair" residents in institutions have also been studied with varying results (Cohen, Hyland, & Devlin, 1999; Oleson, Torgerud, Bernette, Steiner, & Odiet, 1998).

Stage 3: What Interventions Have Been Found to Be Effective for Persons in the Advanced to Vegetative Disease Stages?

In the advanced disease stages, PWD become increasingly dependent on others for assistance, progressing to a totally dependent state, as found in Table 4.1. Although behavioral symptoms peak during the middle disease stage, problematic vocalizations are often manifested during the later disease stages, presenting additional challenges to providing therapeutic care. Research regarding appropriate care within these basic needs and behavioral symptoms will be described, with the exception of comfort measures, found in chapter 3 by Miller and Talerico.

INTERVENTIONS TO MEET NUTRITIONAL NEEDS

Most studies of eating behaviors and nutritional needs have been descriptive in nature, have been conducted in institutional settings, and have

varied in sample size, ranging from 20 to 457. Findings with institutionalized elders ($N = 457$; 47% PWD) indicate that weight loss was associated
with difficulties in bringing food to the mouth, chewing, and lack of
choice in food selections, with greater weight loss in persons with vascular
dementia compared with persons with Alzheimer dementia (Berkhout,
Cools, & Van Houwelingen, 1998). Some support has been found for
improving intake through increasing the nutritional content of food (Peck,
Cohen, & Mulvihill, 1990), exploiting dietary preferences for sweet foods
(Mungas et al., 1990), the use of consistent interaction with the same
caregiver during feeding (Athlin & Norberg, 1998; Van Ort & Phillips,
1992), and the relevance of environmental effects on behaviors during
eating (Durnbaugh, Haley, & Roberts, 1996; Goddaer & Abraham, 1994).
In one randomized trial ($N = 63$; mean MMSE = 6.4) testing the effects
of skill training on ADL performance, including eating behaviors, improvements in performance were found, although the long-term effects of this
intensive (2.5 hours/day; 5 days/week; 20 weeks) intervention were not
evaluated (Tappen, 1994). In a review of feeding difficulties in PWD,
Watson (1993) notes that few empirical studies have been conducted
supporting interventions for improvement in nutrition, with most studies
being hampered by measurement of eating behaviors rather than amount
of food eaten. A later review by McGillivray and Marland (1999) concluded
that progress had been made in identifying difficulties with assisting PWD
during eating: task-centered approach, inconsistency in caregivers, induced
dependency, environmental distractors, and lack of staff training and empa-
thy toward PWD. The authors identify support for adopting a primary
nursing approach, increased staff education, environment modification,
and improved assessment of the quality of care provided.

In studies of nutrition supplied through tube feedings, including naso-
gastric, gastrostomy, and jejunostomy tubes, weight increases were found
for 48% of intubated PWD ($n = 52$) versus 17% of nonintubated PWD
($n = 52$), with significantly higher rates of aspiration pneumonia in the
intubated (58%) versus nonintubated (17%) group. No significant differences were found for decubitus ulcers or restraint use, although there was
a trend toward higher rates of both in intubated PWD (Peck et al., 1990).
In a review of the literature (15 reviewed studies) with mixed populations,
high rates of mortality were found, ranging from 8% mortality at one month
to 64% mortality by one year, with adverse effects including aspiration
pneumonia (1%–66.6%), occlusion (29%–34.7%), leaking (13%–20%),
and local infection (4.3%–16%) (Finucane, Christmas, & Travis, 1999).
The authors concluded there was no evidence that tube feedings improved
clinically important outcomes of prolonging survival, prevention of aspira-

tion pneumonia, improving function, providing palliation, or reducing the risk of infection. Although negative effects of tube feedings have been identified, few prospective studies have been conducted to examine a variety of personal and environmental variables (staff competency, consistency in procedures, comorbidity factors) predicting outcomes over time, making conclusions about the effectiveness of tube feedings tenuous at present.

INTERVENTIONS TO IMPROVE ELIMINATION AND SKIN INTEGRITY

Considerable progress has been demonstrated in the area of improving urinary incontinence (UI) for PWD, with nurses conducting and/or contributing to much of the key research in this area. The AHCPR Clinical Practice Update (Fantl et al., 1996) presents an excellent critical review of the research literature, along with recommendations for care. Studies of UI interventions for PWD have involved intensive staff education (Colling, Ouslander, Hadley, Eisch, & Campbell, 1992), assessment of staff response to the interventions (Lekan-Rutledge, Palmer, & Belyea, 1998), individualized care plans (Schnelle, Cruise, Alessi, Al-Samarrai, & Ouslander, 1998), built-in quality control measures for institutional settings (Remsburg, Palmer, Langford, & Mendelson, 1999; Schnelle, Newman, et al., 1993), and consideration of the relative costs and benefits of implementation (Cummings, Holt, Van der Sloot, Moore, & Griffiths, 1995). Many of the studies are based on the seminal research of Schnelle and colleagues (1989) who described a prompted voiding intervention that assists in identifying PWD most appropriate for toileting.

Much of the research on preserving skin integrity has been centered around care for pressure ulcers; such research has been conducted by nurse researchers and has been appropriately focused on interventions for prevention, rather than treatment (Vap & Dunaye, 2000). Although pressure ulcers have not been studied extensively specific to PWD, the prevalence of the known major risk factors (impaired mobility, incontinence, poor nutrition) are well documented in this population. The AHCPR has published Clinical Practice Guidelines for the prevention and treatment of pressure ulcers (Bergstrom et al., 1992, 1994) and The University of Iowa Gerontology Nursing Research Center (Lyons & Specht, 1999) has developed research-based protocols available on the web site for use with this population. See chapter 2 by Lyder in this volume.

INTERVENTIONS TO DECREASE PROBLEMATIC VOCALIZATIONS

Problematic vocalizations (PVs) are often considered separately from other behavioral symptoms in PWD as they tend to occur in the later disease stages, are often associated with discomfort, distress, or isolation, and tend to be resistant to interventions. Findings from descriptive studies indicate that PVs are associated with limited walking ability, incontinence, impaired communication ability, and constant requests for help (Cariaga, Burgio, Flynn, & Martin, 1991; Cohen-Mansfield, Werner, & Marx, 1990; Cohen-Mansfield, Marx, & Werner, 1993; Schnelle, Ouslander, Simmons, Alessi, & Gravel, 1993). Studies have supported the association between increased PVs and cognitive impairment, with sample sizes ranging from 24 to 408 (Beck, Rossby, & Baldwin, 1991; Cohen-Mansfield, Marx, & Rosenthal, 1990; Cohen-Mansfield, Werner, & Marx, 1990; Reisberg, 1996). Physiological variables, such as discomfort states, are reported as being associated with PVs, with increased signs of discomfort (PVs) being associated with fever in 20 PWD (Hurley, Volicer, Hanrahan, Houde, & Volicer, 1992), PVs during caregiving routines in PWD with musculoskeletal disorders (Cohen-Mansfield, Werner, & Marx, 1990; Hurley et al., 1992), restraint use during care tasks (Burgio et al., 1994; Cohen-Mansfield, Marx, & Werner, 1993; Kikuta, 1991), and early symptoms of infective processes (Algase et al., 1996). In a recent study of 97 PWD (mean MMSE = 7.7) in three nursing homes, Beck and Vogelpohl (1999) found that nearly half (48%) of all disruptive behaviors were PVs, with PVs being significantly related to physically aggressive behaviors, such as scratching and pinching. Being male, having a disoriented sleep pattern, and negative affect accounted for 39% of the variance in PVs. Findings from a smaller study ($N = 19$ PWD) by Holst, Hallberg, and Gustafson (1997) support the relationship between PVs and personal characteristics, with extroverted, neurotic, and controlling-of-emotions personality characteristics (as measured by proxy ratings of previous personality traits) being associated with PWD displaying PV behaviors, supporting the work of Kolanowski and colleagues (1994) indicating a relationship between premorbid neuroticism and aggressive behaviors ($r = .62$).

Studies specific to PWD in advanced disease stages support the persistence of other behavioral symptoms into the latter disease stages. Behavioral symptoms (physically aggressive, physically nonaggressive, vocally agitated, and vocally aggressive) were found to be associated with cognitive status (beta = −.237 to −.346, higher MMSE scores predicting lower levels of behavioral symptoms) (Beck et al., 1998), use of restraints (beta = .19), antipsychotic medications (beta = .18), antidepressant medications (beta = −.219), and placement on a secured unit (beta = .32) with PWD displaying an average of 9.5 problem behaviors (Ryden et al., 1999). In the reports of intervention studies on problem behaviors in PWD ($N = 31$), a modified environment during bathing has been found to result in decreases in problem behaviors (Whall et al., 1997); tailored interventions (10–14 days) resulted in reduced PVs in 3 of 12 PWD (Doyle, Zapparoni, O'Connor, & Runci, 1997), "white noise" treatments resulted in a 23% reduction in verbal agitation in nursing home residents (Burgio, Scilley, Hardin, Hsu, & Yancey, 1996), while participation in a wellness group (relaxation and sensory awareness exercises) resulted in decreased problem behaviors in treatment group participants (Lantz, Buchalter, & McBee, 1997). Positive effects of a family visit education program on problem behaviors and depression have been found ($N = 65$; 5 nursing homes) (McCallion, Toseland, & Freeman, 1999), along with increases in self care and decreases in problem behaviors ($N = 47$; community-dwelling PWD) associated with behavioral and family education interventions (Burgener et al., 1998), and improvements in problem behaviors ($N = 27$; 4 nursing homes) following the institution of Simulated Presence Therapy using tape-recorded messages (Woods & Ashley, 1995). Overall, studies of behavioral symptoms in PWD in the advanced disease stages support the existence of behavioral symptoms well into the latter disease stages, especially PVs; the relationship of PV's and aggressive behaviors to a variety of personal, environmental, and treatment factors; and the potential of care interventions for reducing aggressive and agitated behaviors. The need continues, however, for controlled trials with adequate sample sizes to test interventions to alleviate factors contributing to the development of PVs such as discomfort and isolation.

INTERVENTIONS PROMOTING THE CONTINUATION OF SELF, ENGAGEMENT, AND GENERAL OUTCOMES

Studies addressing a variety of care outcomes in PWD have used qualitative, descriptive, one-group, pretest–posttest, and quasi-experimental designs, and have been conducted in institutional settings. Sample sizes ranged from 4 to 23 for qualitative studies and 10 to 112 for quantitative studies, with all participants being described in the late or advanced stages of dementia (MMSE mean ranges from 0.6 to 8.9). A persistent sense of self, awareness of cognitive changes, and attempts to explain changes in the self have been identified in PWD ($N = 23$) (Tappen, Roach, Applegate, & Stowell, 2000) and assessments of self-care, social, interactional, and interpretive abilities were found to be retained in 112 male veterans (Wells & Dawson, 2000).

A variety of caregiving approaches (29 interventions) have been identified as alternatives to restraint use, including social, psychological, functional, behavioral, environmental, medical, and cognitive domains (Taft, 1995), whereas a small group sensory-motor activity ($N = 4$) has been found to foster attention, participation, and communication in participants (Pulsford, Rushforth, & Connor, 2000). Improvement in depression and mental status ($N = 14$ PWD) have been found following introduction of a 5-month computer service (McContha, McContha, & Dermigny, 1994), whereas increases in communication skills ($N = 30$; 15 per group) were noted in PWD who were randomly assigned to a 10-week structured walking intervention (Friedman & Tappen, 1991), and decreases in sun-downing behaviors and afternoon agitation ($N = 10$) and increased body movement ($N = 12$) were noted as a result of a bright light intervention (Hopkins, Rindlisbacher, & Grant, 1992; Satlin, Volicer, Ross, Herz, & Campbell, 1992). Increases in engagement behaviors have been found in several studies, including increases in engagement related to number of senses stimulated in a descriptive study of multimodal sensory activities ($N = 23$) (Kovach & Magliocco, 1998); increased engagement, changes in heart rate, lowered noise levels, increased orientation to day of the week, and decreased restraint use following introduction of a canine companion program (Katsinas, 2000; Walsh, Mertin, Verlander, & Pollard, 1995), and increased participation in morning care routines following either a skill elicitation or habit training intervention in 84 nursing home residents (Rogers et al., 1999). Only one study reported negative findings, with Robichaud, Hebert, and Desrosiers (1994) finding no effect of a sensory integration intervention on problem behaviors and ADL performance in 43 PWD residing in 3 nursing homes. Descriptive studies support the persistence of self and awareness, even in the late disease stages. Although a number of interventions (computer services, structured walking pro-grams, light therapy) have been identified to increase positive outcomes in PWD in the later disease stages, few interventions have been tested in controlled studies with adequate sample sizes. As some interventions are low cost and require minimal resources (light therapy, computer services, canine companion), the cost/outcome benefits alone may justify the imple-mentation of these interventions in the clinical setting until empirical support for the interventions can be realized.

CONCLUSIONS

In assessing interventions and support for care of PWD throughout the disease process, a few care issues were identified which were not addressed in the research literature and are understood clinically to be unalterable at present. For example, although descriptive studies have begun to identify factors associated with risks in driving for PWD, interventions to effectively manage the risks, loss to PWD, and family stress associated with continued driving or the driving termination process have not been tested. Although descriptive studies have examined the incidence of inappropriate sexual behaviors, no studies were found addressing appropriate care for persons expressing these behaviors or the disrobing behaviors common in PWD in the middle disease stages (Zeiss, Davies, & Tinklenberg, 1991). In both the early and middle disease stages, PWD also often repeat questions or *stories* concerning their life, causing frustration in caregivers and frequent contacts, with care approaches to effectively manage this behavior being in the early testing stages. Pharmacological interventions used to treat related care needs, such as depression associated with loss in PWD, have not been effective in assisting with these specific care issues. Testing of interventions to effectively mange these concerns for both PWD and their family caregivers continues to be one priority for future research.

Although specific gaps in the extant literature were noted within each disease stage, some general conclusions can be reached regarding this global area of study. Problems with the conceptual and operational definitions of behavioral symptoms continue, despite the understanding that PWD are capable of offering valid information regarding their own perspective and needs well into the later disease stages. Generally, randomized trials have suffered from the use of raters not blinded to group placement, selection of participants without assuring a baseline level of the target outcome (i.e., problem behaviors, depression), and lack of evaluation of long-term outcomes, making conclusions about the effectiveness of an intervention over time impossible. Many studies continue to rely on caregiver (staff) ratings of behaviors and outcomes without adequate assurance of the reliability and validity of these ratings. With a few exceptions, sample sizes for clinical trials were small, increasing the risk of Type II error. Often, a single global measure of the target outcome was used, increasing the risk of measurement error and threats to validity. Based on descriptive data, inclusion of more varied predictors, including pharmacological treatments, may increase explained variance in outcomes, especially use of psychotropic medications. The vast majority of studies, regardless of design, have been conducted in institutional settings, although it is estimated that 85% to 90% of all PWD continue to reside in the home or community setting. Finally, a need continues to reconceptualize care outcomes from a positive perspective—not just elimination of behaviors found to be difficult for caregivers, but rather the development of positive behaviors and outcomes, such as QOL. A need continues for studies testing positive interventions, such as exercise and companion programs, especially at later disease stages. Even though the efficacy for some well-established interventions (validation and reminiscence therapy) is assumed, evidence supporting the long-term effectiveness of these interventions, especially at the various disease stages, is lacking. Therefore, to effectively evaluate the cost-effectiveness of care interventions, the long-term outcomes and total costs should be inherent in the study design. The need for knowledge-driven interventions in these identified areas is critical, considering the growing population of PWD and the disastrous effects of the disease on the person and family.

While gaps in the research are evident, effective care interventions were identified at each disease stage. In the early disease stages, cognitive-behavioral and memory enhancing therapies positively impacted cognitive performance and memory, while behavioral therapies were found to alleviate depressive symptomatology. In the middle disease stages, a variety of behavioral (e.g., use of recreational items, sensory stimulation) and environmental (e.g., bright lights, rocking chairs) therapies hold promise for alleviating behavioral symptoms, while functioning has been positively affected by environmental modification and staff education interventions. Continued maintenance of activities has also been associated with structured interventions (e.g., use of stimulus objects, Montessori-type activities), although this area of study has suffered from a lack of systematic evaluation. In the later disease stages, positive nutritional outcomes have been associated with environmental modification during meals, consistency in caregivers, and increasing nutritional value of foods, while the positive effects of tube feedings remains equivocal. Well-developed interventions were found for treatment of urinary incontinence and skin impairment, while behavioral symptoms have been alleviated through a variety of environmental, group, and individual therapies. These positive findings provide a sound basis for development of future studies and interventions for PWD across the disease progression.

REFERENCES

Abraham, I. L., & Reel, S. J. (1992). Cognitive nursing interventions with long-term care residents: Effects on neurocognitive dimensions. *Archives of Psychiatric Nursing, 6,* 356–365.

Algase, D. L., Beck, C., Kolanowski, A., Whall, A., Berent, S., Richards, K., & Beattie, E. (1996). Need-driven dementia-compromised behavior: An alternative view of disruptive behavior. *American Journal of Alzheimer's Disease, 11*(6), 10–19.

American Psychiatric Association. (1997). Practice guidelines for the treatment of patients with Alzheimer's disease and other dementias of late life. *American Journal of Psychiatry, 145*(Suppl. 5), 1–39.

Arkin, S. M. (1991). Memory training in early Alzheimer's disease: An optimistic look at the field. *American Journal of Alzheimer's Care and Related Disorders & Research, 6*(4), 17–25.

Arkin, S. M. (1997). Alzheimer memory training: Quizzes beat repetition, especially with more impaired. *American Journal of Alzheimer's Disease, 12,* 147–158.

Arkin, S. M. (1998). Alzheimer memory training: Positive results replicated. *American Journal of Alzheimer's Disease, 13,* 102–104.

Aronstein, Z., Olsen, R., & Schulman, E. (1996). The nursing assistant's use of recreational interventions for behavioral management of residents with Alzheimer's disease. *American Journal of Alzheimer's Disease, 11*(3), 26–31.

Athlin, E., & Norberg, A. (1998). Interaction between patients with severe dementia and their caregivers during feeding in a task-assignment versus a patient-assignment care system. *European Nurse, 3,* 215–227.

Bair, B., Toth, W., Johnson, M. A., Rosenberg, C., & Hurdle, J. F. (1999). Interventions for disruptive behaviors: Use and success. *Journal of Gerontological Nursing, 14*(1), 13–21.

Baldelli, M. V., Pirani, A., Motta, M., Abati, E., Mariani, E., & Manzi, V. (1993). Effects of reality orientation therapy on elderly patients in the community. *Archives of Gerontology and Geriatrics, 17,* 211–218.

Beck, C., Frank, L., Chumbler, N. R., O'Sullivan, P., Vogelpohl, T. S., Rasin, J., Walls, R., & Baldwin, B. (1998). Correlates of disruptive behavior in severely cognitively impaired nursing home residents. *Gerontologist, 38,* 189–198.

Beck, C., Heacock, P., Mercer, S. O., Walls, R. C., Rapp, C. G., & Vogelpohl, T. S. (1997). Improving dressing behavior in cognitively impaired nursing home residents. *Nursing Research, 46,* 126–132.

Beck, C., Heithoff, K., Baldwin, B., Cuffel, B., O'Sullivan, P., & Chumbler, N. R. (1997). Assessing disruptive behavior in older adults: The disruptive behavior scale. *Aging and Mental Health, 1*(1), 71–79.

Beck, C., Rossby, L., & Baldwin, B. (1991). Correlates of disruptive behavior in cognitively impaired elderly nursing home residents. *Archives of Psychiatric Nursing, 5,* 281–291.

Beck, C. K., Cronin-Stubbs, D., Buckwalter, K. C., & Rapp, C. G. (1999). Managing cognitive impairment and depression in the elderly. In A. S. Hinshaw, S. L. Feetham, & J. L. F. Shaver (Eds.), *Handbook of clinical nursing research.* Thousand Oaks, CA: Sage.

Beck, C. K., & Shue, V. M. (1994). Interventions for treating disruptive behavior in demented elderly people. *Nursing Clinics of North America, 29*(1), 143–155.

Beck, C. K., & Vogelpohl, T. S. (1999). Problematic vocalizations in institutionalized individuals with dementia. *Journal of Gerontological Nursing, 25*(9), 17–26.

Bergstrom, N., Allman, R. M., et al. (1992). *Pressure ulcers in adults: Prediction and prevention. Clinical Practice Guideline, No. 3.* AHCPR Publication No. 92-0047.

Rockville, MD: U.S. Department of Health and Human Services, Public Health Service, Agency for Health Care Policy and Research.

Bergstrom, N., Bennett, M. A., et al. (1994). *Pressure ulcer treatment. Clinical Practice Guideline, No. 15.* AHCPR Publication No. 95-0652. Rockville, MD: U.S. Department of Health and Human Services, Public Health Service, Agency for Health Care Policy and Research.

Berkhout, A. M. M., Cools, H. J. M., & Van Houwelingen, H. C. (1998). The relationship between difficulties in feeding oneself and loss of weight in nursing-home patients with dementia. *Age and Ageing, 27,* 637–641.

Bourgeois, M. S., Burgio, L. D., Schulz, R., Beach, S., & Palmer, B. (1997). Modifying repetitive verbalizations of community-dwelling patients with AD. *Gerontologist, 37*(1), 30–39.

Brashear, A., Unverzagt, F. W., Kuhn, E. R., Glazier, B. S., Farlow, M. R., Perkins, A. J., & Hui, S. L. (1998). Impaired traffic sign recognition in drivers with dementia. *American Journal of Alzheimer's Disease, 13,* 131–137.

Brehm, J. W. (1966). *A theory of psychological reactance.* New York: Academic Press.

Brehm, J. W., & Brehm, S. S. (1981). *Psychological reactance: A theory of freedom and control.* New York: Academic Press.

Brotons, M., Koger, S. M., & Pickett-Cooper, P. (1997). Music and dementia: A review of literature. *Journal of Music Therapy, 34,* 204–245.

Buckwalter, K. C., Stolley, J. M., & Farran, C. J. (1999). Managing cognitive impairment in the elderly: Conceptual, intervention, and methodological issues. *Online Journal of Nursing Synthesis, 6*(10).

Buettner, L. L. (1999). Simple pleasures: A multilevel sensorimotor intervention for nursing home residents with dementia. *American Journal of Alzheimer's Disease, 14*(1), 41–52.

Burgener, S., Bakas, T., Murray, C., Dunahee, J., & Tossey, S. (1998). Effective caregiving approaches for patients with Alzheimer's disease. *Geriatric Nursing, 19,* 121–126.

Burgener, S. C., & Chiverton, P. (1992). Conceptualizing psychological well-being in cognitively impaired older persons. *Image: Journal of Nursing Scholarship, 24,* 209–213.

Burgener, S. C., & Dickerson-Putman, J. (1999). Assessing the patient in the early stages of irreversible dementia: The relevance of patient perspectives. *Journal of Gerontological Nursing, 25*(2), 33–41.

Burgener, S. C., Jirovec, M., Murrell, L., & Barton, D. (1992). Caregiver and environmental variables related to difficult behaviors in institutionalized, demented elderly persons. *Journal of Gerontology, 47,* P242–P249.

Burgio, L. D., Scilley, K., Hardin, J. M., Janosky, J., Bonino, P., Slater, S. C., & Engberg, R. (1994). Studying disruptive vocalization and contextual factors in the nursing home using computer-assessed real time observations. *Journal of Gerontology: Psychological Sciences, 51,* P364–P373.

Burgio, L., Scilley, K., Hardin, J. M., Hsu, C., & Yancey, J. (1996). Environmental "white noise": An intervention for verbally agitated nursing home residents. *Journal of Gerontology B, 51B,* 364–373.

Burnside, I., & Haight, B. (1994). Reminiscence and life review: Therapeutic interventions for older people. *Nurse Practitioner, 19*(4), 55–61.

Byrd, M. (1990). The use of visual imagery as a mnemonic device for healthy elderly and Alzheimer's disease patients. *American Journal of Alzheimer's Care and Related Disorders & Research, 5*(2), 10–15.

Camberg, L., Woods, P., Ooi, W. L., Hurley, A., Volicer, L., Ashley, J., Odenheimer, G., & McIntyre, K. (1999). Evaluation of simulated presence: A personalized approach to enhance well-being in persons with Alzheimer's disease. *Journal of the American Geriatrics Society, 47,* 446–452.

Camp, C. J., Judge, K. S., Bye, C. A., Fox, K. M., Bowden, J., Bell, M., Valencic, K., & Matter, J. M. (1997). An intergenerational program for person with dementia using Montessori methods. *Gerontologist, 37,* 688–692.

Cariaga, J., Burgio, L. K., Flynn, W., & Martin, D. (1991). A controlled study of disruptive vocalization among geriatric residents in nursing homes. *Journal of the American Geriatrics Society, 39,* 501–507.

Casby, J. A., & Holm, M. B. (1994). The effect of music on repetitive disruptive vocalizations of persons with dementia. *American Journal of Occupational Therapy, 48,* 883–889.

Clark, M. E., Lipe, A. W., & Bilbrey, M. (1998). Use of music to decrease aggressive behaviors in people with dementia. *Journal of Gerontological Nursing, 24*(7), 10–17.

Cohen, J. (1988). *Statistical power analysis for the behavioral sciences.* Hillsdale, NJ: Lawrence Erlbaum.

Cohen, C. I., Hyland, K., & Devlin, M. (1999). An evaluation of the use of the natural helping network model to enhance the well-being of nursing home residents. *Gerontologist, 39,* 426–433.

Cohen-Mansfield, J., Marx, M. S., & Rosenthal, A. S. (1989). A description of agitation in a nursing home. *Journal of Gerontology, 44,* 77–84.

Cohen-Mansfield, J., Marx, M. S., & Rosenthal, A. S. (1990). Dementia and agitation in nursing home residents: How are they related? *Psychology & Aging, 5*(1), 3–8.

Cohen-Mansfield, J., Marx, M. S., & Werner, P. (1993). Restraining cognitively impaired nursing home residents. *Nursing Management, 24,* 112Q–112W.

Cohen-Mansfield, J., & Werner, P. (1998). The effects of an enhanced environment on nursing home residents who pace. *Gerontologist, 38,* 199–208.

Cohen-Mansfield, J., Werner, P., & Marx, M. S. (1990). Screaming in nursing home residents. *Journal of the American Geriatrics Society, 38,* 785–792.

Colling, J., Ouslander, J., Hadley, B. J., Eisch, J., & Campbell, E. (1992). The effects of patterned urge response toileting (PURT) on urinary incontinence among nursing home residents. *Journal of the American Geriatrics Society, 40,* 135–141.

Colling, K. B. (1999a). Passive behaviors in Alzheimer's disease: A descriptive analysis. *American Journal of Alzheimer's Disease, 14*(1), 27–40.

Colling, K. B. (1999b). Passive behaviors in dementia. *Journal of Gerontological Nursing, 25*(9), 27–32.

Cummings, V., Holt, R., Van der Sloot, C., Moore, K., & Griffiths, D. (1995). Costs and management of urinary incontinence in long-term care. *Journal of Wound, Ostomy, and Continence Nursing, 22,* 193–198.

Dashiell, J., & Kirk, T. (1989). Alzheimer's disease: A current perspective. *Caring, 5*(8), 5–10.

Davis, L. L., Buckwalter, K., & Burgio, L. (1997). Measuring problem behaviors in dementia: Developing a methodological agenda. *Advances in Nursing Science, 20*(1), 40–55.

Dawson, P., Wells, D. L., & Kline, K. (1993). *Enhancing the abilities of persons with Alzheimer's and related dementias: A nursing perspective.* New York: Springer Publishing Co.

Day, K., Carreon, K., & Stump, C. (2000). The therapeutic design of environments for people with dementia: A review of the empirical research. *Gerontologist, 40,* 397–416.

Doyle, C., Zapparoni, T., O'Connor, D., & Runci, S. (1997). Efficacy of psychosocial treatment of noisemaking in severe dementia. *International Psychogeriatrics, 9,* 405–422.

Draper, B. (1999). The diagnosis and treatment of depression in dementia. *Psychiatric Services, 50,* 1151–1153.

Droes, R. M., Breebaart, E., Ettema, T. P., van Tilburg, W., & Mellenbergh, G. J. (2000). Effect of integrated family support versus day care only on behavior and mood of patients with dementia. *International Psychogeriatrics, 12,* 99–115.

Duncan, B. A., & Siegal, A. P. (1998). Early diagnosis and management of Alzheimer's disease. *Journal of Clinical Psychiatry, 59*(Suppl. 9), 15–21.

Durnbaugh, T., Haley, B., & Roberts, S. (1996). Assessing problem feeding behaviors in mid-stage Alzheimer's disease. *Geriatric Nursing, 17*(2), 63–67.

Dyer, C. B., Pavilik, V. N., Murphy, K. P., & Hyman, D. J. (2000). The high prevalence of depression and dementia in elder abuse or neglect. *Journal of American Geriatrics Society, 48,* 205–208.

Erikson, E. (1963). *Childhood and society.* New York: Norton.

Evans, D. A., Frankenstein, H. H., Albert, M. S., Scheer, P. A., Cook, N. R., Chown, M. J., Hebert, L. E., Hennekens, C. H., & Taylor, J. O. (1989). Prevalence of Alzheimer's disease in a community population of older persons. *Journal of the American Medical Association, 262,* 2551–2556.

Fantl, J. A., Newman, D. K., Colling, J., DeLancey, J. O. L., Keeys, C., Loughery, R., McDowell, B. J., Norton, P., Ouslander, J., Schnelle, J., Staskin, D., Tries, J., Urich, V., Vitousek, S. H., Weiss, B. D., & Whitmore, K. (1996). *Urinary incontinence in adults: Acute and chronic management. Clinical Practice Guideline, No. 2, 1996 Update.* AHCPR Publication No. 96-0682. Rockville, MD: U.S. Department of Health and Human Services. Public Health Service, Agency for Health Care Policy and Research.

Feil, N. (1993). *The validation breakthrough: Simple techniques for communicating with people with Alzheimer's type dementia.* Baltimore, MD: Health Professions.

Ferrario, E., Cappa, G., Molaschi, M., Rocco, M., & Fabris, F. (1991). Reality orientation therapy in institutionalized elderly patients: Preliminary results. *Archives of Gerontology and Geriatrics* (Suppl. 2), 139–142.

Finucane, T. E., Christmas, C., & Travis, K. (1999). Tube feeding in patients with advanced dementia. A review of the evidence. *Journal of the American Medical Association, 282,* 1365–1369.

Foley, D. J., Masaki, K. H., Ross, G. W., & White, L. R. (2000). Driving cessation in older men with incident dementia. *Journal of the American Geriatrics Society, 48,* 928–930.

Fopma-Loy, J., & Austin, J. K. (1993). An attributional analysis of formal caregivers' perceptions of agitated behavior of a resident with Alzheimer's disease. *Archives of Psychiatric Nursing, 7,* 217–225.

Frey, L. W., Leach, L., Nelson, N., Pirozzolo, F. J., & Mahurin, R. (1991). Improved neuropsychological test scores in Alzheimer disease patients after ecologically sensitive, cognitive interventions: A pilot study. *American Journal of Alzheimer's Care and Related Disorders & Research,* 34–39.

Friedman, R., & Tappen, R. M. (1991). The effects of planned walking on communication in Alzheimer's disease. *Journal of the American Geriatrics Society, 39,* 650–654.

Gerber, G. J., Prince, P. N., Snider, H. G., Atchison, K., Dubois, L., & Kilgour, J. A. (1991). Group activity and cognitive improvement among patients with Alzheimer's disease. *Hospital and Community Psychiatry, 42,* 843–846.

Gerdner, L. A., & Buckwalter, K. C. (1994). Assessment and management of agitation in Alzheimer's patients. *Journal of Gerontological Nursing, 20*(4), 11–20.

Gerdner, L. A., & Swanson, E. A. (1993). Effects of individualized music on confused and agitated elderly patients. *Archives of Psychiatric Nursing, 7,* 284–291.

Goddaer, J., & Abraham, I. L. (1994). Effects of relaxing music on agitation during meals among nursing home residents with severe cognitive impairment. *Archives of Psychiatric Nursing, 8,* 150–158.

Hall, G. R., & Buckwalter, K. C. (1987). Progressively lowered stress threshold: A conceptual model for care of adults with Alzheimer's disease. *Archives of Psychiatric Nursing, 1,* 399–406.

Hall, G. R. (1994). Caring for people with Alzheimer's disease using the conceptual model of Progressively Lowered Stress Threshold in the clinical setting. *Nursing Clinics of North America, 29*(1), 129–141.

Hoeffer, B., Rader, J., McKenzie, D., Lavelle, M., & Stewart, B. (1997). Reducing aggressive behavior during bathing cognitively impaired nursing home residents. *Journal of Gerontological Nursing, 23*(5), 16–23.

Holmberg, S. K. (1997). Evaluation of a clinical intervention for wanderers on a geriatric nursing unit. *Archives of Psychiatric Nursing, 11*(1), 21–28.

Holst, G., Hallberg, I., & Gustafson, L. (1997). The relationship of vocally disruptive behavior and previous personality in severely demented institutionalized patients. *Archives of Psychiatric Nursing, 11,* 147–154.

Hopkins, R. W., Rindlessbacher, P., & Grant, N. T. (1992). An investigation of the sundowning syndrome and ambient light. *American Journal of Alzheimer's Care and Related Disorders & Research, 7,* 22–27.

Huber, T. J., & Dietrich, D. E. (1999). Possible use of amantadine in depression. *Pharmacopsychiatry, 32*(2), 47–55.

Hughes, C., Berg, I., Danzinger, W., Coben, L., & Martin, R. (1982). A new clinical scale for the staging of dementia. *British Journal of Psychiatry, 140,* 566–572.

Hurley, A. C., Volicer, B. J., Hanrahan, P. A., Houde, S., & Volicer, L. (1992). Assessment of discomfort in advanced Alzheimer patients. *Research in Nursing and Health, 15,* 369–377.

Hutchinson, S. A., & Marshall, M. (2000). Responses of family caregivers and family members with Alzheimer's disease to an activity kit: An ethnographic study. *Journal of Advanced Nursing, 31*(1), 44–50.

International Psychogeriatric Association. (2000). *Primary care management of behavioral and psychological symptoms of dementia: Modules 1-8.* Northfield, IL: Author.

Judge, K. S., Camp, C. J., & Orsulic-Jeras, S. (2000). Use of Montessori-based activities for clients with dementia in adult day care: Effects on engagement. *American Journal of Alzheimer's Disease, 15*(1), 42–46.

Katsinas, R. (2000). The use and implications of a canine companion in a therapeutic day program for nursing home residents with dementia. *Activities, Adaptation & Aging, 25*(1), 13–30.

Kayser-Jones, J. (1989). The environment and quality of life in long-term care institutions. *Nursing and Health Care, 10,* 125–130.

Kayser-Jones, J. (1991). The impact of the environment on the quality of care in nursing homes: A social-psychological perspective. *Holistic Nursing Practice, 5*(3), 29–38.

Kikuta, S. C. (1991). Clinically managing disruptive behavior on the ward. *Journal of Gerontological Nursing, 17*(8), 4–8, 44–45.

Kim, E. J., & Buschmann, M. T. (1999). The effect of expressive physical touch on patients with dementia. *International Journal of Nursing Studies, 36,* 235–243.

Kitwood, T., & Bredin, K. (1992). A new approach to the evaluation of dementia care. *Journal of Advances in Health and Nursing Care, 1*(5), 41–60.

Kitwood, T. (1997). *Dementia reconsidered: The person comes first.* Philadelphia: Open University Press.

Koger, S. M., & Brotons, M. (1999). Music therapy for dementia symptoms. *The Cochrane Library, 4,* 1–19.

Kolanowski, A. M. (1995a). Disturbing behaviors in demented elders: A concept synthesis. *Archives of Psychiatric Nursing, 9,* 188–194.

Kolanowski, A. M. (1995b). Aggressive behaviors in institutionalized elders: A theoretical framework. *American Journal of Alzheimer's Disease, 10*(2), 23–29.

Kolanowski, A. M. (1999). An overview of the need-driven, dementia-compromised behavior model. *Journal of Gerontological Nursing, 25*(9), 7–9.

Kolanowski, A. M., Hurwitz, S., Taylor, L. A., Evans, L., & Strumpf, N. (1994). Contextual factors associated with disturbing behaviors in institutionalized elders. *Nursing Research, 43*(2), 73–79.

Kovach, C. R., & Magliocco, J. S. (1998). Late-stage dementia and participation in therapeutic activities. *Applied Nursing Research, 11,* 167–173.

Lantz, M. S., Buchalter, E. N., & McBee, L. (1997). The wellness group: A novel intervention for coping with disruptive behavior in elderly nursing home residents. *Gerontologist, 37,* 551–556.

Lawton, M. P. (1983). The dimensions of well being. *Experimental Aging Research, 9,* 65–72.

Lawton, M. P., & Rubinstein, R. L. (2000). Introduction. In M. P. Lawton & R. L. Rubinstein (Eds.), *Interventions in dementia care: Toward improving quality of life.* New York: Springer Publishing Co.

Lekan-Rutledge, D., Palmer, M. H., & Belyea, M. (1998). In their own words: Nursing assistants' perceptions of barriers to implementation of prompted voiding in long-term care. *Gerontologist, 38,* 370–378.

Lindenmuth, G. F., & Moose, B. (1990). Improving cognitive abilities of elderly Alzheimer's patients with intense exercise therapy. *The American Journal of Alzheimer's Care and Related Disorders & Research, 5*(1), 31–33.

Lindenmuth, G. F., Patel, M., & Chang, P. K. (1992). Effects of music on sleep in healthy elderly and subjects with senile dementia of the Alzheimer's type. *The American Journal of Alzheimer's Care and Related Disorders & Research, 7*(2), 13–20.

Lopez, O. L., Wisniewski, S. R., Becker, J. T., Boller, F., & DeKosky, S. T. (1999). Psychiatric medication and abnormal behavior as predictors of progression in probable Alzheimer disease. *Archives of Neurology, 56,* 1266–1272.

Lyketsos, C. G., Steele, C., Baker, L., Galik, E., Kopunek, S., Steinberg, M., & Warren, A. (1997). Major and minor depression in Alzheimer's disease: Prevalence and impact. *Journal of Neuropsychiatry & Clinical Neurosciences, 9,* 556–561.

Lyman, K. A. (1989). Bringing the social back in: A critique of the biomedicalization of dementia. *Gerontologist, 29,* 597–606.

Lyons, S. S., & Specht, J. K. S. (1999). *Research-based protocol: Prompted voiding for persons with urinary incontinence.* Iowa City, IA: University of Iowa Gerontological Nursing Interventions Research Center, Research Development and Dissemination Core.

MacDonald-Connolly, D., Pedlar, D., MacKnight, C., Lewis, C., & Fisher, J. (2000). Guidelines for stage-based supports in Alzheimer's care: The FAST-ACT. *Journal of Gerontological Nursing, 26*(11), 34–45.

Maxfield, M. C., Lewis, R. E., & Cannon, S. (1996). Training staff to prevent aggressive behavior of cognitively impaired elderly patients during bathing and grooming. *Journal of Gerontological Nursing, 22*(1), 37–43.

Mayers, K., & Griffin, M. (1990). The Play Project: Use of stimulus objects with demented patients. *Journal of Gerontological Nursing, 16*(1), 32–37.

McCallion, P., Toseland, R. W., & Freeman, K. (1999). An evaluation of a family visit education program. *The Journal of the American Geriatrics Society, 47,* 203–214.

McContha, D., McContha, J. T., & Dermigny, R. (1994). The use of interactive computer services to enhance the quality of life for long-term care residents. *Gerontologist, 34,* 553–556.

McDougall, G. J. (1995). Metamemory and depression in cognitively impaired elders. *Nursing Research, 44*(5), 306–311.

McGillivray, T., & Marland, G. R. (1999). Assisting demented patients with feeding: Problems in a ward environment. A review of literature. *Journal of Advanced Nursing, 29,* 608–614.

Meddaugh, D. I. (1990). Reactance: Understanding aggressive behavior in long-term care. *Journal of Gerontological Nursing, 28*(4), 28–33.

Migliorelli, R., Teson, A., Sabe, L., Petracchi, M., Leiguarda, R., & Starkstein, S. E. (1995). Prevalence and correlates of dysthymia and major depression among patients with Alzheimer's disease. *American Journal of Psychiatry, 152*(1), 37–44.

Moniz-Cook, E., Gibson, A., Win, T., & Wang, M. (1998). A preliminary study of the effects of early intervention with people with dementia and their families in a memory clinic. *Aging and Mental Health, 2,* 199–211.

Morhardt, D., & Johnson, N. (1998, November). *Effects of memory loss support groups for persons with early stage dementia and their families.* Paper presented at the meeting of the Gerontological Society of America, Philadelphia.

Morrissey, M., & Biela, C. (1997). Snoezelen: Benefits for nursing older clients. *Nursing Standard, 12*(3), 38–40.

Morton, I., & Bleathman, C. (1991). The effectiveness of validation therapy in dementia—a pilot study. *International Journal of Geriatric Psychiatry, 6,* 327–330.

Mungas, D., Cooper, J. K., Weiler, P. G., Gietzen, D., Franzi, C., & Bernick, C. (1990). Dietary preference for sweet foods in patients with dementia. *Journal of the American Geriatrics Society, 38,* 999–1007.

Namazi, K. H., & Johnson, B. D. (1992a). Dressing independently: A closet modification model for Alzheimer's disease patients. *American Journal of Alzheimer's Care and Related Disorders & Research, 7*(1), 22–28.

Namazi, K. H., & Johnson, B. D. (1992b). How familiar tasks can enhance concentration in Alzheimer's disease patients. *American Journal of Alzheimer's Care and Related Disorders & Research, 7*(1), 35–40.

Neal, M., & Briggs, M. (2000). Validation therapy for dementia [on-line]. *Cochrane Library, 3.* Available: http://gateway1.ovid.com/ovidweb.cgi [Retrieved April 29, 2001].

Oleson, M., Torgerud, R., Bernette, D., Steiner, P., & Odiet, M. (1998). Improving nursing home quality of life: Residents helping residents. *American Journal of Alzheimer's Disease, 13,* 138–145.

Onega, L. L., & Abraham, I. L. (1998). Differentiated nursing assessment of depressive symptoms in community-dwelling elders. *Nursing Clinics of North America, 33,* 407–416.

Peck, A., Cohen, C. E., & Mulvihill, M. N. (1990). Long-term enteral feeding of aged demented nursing home patients. *Journal of the American Geriatrics Society, 38,* 1195–1198.

Perrin, T. (1997). Occupational need in severe dementia: A descriptive study. *Journal of Advanced Nursing, 25,* 934–941.

Phillips, L. R., & Ayres, M. (1999). Supportive and nonsupportive care environments for the elderly. In A. S. Hinshaw, S. L. Feetham, & J. L. F. Shaver (Eds.), *Handbook of clinical nursing research* (pp. 599–627). Thousand Oaks, CA: Sage.

Pulsford, D. (1997). Therapeutic activities for people with dementia—what, why . . . and why not? *Journal of Advanced Nursing, 26,* 704–709.

Pulsford, D., Rushforth, D., & Connor, I. (2000). Woodlands therapy: An ethnographic analysis of a small-group therapeutic activity for people with moderate or severe dementia. *Journal of Advanced Nursing, 32,* 650–657.

Quayhagen, M. P., & Quayhagen, M. (1996). Discovering life quality in coping with dementia. *Western Journal of Nursing Research, 18,* 120–135.

Quayhagen, M. P., Quayhagen, M., Corbeil, R. R., Hendrix, R. C., Jackson, J. E., Snyder, L., & Bower, D. (2000). Coping with dementia: Evaluation of four nonpharmacologic interventions. *International Psychogeriatrics, 12,* 249–265.

Rao, V., & Lyketsos, C. G. (2000). The benefits and risks of ECT for patients with primary dementia who also suffer from depression. *International Journal of Geriatric Psychiatry, 15,* 729–735.

Reisberg, B. (1986). Dementia: A systematic approach to identifying reversible causes. *Geriatrics, 41,* 30–36, 39, 42–46.

Reisberg, B. (1988). Functional assessment staging (FAST). *Psychopharmacology Bulletin, 24,* 653–659.

Reisberg, B. (1996). Behavioral intervention approaches to the treatment and management of Alzheimer's disease: A research agenda. *International Psychogeriatrics,*
8(Suppl.), 38–44.

Remsburg, R. E., Palmer, M. H., Langford, A. M., & Mendelson, G. F. (1999). Staff
compliance with and ratings of effectiveness of a prompted voiding program in
a long-term care facility. *Journal of Wound, Ostomy, and Continence Nursing,*
26, 261–269.

Rheaume, Y. L., Manning, B. C., Harper, D. G., & Volicer, L. (1998). Effect of light
therapy upon disturbed behaviors in Alzheimer's patients. *American Journal of*
Alzheimer's Disease, 13, 291–295.

Robichaud, L., Hébert, R., & Desrosiers, J. (1994). Efficacy of a sensory integration
program on behaviors of inpatients with dementia. *American Journal of Occupational Therapy, 48,* 355–360.

Rogers, J. C., Holm, M. B., Burgio, L. D., Granieri, E., Hsu, C., Hardin, J. M., &
McDowell, B. J. (1999). Improving morning care routines of nursing home
residents with dementia. *Journal of the American Geriatrics Society, 47,*
1057–1057.

Rovner, B. W., Steele, C. D., Shmuely, Y., & Folstein, M. F. (1996). A randomized
trial of dementia care in nursing homes. *Journal of the American Geriatrics*
Society, 44(1), 7–13.

Rowe, M., & Alfred, D. (1999). The effectiveness of slow-stroke massage in diffusing
agitated behaviors in individuals with Alzheimer's disease. *Journal of Gerontological Nursing, 25*(6), 22–34.

Ryden, M. (1998). A theory of caring and dementia. *American Journal of Alzheimer*
Disease, 13(4), 203–207.

Ryden, M. B., Feldt, K. S., Oh, H. L., Brand, K., Warne, M., Weber, E., Nelson,
J., & Gross, C. (1999). Relationships between aggressive behavior in cognitively
impaired nursing home residents and use of restraints, psychoactive drugs, and
secured units. *Archives of Psychiatric Nursing, 13,* 170–178.

Saitlin, A., Volicer, L., Ross, V., Herz, L., & Campbell, S. (1992). Bright light treatment
of behavioral and sleep disturbances in patients with Alzheimer's disease. *American Journal of Psychiatry, 149,* 1028–1032.

Schnelle, J. F., Cruise, P. A., Alessi, C. A., Al-Samarrai, N., & Ouslander, J. G. (1998).
Individualizing nighttime incontinence care in nursing home residents. *Nursing*
Research, 47, 197–204.

Schnelle, J. F., Newman, D., White, M., Abbey, J., Wallston, K. A., Fogarty, T., &
Ory, M. G. (1993). Maintaining continence in nursing home residents through
the application of industrial quality control. *Gerontologist, 33,* 114–121.

Schnelle, J. F., Ouslander, J. G., Simmons, S. F., Alessi, C. A., & Gravel, M. D.
(1993). The nighttime environment, incontinence care, and sleep disruption in
nursing homes. *Journal of the American Geriatrics Society, 41,* 910–914.

Schnelle, J. F., Traughber, B., Sowell, V. A., Newman, D. R., Petrilli, C. O., & Ory,
M. (1989). Prompted voiding treatment of urinary incontinence in nursing home
patients: A behavioral management approach for nursing home staff. *Journal of*
the American Geriatrics Society, 37, 1051–1057.

Small, G. W., Rabins, P. V., Barry, P., Buckholtz, N. S., DeKosky, S. T., Ferris, S.
H., Finkel, S. I., Gwyther, L. P., Khachaturian, Z. S., Lebowitz, B. D., McRae,

T. D., Morris, J. C., Oakley, F., Schneider, L. S., Streim, J. E., Sunderland, T., Teri, L. A., & Tune, L. E. (1997). Diagnosis and treatment of Alzheimer disease and related disorders: Consensus statement of the American Association for Geriatric Psychiatry, the Alzheimer's Association, and the American Geriatrics Society. *Journal of American Medical Association, 278,* 1363–1371.

Snyder, M., Egan, E. C., & Burns, K. R. (1995). Interventions for decreasing agitation behaviors in persons with dementia. *Journal of Gerontological Nursing, 21*(7), 34–40.

Spector, A., Davies, S., Woods, B., & Orrell, M. (2000). Reality orientation for dementia: A systematic review of the evidence of effectiveness from randomized controlled trials. *Gerontologist, 40,* 206–212.

Spector, A., Orrell, S. A., Davies, S., & Woods, R. T. (2000). Reminiscence therapy for dementia [on-line]. *Cochrane Library, 4.* Available: http://gateway1.ovid.com/ovidweb.cgi [Retrieved May 8, 2001].

Swanson, K. M. (1991). Empirical development of a middle range theory of caring. *Nursing Research, 40,* 161–166.

Tabloski, P. A., McKinnon-Howe, L., & Remington, R. (1995). Effects of calming music on the level of agitation in cognitively impaired nursing home residents. *The American Journal of Alzheimer's Care and Related Disorders & Research, 10*(1), 10–15.

Taft, L. B. (1995). Interventions in dementia care: Responding to the call for alternatives to restraints. *American Journal of Alzheimer's Disease, 10*(2), 30–38.

Taft, L. B., & Cronin-Stubbs, D. (1995). Behavioral symptoms in dementia: An update. *Research in Nursing and Health, 18,* 143–163.

Taft, L. B., Matthiesen, V., Farran, C. J., McCann, J. J., & Knafl, K. A. (1997). Supporting strengths and responding to agitation in dementia care: An exploratory study. *American Journal of Alzheimer's Disease, 12,* 198–208.

Tappen, R. M. (1994). The effect of skill training functional abilities of nursing home residents with dementia. *Research in Nursing & Health, 17,* 159–165.

Tappen, R. M., Roach, K. E., Applegate, E. B., & Stowell, P. (2000). Effect of a combined walking and conversation intervention on functional mobility of nursing home residents with Alzheimer disease. *Alzheimer Disease and Associated Disorders, 14,* 196–201.

Teri, L. (1994). Behavioral treatment of depression in patients with dementia. *Alzheimer Disease and Associated Disorders, 8*(Suppl. 3), 66–74.

Teri, L., Logsdon, R., Uomoto, J., & McCurry, S. M. (1997). Behavioral treatment of depression in dementia patients: A controlled clinical trial. *Journal of Gerontology: Psychological Sciences, 52B*(4), P159–P166.

Thorpe, L., Middleton, J., Russell, G., & Stewart, N. (2000). Bright light therapy for demented nursing home patients with behavioral disturbance. *American Journal of Alzheimer's Disease, 15*(1), 18–26.

Topp, R., & Burgener, S. C. (1993, November). *The effect of exercise upon Alzheimer's patients and their primary caregiver: A pilot study.* Paper presented at the meeting of Sigma Theta Tau International, Indianapolis, IN.

Toseland, R. W., Diehl, M., Freeman, K., Manzanares, T., Naleppa, M., & McCallion, P. (1997). The impact of validation group therapy on nursing home residents with dementia. *Journal of Applied Gerontology, 16*(1), 31–50.

Van Ort, S., & Phillips, L. (1992). Feeding nursing home residents with Alzheimer's disease. *Geriatric Nursing, 13,* 249–253.

Vap, P. W., & Dunaye, T. (2000). Pressure ulcer risk assessment in long-term care nursing. *Journal of Gerontological Nursing, 26*(6), 37–45.

Visser, P. J., Verhey, F., Ponds, R., Kester, A., & Jolles, J. (2000). Distinction between preclinical Alzheimer's disease and depression. *Journal of the American Geriatrics Society, 48,* 479–484.

Walsh, P. G., Mertin, P. G., Verlander, D. F., & Pollard, C. F. (1995). The effects of a "pets as therapy" dog on persons with dementia in a psychiatric ward. *Australian Occupational Therapy Journal, 42,* 161–166.

Watson, N. M., Wells, T. J., & Cox, C. (1998). Rocking chair therapy for dementia patients: Its effects on psychosocial well-being and balance. *American Journal of Alzheimer's Disease, 13,* 296–308.

Watson, R. (1993). Measuring feeding difficulty in patients with dementia: Perspectives and problems. *Journal of Advanced Nursing, 18*(4), 25–31.

Weinrich, S., Egbert, C., Eleazer, G. P., & Haddock, K. S. (1995). Agitation: Measurement, management, and intervention *Psychiatric Nursing, 9,* 251–160.

Wells, D. L., & Dawson, P. (2000). Description of retained abilities in older persons with dementia. *Research in Nursing & Health, 23,* 158–166.

Wells, D. L., Dawson, P., Sidani, S., Craig, D., & Pringle, D. (2000). Effects of an abilities-focused program of morning care on residents who have dementia and on caregivers. *Journal of the American Geriatrics Society, 48,* 442–449.

Whall, A. L., Gillis, G. L., Yankou, D., Booth, D. E., & Beel-Bates, C. A. (1992). Disruptive behavior in elderly nursing home residents: A survey of nursing staff. *Journal of Gerontological Nursing, 18*(10), 13–17.

Whall, A. N., Black, M. E., Groh, C. J., Yankou, D. J., Kupferschmid, B. J., & Foster, N. (1997). The effect of natural environments upon agitation and aggression in late stage dementia patients. *American Journal of Alzheimer's Disease, 12,* 216–220.

Witucki, J. M., & Twibell, R. S. (1997). The effect of sensory stimulation activities on the psychological well-being of patients with advanced Alzheimer's disease. *American Journal of Alzheimer's Disease, 12*(1), 10–15.

Woods, P., & Ashley, J. (1995). Simulated presence therapy: Using selected memories to manage problem behaviors in Alzheimer's disease patients. *Geriatric Nursing, 16,* 9–14.

Yale, R. (1998, November). *Support groups for newly diagnosed, early stage Alzheimer's patients: How patients manage their concerns.* Paper presented at the meeting of the Gerontological Society of America, Philadelphia.

Zanetti, O., Fisoni, G. B., DeLeo, D., Buono, M. D., Bianchetti, A., & Trabucchi, M. (1995). Reality orientation therapy in Alzheimer's disease: Useful or not? A controlled study. *Alzheimer Disease and Associated Disorders, 9,* 132–138.

Zanetti, O., Binetti, G., Magni, E., Rozzini, L., Bianchetti, A., & Trabucchi, M. (1997). Procedural memory stimulation in Alzheimer's disease: Impact of a training programme. *Acta Neurologica Scandinavica, 95,* 152–157.

Zeiss, A. M., Davies, H. D., & Tinklenberg, J. R. (1991). An observational study of sexual behavior in demented male patients. *Journal of Gerontology, 51A,* M325–M329.

PART II

Settings for Elder Care

Chapter 5

Transitional Care of Older Adults

MARY D. NAYLOR

ABSTRACT

This chapter reviews 94 published research reports on transitional care of older adults by nurse researchers and researchers from other disciplines. Reports were identified through searches of MEDLINE, CINAHL, HealthSTAR, Sociological Abstracts and PsycINFO using combinations of the following search terms: *transitional care, discharge planning, care coordination, case management, continuity of care, referrals, postdischarge follow-up, patient assessment, patient needs, interventions*, and *evaluation*. Reports were included if published between 1985 and 2001, if conducted on samples age 55 and older, if relevant to nursing research, and if published in English. Intervention studies had to have a control or comparison group and a test for statistical significance. Four key findings from this review were identified. A high proportion of elders and their caregivers report substantial unmet transitional care needs, with the need for information and increased access to services consistently among the top priorities. Differences in expectations between and among patients, families, and health care providers, and the need for increased patient and family involvement in decision making, are common themes in discharge planning studies. Gaps in communication have been identified through the discharge planning process. Evidence about the effects of innovations in transitional care on quality and cost outcomes is sparse. Four main recommendations are made. Differences in older adults' transitional care needs based on race, ethnicity, and educational level, with attention to potential disparities, require further study. Studies of strategies to promote effective involvement of patients and families in decision making throughout discharge planning are needed. The development and testing of referral and other information systems designed to promote the transfer of accurate and complete information across sites of care should be a research focus. A priority for future research should be continued study of strategies to improve transitional care outcomes of older adults and their caregivers.

Keywords: transitional care, continuity of care, discharge planning, postdischarge/home follow-up, case management

In recent years, fundamental changes in the delivery and financing of health care for older adults have stimulated the growth and development of a new line of health care services and environments known as transitional care (Aaron & Reischauer, 1995; Moon & Davis, 1995). Medicare's Prospective Payment System and the movement to managed care have provided incentives for services and sites of care that prevent or minimize the use of costly acute care services. The result is an increased demand for subacute, postacute, and rehabilitative services and a beginning appreciation of the importance of models of care that promote continuity. Transitional care has emerged to bridge the gaps between and among a diverse range of providers, services, and sites, caring for the vastly growing population of older adults in America.

Transitional care is a term that encompasses a broad range of services and environments designed to promote the safe and timely transfer of patients from one level of care to another (e.g., acute to subacute) or from one type of setting to another (e.g., hospital to home) (Brooten & Naylor, 1999). Similarly, *continuity of care* is a multidimensional term used to describe a variety of relationships between patients and the delivery of health care. This concept incorporates accurate and complete communication of patient information between and among providers and across settings, and the availability of a constant point person to help negotiate an exceedingly complex system with a goal of seamlessness in transitions (Fletcher, O'Malley, Fletcher, Earp, & Alexander, 1984; Ruane & Brody, 1987).

The following question guided a review of the state of the science related to the area of transitional care: What is known about the effectiveness of existing processes of care and innovative interventions designed to address the needs of elders and their caregivers who are making transitions across settings or from one level of care to another?

At-Risk Older Adults

In the aggregate, older adults are disproportionately heavy users of the most costly health services including hospitalization, nursing home, and home health care. Although they represent less than 13% of the population, older adults account for more than 35% of total health care expenditures (National Center for Health Statistics, 1999). Medicare pays for a substantial amount of these expenditures, which amounted to $306 billion in 1998 (Health Care Financing Administration, 1999). Thus, considerable interest has focused on Medicare's outlays for health services consumption by this population.

From what is known about the effectiveness of existing processes of care and interventions, it is apparent that continued development of transitional care services and sites should be informed by study findings that have examined the unique needs of older patients, the nature and intensity of services needed to achieve positive patient and caregiver outcomes, the types and level of providers needed, and the associated costs. Knowledge generated from examining existing and emerging models of care is also necessary to understand the critical elements needed to assure that transitional care services are designed to achieve the highest quality and most cost-effective outcomes for this vulnerable population.

METHOD

A search for studies published since 1985 that describe the needs of elders as they make transitions from one level of care or one setting to another, and that examine existing processes of transitional care or empirically test transitional care innovations was conducted. In the aforementioned databases, combinations of the following key words were used: *transitional care*, *discharge planning*, *care coordination*, *case management*, *continuity of care*, *referrals*, *postdischarge follow-up*, *patient assessment*, *patient needs*, *interventions*, and *evaluation*. While caregivers were not the main focus of this search, a number of studies included them. In this paper, this term applies to informal caregivers only, such as family members or friends. Acceptable studies were published between 1985 and 2001 and focused on the age 55 and older population. Intervention studies had to have a control or comparison group and a test for statistical significance. This search yielded 94 articles for analysis.

The organizing framework selected for the presentation of the findings is the nursing process. This framework was selected because it encompasses the major stages of assuring high-quality and cost-effective service delivery including: needs assessment, planning, implementation, and evaluation. Guided by this framework, the following section summarizes the major findings.

A number of largely descriptive studies, relying primarily on surveys and/or interviews and involving a diverse range of typically small samples have increased our understanding of the needs of patients and their caregivers as they make the difficult transition from hospital to home or nursing home. Studies of the nature of the experience of older adults and their caregivers during important transitions have relied primarily on qualitative methods employing in-depth interviews with small samples. The research designs for the few intervention studies identified through this search were primarily quasi-experimental or prospective randomized clinical trials (RCTs).

RESULTS

Needs Assessment

Multiple transitions are the norm, especially among that segment of the population of elders living with complex chronic illnesses, deteriorating health status, and changing care needs. Because of recent changes in health care, there have been substantially greater care needs of patients making transitions to nursing homes or discharged to home following hospitalization (Shaughnessy & Kramer, 1990). In general, elders and their caregivers report a high proportion of unmet needs in the period immediately following hospital discharge (Jones, Densen, & Brown, 1989; Mistiaen, Duijnhouwer, Wijkel, de Bont, & Veeger, 1997; Wolock, Schlesinger, Dinerman, & Seaton, 1987). Major problems reported by patients and/or caregivers include managing the illness (e.g., symptoms/complications, and treatments), personal care needs, and lack of knowledge and skills (Bowman, Howden, Allen, Webster, & Thompson, 1994; Bull & Jervis, 1997; Jones et al., 1989; Lough, 1996; Naylor, Bowles, & Brooten, 2000; Tierney, Closs, Hunter, & Macmillan, 1993).

Regardless of the reason for hospitalization, discharge priorities consistently identified include the need for information, increased access to essential health and social services and resources, and enhanced emotional support (Bowman et al., 1994; Boyle, Nance, & Passau-Buck, 1992; Bull & Jervis, 1997; Gustafson, Arora, Nelson, & Boberg, 2001; Hughes, Hodgson, Muller, Robinson, & McCorkle, 2000; Jacobs, 2000; Lough, 1996; Mistiaen et al., 1997; Tierney et al., 1993; Weaver, Perloff, & Waters,

1998; Wolock et al., 1987). Studies that have explored the influence of sociodemographic, clinical, and decision-making factors influencing patient and caregiver needs are sparse (Bubela et al., 1990). Findings from the few studies that addressed the issue of timing found that 4 to 6 weeks postdischarge represents a critical period when many elders are at highest risk for poor postdischarge outcomes following hospital discharge (Fethke & Smith, 1991; Naylor et al., 1994; Naylor et al., 1999).

A few instruments have been designed to strengthen assessment of the needs of elders making the transition from hospital to another setting and predict their outcomes; additional testing to assess their reliability and validity is needed (Blaylock & Cason, 1992; Naughton, Saltzman, Priore, Reedy, & Mylotte, 1999; Reuben et al., 1992; Sager et al., 1996; Satish, Winograd, Chavez, & Bloch, 1996). Similarly, investigators have attempted to identify predictors of need for postdischarge services. Increased functional deficits, decreased social support, and longer lengths of hospital stay are patient characteristics consistently predicting home health service use following hospital discharge (Bull, 1994a; Kane et al., 1996; Narsavage & Naylor, 2000; Solomon et al., 1993). An examination of system characteristics found that referrals to home health are heavily influenced by the hospitals' long-term care arrangements and by conditions in the local market (Kenney, 1993).

Data generated from examining elders' hospital discharge experience from the perspectives of patients, families, and nurses have generated a few consistent themes. From patients' and families' perspectives, these include diversity of discharge readiness, support for patients but little for families, limited knowledge of community resources, and a general lack of involvement of patients and families in decision making (Congdon, 1994; Magilvy & Congdon, 2000). A lack of coordination of team members in the discharge planning process contributed to nurses' confusion and distress (Congdon, 1994).

Transition to nursing home life for elders is part of a process (Dellasega & Nolan, 1997) that seems to occur in phases that begin with feeling overwhelmed and progresses over time to initial acceptance (Wilson, 1997). Themes identified from studies of caregivers actively involved in the process of placing an older adult in a nursing home include uncertainty, a sense of turmoil, surrendering to system, urgency, and validation (Penrod & Dellasega, 1998; Rodgers, 1997). Themes identified from examining the nursing home placement experiences of African American and European American caregivers included relief and reinvolvement, regrets and losses, and a continuing caregiver role (Fink & Picot, 1995).

Planning

Findings from Jewell's (1993) qualitative study revealed a distinctive discharge process beginning at hospital admission and ending at discharge with discharge planning a separate component of the process. Expectations play an important role in preparing elders and caregivers for major transitions. In general, findings from studies that have examined differences in expectations reveal a substantial lack of agreement between patients/families and health professionals related to patients' health status and problems in self-care during and following hospitalization (Bull, 1994a; Reiley et al., 1996; Rose, Bowman, & Kresevic, 2000). For example, nurses were found to underestimate patients' postdischarge functional abilities and overestimate patients' understanding of the postdischarge treatment plan (Reiley et al., 1996).

Level of involvement of patients and caregivers in decision making related to transitional care has been the focus of a wide range of studies, with most identifying the need for their increased participation (Coulton, Dunkle, Chow, Haug, & Vielhaber, 1988; Coulton, Dunkle, Haug, Chow, & Vielhaber, 1989; Forbes & Hoffart, 1998; Jewell, 1996; Kadushin & Kulys, 1994). Patients' perceptions of the decision-making process related to posthospital care ranged from certainty about outcomes and family support for decision making to feelings of being rushed, unable to fulfill role in decision making, and restricted in choices (Coulton et al., 1988; Jewell, 1996). Elderly patients discharged from an acute hospital vary in their reactions to the decision making process and the degree to which they exert control over decisions. Perceived lack of control over the decision has been associated with psychological distress for patients with high levels of internal locus of control, but not for those whose expectations of internal control are low (Coulton et al., 1989). Similarly, loss of control was threatening to the sense of self among elders making the decision to use both institutional and community-based long term care services (Forbes & Hoffart, 1998).

Common themes emerging from studies of the decision-making process used by caregivers in placing an elder in a nursing home include the perspectives that such a decision conflicted with perception of the role of caregiver and that it was often a singular process with advice from health professionals often viewed as inadequate and sometimes detrimental (Dellasega & Mastrian, 1995). Caregivers' attitudes related to institutional care were found to be at least as important as elders' physical and emotional health in determining which elders are placed in a nursing home following a health crisis (Deimling & Poulshock, 1985).

While health professionals, especially nurses, recognize the need for patient and family involvement in decision making related to posthospital care, study findings suggest that they sometimes view patients as being both passive and reluctant participants (Jewell, 1996). In other sites, however, nurses may not fully understand the importance of their own involvement in the discharge experience. Examination of the nature of planning to prepare older adults for discharge following ambulatory procedures revealed that no effort had been made to adapt discharge planning practices to the unique needs of this patient group (Tappen, Muzic, & Kennedy, 2001). Furthermore, nurses in this setting viewed discharge planning as ancillary to their role.

Essential characteristics of quality discharge planning have been examined. Both patients and health care professionals have identified effective communication (Bull, 1994b) and the use of highly formalized structures such as a focused admission assessment and postdischarge follow-up program (Haddock, 1991) as key components of successful discharge planning. In contrast, Feather (1993) found that power, defined as the influence of the discharge planner and physician, had the strongest independent effect on discharge planning effectiveness. Open communication and collaboration with social workers, and problem solving with physicians have been identified by nurses as important to effective discharge planning (Hansen, Bull, & Gross, 1998).

Despite a strong relationship between good communication and patient and caregiver satisfaction with care planning, available evidence demonstrates that there are multiple consistent breakdowns in the transfer of information needed to assure a quality transition. Study findings suggest that many elders who may benefit from home health referrals following hospital discharge do not receive them (Castro, Anderson, Hanson, & Helms, 1998). For elders who do receive them, findings suggest that essential data are often missing (Anderson & Helms, 1993; Anderson & Helms, 1995; Anderson & Helms, 1998a; Anderson & Helms, 1998b; Anderson, Helms, Black, & Myers, 2000). For example, Anderson and Helms (1998a) compared the communication exchanged between staff in hospitals with staff in extended care facilities (ECFs) and home care agencies and found that hospital referrals transferred approximately three-quarters of the recommended information to extended care facilities (ECFs) and about half of the recommended data to home health agencies. In general, such referral data pay greater attention to the patient's background and medical care needs and much less emphasis on nursing and psychosocial care needs. More information tends to be provided by larger hospitals and specialty units to proprietary rather than not-for-profit ECFs (Anderson & Helms, 1998a).

Patient and system factors that impede quality discharge planning have received limited attention. Proctor and Morrow-Howell (1990) identified factors that complicated planning for 61% of cases examined. Financial impediments followed by patient confusion and problems with patients and families were associated with delays in discharge and adequacy of plans. Additional study of the nature of systems' constraints affecting discharge planning yielded the following: insufficient time and resources, lack of information and health professionals' ageism (Bull & Kane, 1996).

Implementation

Despite evidence suggesting their potential, very few reports of interventions aimed at preventing hospitalization or nursing home placement were found. Preventive home visits to elders, age 75 and older, provided by either a nurse or physician resulted in a significant reduction in the number of hospital admissions, especially readmissions in the intervention compared with a control group (Hendricksen, Lund, & Stromgard, 1989). A treatment consisting of individual and family counseling and support groups targeted at spouse caregivers of Alzheimer disease patients resulted in less than half as many nursing home placements for the treatment group as the control group (Mittleman et al., 1993).

Newly admitted nursing home residents who received evidence-based protocols implemented by advanced practice nurses (APNs) experienced significantly greater improvement or less decline in incontinence, pressure ulcers, and aggressive behavior compared with residents receiving usual care, suggesting that such science-based protocols implemented by clinical experts may improve outcomes for elders making this difficult transition (Ryden et al., 2000).

Consultative and unit-based interventions have generally been unsuccessful in improving functional outcomes among hospitalized older adults (Fretwell et al., 1990; Reuben et al., 1992; Saltz, McVey, Becker, Feussner, & Cohen, 1988). The effects of a multimodal intervention, Acute Care for the Elders (ACE), consisting of a specially designed environment, patient-centered care, and including specific protocols for prevention of disability and rehabilitation and discharge planning have yielded mixed results. In general, ACE interventions improved the process of care and patient and provider satisfaction (Counsell et al., 2000), enhanced performance of ADLs at hospital discharge and decreased discharges to nursing homes (Landefeld, Palmer, Kresevic, Fortinsky, & Kowal, 1995) but had no effect on hospital length of stay or costs (Counsell et al., 2000; Landefeld et al., 1995).

Results of discharge planning innovations among older adults are also mixed. Compared with control patients, some studies that tested structured discharge planning interventions resulted in decreased lengths of hospital stay (Evans & Hendricks, 1993; Farren, 1991; Haddock, 1994; Kennedy, Neidlinger, & Scroggins, 1987), reduced readmissions (Evans & Hendricks, 1993; Haddock, 1991), shortened lengths of stay for readmitted patients, improved patients' preparation to manage care, and continuity in information for patients and caregivers (Bull, Hansen & Gross, 2000a), and contributed to higher levels of satisfaction (Haddock, 1994). In contrast, studies testing these or similar interventions demonstrated no significant differences in hospital length of stay (Evans & Hendricks, 1993; Riegel et al., 1996) or hospital readmission rates (Bull, Hanson, & Gross, 2000a).

A number of studies have tested a broad range of posthospital discharge interventions designed to improve patient outcomes and decrease health care costs. These ranged from high-intensity, long-term postdischarge follow-up (Rubin, Sizemore, Loftis, Adams-Suet, & Anderson, 1992; Oktay & Volland, 1990) to both low-intensity (Dellasega & Zerbe, 2000; Kravitz et al., 1994) and high-intensity, short-term follow-up (Smith et al., 1988; Weinberger, Oddone, & Henderson, 1996). Drawing conclusions from these studies is difficult, given the conflicting findings. The longer-term interventions were typically multidimensional and used a team approach to care. One intervention resulted in significant reductions in hospital days and decreased caregiver stress (Oktay & Volland, 1990) while a similar intervention tested revealed no significant differences in total acute care resource use (Rubin et al., 1992). A relatively low-intensity intervention examining the effects of APN follow-up with rural elders discharged from hospitals decreased the number of work days missed by caregivers but had no effect on readmissions and emergency department visits (Dellasega & Zerbe, 2000). Postdischarge assessment and follow-up by an APN improved identification of potentially reversible clinical problems (Kravitz et al., 1994). Patients receiving high-intensity, short-term follow-up demonstrated increased postdischarge outpatient contacts (Smith et al., 1988) and improved patient satisfaction (Weinberger et al., 1996), but either no differences in hospital readmission rates or even increased use of this costly resource (Weinberger et al., 1996).

A variety of transitional care interventions, those that cut across settings and levels of care, have been the focus of relatively few studies. A low intensity discharge planning and post-discharge follow-up intervention provided by a nurse case manager improved adherence to scheduled outpatient visits but had no effect on readmission rates or ED use. Higher intensity, nurse-centered, multidimensional interventions have demonstrated greater promise in reducing costly resource utilization. Rich and colleagues (1995) examined the effects of conventional care supplemented by a nurse-directed interdisciplinary team on the outcomes of heart failure patients. At 90 days posthospital discharge, reductions in hospital readmissions (including all-cause and heart failure related) and in the number of patients with multiple readmissions were demonstrated compared with the control group.

Building on the findings from an earlier studies testing the effects on patient and cost outcomes of a APN-directed comprehensive discharge planning protocol that demonstrated short-term reductions in hospital readmissions and charges for postdischarge health services (Naylor, 1990; Naylor et al., 1994), the effects of a comprehensive discharge planning and home follow-up protocol designed specifically for high-risk elders and implemented by APNs were examined. At 24 weeks after the index hospital discharge and compared with the control group, the intervention group had fewer total rehospitalizations and fewer patients with multiple readmissions; the intervention generated an estimated mean per patient savings of $3,000 (in Medicare reimbursements) for postdischarge health services (Naylor et al., 1999). The effects of this intervention differed between medical vs. surgical patients. Medical patients had fewer multiple readmissions and a reduced number of hospitalization days through the 24-week period while surgical patients had fewer readmissions through 6 weeks postdischarge (Naylor & McCauley, 1999).

Evaluation

The appropriateness of transitioning elders from one setting to another has received very little attention. Guided by a structured review of medical records, clinical experts assessed that 36% of the transfers of elders from a nursing home to the emergency department and 40% of transfers to the hospital were inappropriate, in that the resident could have been cared for safely at a lower level of care (Saliba et al., 2000).

More attention has been devoted to assessing the effectiveness of existing care processes once transfer has occurred. The adequacy of discharge plans in meeting elders' posthospital needs has been the subject of a few studies (Cummings, 1999; Mamon et al., 1992; Oktay & Volland, 1990; Proctor & Morrow-Howell, 1990; Proctor, Morrow-Howell, & Kaplan, 1996). While virtually all patients reported one or more care needs in the immediate postdischarge period, approximately one-third of the patients in the study samples were found to have unmet needs (Mamon et al., 1992; Oktay & Volland, 1990). Inadequate implementation in one or more components of the discharge plan for more than one-third of the patients was found to be associated with unmet needs and less than adequate care (Cummings, 1999; Proctor et al., 1996), as well as hospital readmissions (Cummings, 1999).

Patient and family member satisfaction with traditional discharge planning has consistently been linked with their degree of involvement in the decision-making process; increased involvement resulted in enhanced satisfaction (Bull, Hansen, & Gross, 2000b; Cox, 1996; Proctor, Morrow-Howell, Albaz, & Weir, 1992). In addition, patient satisfaction has been associated with their physical health status at discharge and social support networks while family members' satisfaction has been correlated with patients' discharge destination and length of hospital stay (Proctor et al., 1992). Greater family participation in discharge planning was associated with increased satisfaction with care, feelings of preparedness and perception of care continuity (Bull, Hansen, & Gross, 2000c). Family caregivers who were more involved in this process also reported better health and were more accepting of the caregiver role (Bull, Hansen, et al., 2000c). Despite variability in the nature of factors influencing patient and caregiver satisfaction, no patient-caregiver differences in overall satisfaction with the discharge planning process have been identified (Bull, Hansen, et al., 2000c).

Assisting most elders to meet their needs following hospitalization is the responsibility of family members (Weaver et al., 1998). The caregiver-patient relationship has been found to be more important than coresidence patterns or patient demands in explaining assistance from secondary caregivers (Given, Given, Stommel, & Lin, 1994). However, little is known about the effects of providing assistance over an episode of illness on caregivers' health and stress levels.

Access to needed formal health care services following hospital discharge including follow-up physician services, outpatient services, and home care has been found to be problematic, especially for select Medicare subgroups (Moy & Hogan, 1993; Pohl, Collins, & Given, 1995). Studies of the discharge destination of Medicare beneficiaries following hospitalization revealed that almost 40% leave the hospital for a place different from where they came, adding yet another major transition to an already stressed patient and family (Morrow-Howell & Proctor, 1994). Still others receive formal health care services in their homes.

Findings related to the outcomes of these diverse forms of follow-up care are limited and inconclusive (Benjamin, Fox, & Swan, 1993; Bull, 1994a; Dansky, Milliron, et al., 1996; Kane et al., 2000; Naylor et al., 1999). Patients discharged to nursing homes following hospital discharge fared worst and those sent home with home health or to a rehabilitation setting fared best (Kane et al., 2000), suggesting that better decision making regarding discharge destination may contribute to improved patient outcomes. Outcomes of placement in subacute care settings have been found to differ based on the patient's primary health problem. For example, hip fracture patients may do better in skilled nursing facilities (SNFs), while stroke patients may achieve better outcomes in rehabilitation settings (Kramer et al., 1997).

When compared with elders who had no formal home health follow-up, elders who received these services following hospital discharge were less likely to report health problems or complications (Dansky, Dellasega, Shellenbarger, & Russo, 1996) or be readmitted (Bull, 1994a). However, Naylor and colleagues (1999) found that the readmission rate within 6 months for those who received traditional home health services immediately following hospital discharge was one in two compared with one in five for those who received a discharge planning and home follow-up protocol implemented by APNs. Receipt of home health services has been associated with improvement in ADLs (Stewart, Blaha, Weissfeld, & Yuan, 1995). Satisfaction with home care services was found to be positively associated with the receipt of information about medications, equipment and supplies, and self-care (Weaver et al., 1998). Only one instrument designed to measure the multidimensional concept of continuity of elder's post-hospital care was found in this search; additional testing of its validity and reliability is needed (Bull, Luo, & Maruyama, 2000).

The potential of improved allocation of home care services in producing net long-term care cost savings has been explored. Findings suggest that overall cost neutrality or even cost savings through reducing nursing home use is feasible, but a more medically oriented service mix coupled with more efficient targeting of these services is needed to achieve this goal (Greene, Ondrich, & Laditka, 1998).

DISCUSSION

This state-of-the-science review was designed to answer a major question related to transitional care for older adults: What is known about the effectiveness of existing processes of care and innovative interventions designed to address the needs of elders and their caregivers who are making transitions across settings or from one level of care to another?

Effectiveness of Existing and Innovative Transitional Care Processes

This section of the review centered on patients' needs; those of their caregivers were not a primary focus. Consequently, work that may have strengthened understanding about the effectiveness of traditional and innovative transitional care from the important perspective of caregivers may not be included.

Numerous studies conducted with a range of methodological rigor have contributed to our understanding of older adults' needs as they make difficult care transitions. In general, a high proportion of elders and their caregivers have reported substantial unmet needs, with the need for information and increased access to health and social services consistently among the top priorities. Increased attention needs to be paid to differences in older adults' needs based on educational level, race, and ethnicity. Potential racial and ethnic disparities in access to transitional care services require further study.

Differences in expectations between patients, families, and health care providers, and the need for increased patient and family involvement in decision making, are common themes in studies examining the discharge process. Reinforcement of the importance of such involvement is its consistent linkage with patient and caregiver satisfaction. Studies of strategies to promote effective involvement are needed.

Effective communication has emerged as a critical element in quality discharge planning. Yet, gaps in communication have been identified throughout the process, contributing to unmet needs and potential errors and adverse clinical events. Future research should focus on the development and testing of referral and other information systems that are designed to promote the transfer of accurate and complete patient information across sites of care.

Despite considerable development of different forms of transitional care, evidence about their effects on patient quality and cost of care is sparse. For example, we know very little about the effectiveness of specially designed transitional care units or subacute care units. In addition, there are a number of innovations common in other countries such as day hospitals or hospitals at home that have received little attention in the United States.

A priority for future research should be continued study of strategies to prevent institutionalization of high-risk older adults. Multidimensional interventions that cut across settings and levels of care have demonstrated promise in improving transitions from hospital to home. The potential of such strategies to improve outcomes for those transitioning to and from nursing homes warrants further study.

In summary, transitional care, a relatively new area of the health care market that is likely to grow dramatically with the aging population, represents a tremendous opportunity for nurses. Nurse researchers are well positioned to lead the way in advancing through science the creation of services and environments that embrace values that are at the core of this profession—patient/caregiver-centered care, communication and collaboration, and continuity.

ACKNOWLEDGMENT

The author gratefully acknowledges the invaluable contributions provided by Lenore R. Wilkas, M.A.L.S., and Carol Lynn LaTorre, M.B.A., B.S.N. student.

REFERENCES

Aaron, H. J., & Reischauer, R. D. (1995). The Medicare reform debate: What is the next step? *Health Affairs, 14,* 8–30.

Anderson, M. A., & Helms, L. (1993). Home health care referrals following hospital discharge: Communication in health services delivery. *Hospital & Health Services Administration, 38,* 537–555.

Anderson, M. A., & Helms, L. B. (1995). Communication between continuing care organizations. *Research in Nursing & Health, 18,* 49–57.

Anderson, M. A., & Helms, L. B. (1998a). Extended care referral after hospital discharge. *Research in Nursing & Health, 21,* 385–394.

Anderson, M. A., & Helms, L. B. (1998b). Comparison of continuing care communication. *Image—The Journal of Nursing Scholarship, 30,* 255–260.

Anderson, M. A., Helms, L. B., Black, S., & Myers, D. K. (2000). A rural perspective on home care communication about elderly patients after hospital discharge. *Western Journal of Nursing Research, 22,* 225–243.

Benjamin, A. E., Fox, P. J., & Swan, J. H. (1993). The posthospital experience of elderly Medicare home health users. *Home Health Care Services Quarterly, 14,* 19–35.

Blaylock, A., & Cason, C. L. (1992). Discharge planning: Predicting patients' needs. *Journal of Gerontological Nursing, 18,* 5–10.

Bowman, G. S., Howden, J., Allen, S., Webster, R. A., & Thompson, D. R. (1994). A telephone survey of medical patients 1 week after discharge from hospital. *Journal of Clinical Nursing, 3,* 369–373.

Boyle, K., Nance, J., & Passau-Buck, S. (1992). Post-hospitalization concerns of medical-surgical patients. *Applied Nursing Research, 5,* 122–126.

Brooten, D., & Naylor, M. D. (1999). Transitional environments. In A. S. Hinshaw, S. L. Feethan, & J. L. F. Shaver (Eds.), *Handbook of clinical nursing research* (pp. 641–653). Thousand Oaks, CA: Sage.

Bubela, N., Galloway, S., McCay, E., McKibbon, A., Nagle, L., Pringle, D., Ross, E., & Shamian, J. (1990). Factors influencing patients' informational needs at time of hospital discharge. *Patient Education & Counseling, 16,* 21–28.

Bull, M. J. (1994a). Use of formal community services by elders and their family caregivers 2 weeks following hospital discharge. *Journal of Advanced Nursing, 19,* 503–508.

Bull, M. J. (1994b). Patients' and professionals' perceptions of quality in discharge planning. *Journal of Nursing Care Quality, 8,* 47–61.

Bull, M. J., Hansen, H. E., & Gross, C. R. (2000a). A professional-patient partnership model of discharge planning with elders hospitalized with heart failure. *Applied Nursing Research, 13,* 19–28.

Bull, M. J., Hansen, H. E., & Gross, C. R. (2000b). Predictors of elder and family caregiver satisfaction with discharge planning. *Journal of Cardiovascular Nursing, 14,* 76–87.

Bull, M. J., Hansen, H. E., & Gross, C. R. (2000c). Differences in family caregiver outcomes by their level of involvement in discharge planning. *Applied Nursing Research, 13,* 76–82.

Bull, M. J., & Jervis, L. L. (1997). Strategies used by chronically ill older women and their caregiving daughters in managing posthospital care. *Journal of Advanced Nursing, 25,* 541–547.

Bull, M. J., & Kane, R. L. (1996). Gaps in discharge planning. *Journal of Applied Gerontology, 15*(4), 486–500.

Bull, M. J., Luo, D., & Maruyama, G. M. (2000). Measuring continuity of elders' posthospital care. *Journal of Nursing Measurement, 8,* 41–60.

Castro, J. M., Anderson, M. A., Hanson, K. S., & Helms, L. B. (1998). Home care referral after emergency department discharge. *Journal of Emergency Nursing, 24,* 127–132.

Congdon, J. G. (1994). Managing the incongruities: The hospital discharge experience for elderly patients, their families, and nurses. *Applied Nursing Research, 7,* 125–131.

Coulton, C. J., Dunkle, R. E., Chow, J. C., Haug, M., & Vielhaber, D. P. (1988). Dimensions of post-hospital care decision-making: A factor analytic study. *Gerontologist, 28,* 218–223.

Coulton, C. J., Dunkle, R. E., Haug, M., Chow, J., & Vielhaber, D. P. (1989). Locus of control and decision making for posthospital care. *Gerontologist, 29,* 627–632.

Counsell, S. R., Holder, C. M., Liebenauer, L. L., Palmer, R. M., Fortinsky, R. H., Kresevic, D. M., Quinn, L. M., Allen, K. R., Covinsky, K. E., & Landefeld, C. S. (2000). Effects of a multicomponent intervention on functional outcomes and process of care in hospitalized older patients: A randomized controlled trial of acute care for elders (ACE) in a community hospital. *Journal of the American Geriatrics Society, 48,* 1572–1581.

Cox, C. B. (1996). Discharge planning for dementia patients: Factors influencing caregiver decisions and satisfaction. *Health & Social Work, 21,* 97–104.

Cummings, S. M. (1999). Adequacy of discharge plans and rehospitalization among hospitalized dementia patients. *Health & Social Work, 24,* 249–259.

Dansky, K. H., Dellasega, C., Shellenbarger, T., & Russo, P. C. (1996). After hospitalization: Home health care for elderly persons. *Clinical Nursing Research, 5,* 185–198.

Dansky, K. H., Milliron, M., & Gamm, L. (1996). Understanding hospital referrals to home health agencies. *Hospital & Health Services Administration, 41,* 331–342.

Deimling, G. T., & Poulshock, S. W. (1985). The transition from family in-home care to institutional care. Focus on health and attitudinal issues as predisposing factors. *Research on Aging, 7,* 563–576.

Dellasega, C., & Mastrian, K. (1995). The process and consequences of institutionalizing an elder. *Western Journal of Nursing Research, 17,* 123–140.

Dellasega, C., & Nolan, M. (1997). Admission to care: Facilitating role transition amongst family carers. *Journal of Clinical Nursing, 6,* 443–451.

Dellasega, C. A., & Zerbe, T. M. (2000). A multimethod study of advanced practice nurse postdischarge care. *Clinical Excellence for Nurse Practitioners, 4,* 286–293.

Evans, R. L., & Hendricks, R. D. (1993). Evaluating hospital discharge planning: A randomized clinical trial. *Medical Care, 31,* 358–370.

Farren, E. A. (1991). Effects of early discharge planning on length of hospital stay. *Nursing Economics, 9*(1), 25–30, 63.

Feather, J. (1993). Factors in perceived hospital discharge planning effectiveness. *Social Work in Health Care, 19,* 1–14.

Fethke, C. C., & Smith, I. M. (1991). The critical post-discharge period for older patients leaving a hospital. *Journal of Gerontological Social Work, 16*(3/4), 93–105.

Fink, S. V., & Picot, S. F. (1995). Nursing home placement decisions and post-placement experiences of African-American and European-American caregivers. *Journal of Gerontological Nursing, 21,* 35–42.

Fletcher, R. H., O'Malley, M. S., Fletcher, S. W., Earp, J. A., & Alexander, J. P. (1984). Measuring the continuity and coordination of medical care in a system involving multiple providers. *Medical Care, 22,* 403–411.

Forbes, S., & Hoffart, N. (1998). Elders' decision making regarding the use of long-term care services: A precarious balance. *Qualitative Health Research, 8,* 736–750.

Fretwell, M. D., Raymond, P. M., McGarvey, S. T., Owens, N., Traines, M., Silliman, R. A., & Mor, V. (1990). The Senior Care Study. A controlled trial of a consultative/unit-based geriatric assessment program in acute care. *Journal of the American Geriatrics Society, 38,* 1073–1081.

Given, B. A., Given, C. W., Stommel, M., & Lin, C. S. (1994). Predictors of use of secondary carers used by the elderly following hospital discharge. *Journal of Aging & Health, 6,* 353–376.

Greene, V. L., Ondrich, J., & Laditka, S. (1998). Can home care services achieve cost savings in long-term care for older people? *Journals of Gerontology Series B-Psychological Sciences & Social Sciences, 53B,* S228–S238.

Gustafson, D. H., Arora, N. K., Nelson, E. C., & Boberg, E. W. (2001). Increasing understanding of patient needs during and after hospitalization. *Joint Commission Journal on Quality Improvement, 27,* 81–92.

Haddock, K. S. (1991). Characteristics of effective discharge planning programs for the frail elderly. *Journal of Gerontological Nursing, 17,* 10–14.

Haddock, K. S. (1994). Collaborative discharge planning: Nursing and social services. *Clinical Nurse Specialist, 8,* 248–252.

Hansen, H. E., Bull, M. J., & Gross, C. R. (1998). Interdisciplinary collaboration and discharge planning communication for elders. *Journal of Nursing Administration, 28,* 37–46.

Health Care Financing Administration. (1999). *1999 HCFA statistics.* Baltimore, MD: Author.

Hendriksen, C., Lund, E., & Stromgard, E. (1989). Hospitalization of elderly people: A 3-year controlled trial. *Journal of the American Geriatrics Society, 37,* 117–122.

Hughes, L. C., Hodgson, N. A., Muller, P., Robinson, L. A., & McCorkle, R. (2000). Information needs of elderly postsurgical cancer patients during the transition from hospital to home. *Journal of Nursing Scholarship, 32,* 25–30.

Jacobs, V. (2000). Informational needs of surgical patients following discharge. *Applied Nursing Research, 13,* 12–18.

Jewell, S. (1996). Nuffield Research Award. Elderly patients' participation in discharge decision making: 1. *British Journal of Nursing, 5,* 914–916.

Jewell, S. E. (1993). Discovery of the discharge process: A study of patient discharge from a care unit for elderly people. *Journal of Advanced Nursing, 18,* 1288–1296.

Jones, E. W., Densen, P. M., & Brown, S. D. (1989). Posthospital needs of elderly people at home: Findings from an eight-month follow-up study. *Health Services Research, 24,* 645–664.

Kadushin, G., & Kulys, R. (1994). Patient and family involvement in discharge planning. *Journal of Gerontological Social Work, 22*(3/4), 171–199.

Kane, R. L., Finch, M., Blewett, L., Chen, Q., Burns, R., & Moskowitz, M. (1996). Use of post-hospital care by Medicare patients. *Journal of the American Geriatrics Society, 44,* 242–250.

Kane, R. L., Chen, Q., Finch, M., Blewett, L., Burns, R., & Moskowitz, M. (2000). The optimal outcomes of post-hospital care under medicare. *Health Services Research, 35,* 615–661.

Kennedy, L., Neidlinger, S., & Scroggins, K. (1987). Effective comprehensive discharge planning for hospitalized elderly. *Gerontologist, 27,* 577–580.

Kenney, G. M. (1993). How access to long-term care affects home health transfers. *Journal of Health Politics, Policy & Law, 18,* 937–965.

Kramer, A. M., Steiner, J. F., Schlenker, R. E., Eilertsen, T. B., Hrincevich, C. A., Tropea, D. A., Ahmad, L. A., & Eckhoff, D. G. (1997). Outcomes and costs after hip fracture and stroke: A comparison of rehabilitation settings. *JAMA, 277,* 396–404.

Kravitz, R. L., Reuben, D. B., Davis, J. W., Mitchell, A., Hemmerling, K., Kington, R. S., & Siu, A. L. (1994). Geriatric home assessment after hospital discharge. *Journal of the American Geriatrics Society, 42,* 1229–1234.

Landefeld, C. S., Palmer, R. M., Kresevic, D. M., Fortinsky, R. H., & Kowal, J. (1995). A randomized trial of care in a hospital medical unit especially designed to improve the functional outcomes of acutely ill older patients. *New England Journal of Medicine, 332,* 1338–1344.

Lough, M. A. (1996). Ongoing work of older adults at home after hospitalization. *Journal of Advanced Nursing, 23,* 804–809.

Magilvy, J. K., & Congdon, J. G. (2000). The crisis nature of health care transitions for rural older adults. *Public Health Nursing, 17,* 336–345.

Mamon, J., Steinwachs, D. M., Fahey, M., Bone, L. R., Oktay, J., & Klein, L. (1992). Impact of hospital discharge planning on meeting patient needs after returning home. *Health Services Research, 27,* 155–175.

Mistiaen, P., Duijnhouwer, E., Wijkel, D., de Bont, M., & Veeger, A. (1997). The problems of elderly people at home one week after discharge from an acute care setting. *Journal of Advanced Nursing, 25,* 1233–1240.

Mittelman, M. S., Ferris, S. H., Steinberg, G., Shulman, E., Mackell, J. A., Ambinder, A., & Cohen, J. (1993). An intervention that delays institutionalization of Alzheimer's disease patients: Treatment of spouse-caregivers. *Gerontologist, 33,* 730–740.

Moon, M., & Davis, K. (1995). Preserving and strengthening Medicare. *Health Affairs, 14,* 31–46.

Morrow-Howell, N., & Proctor, E. (1994). Discharge destinations of Medicare patients receiving discharge planning: Who goes where? *Medical Care, 32,* 486–497.

Moy, E., & Hogan, C. (1993). Access to needed follow-up services. Variations among different Medicare populations. *Archives of Internal Medicine, 153,* 1815–1823.

Narsavage, G. L., & Naylor, M. D. (2000). Factors associated with referral of elderly individuals with cardiac and pulmonary disorders for home care services following hospital discharge. *Journal of Gerontological Nursing, 26,* 14–20.

National Center for Health Statistics. (1999). *Health, United States, 1999 with health and aging chartbook.* Hyattsville, MD: Author.

Naughton, B. J., Saltzman, S., Priore, R., Reedy, K., & Mylotte, J. M. (1999). Using admission characteristics to predict return to the community from a post-acute geriatric evaluation and management unit. *Journal of the American Geriatrics Society, 47,* 1100–1104.

Naylor, M., Brooten, D., Jones, R., Lavizzo-Mourey, R., Mezey, M., & Pauly, M. (1994). Comprehensive discharge planning for the hospitalized elderly. A randomized clinical trial. *Annals of Internal Medicine, 120,* 999–1006.

Naylor, M. D. (1990). Comprehensive discharge planning for hospitalized elderly: A pilot study. *Nursing Research, 39,* 156–161.

Naylor, M. D., Brooten, D., Campbell, R., Jacobsen, B. S., Mezey, M. D., Pauly, M. V., & Schwartz, J. S. (1999). Comprehensive discharge planning and home follow-up of hospitalized elders: A randomized clinical trial. *Journal of the American Medical Association, 281,* 613–620.

Naylor, M. D., & McCauley, K. M. (1999). The effects of a discharge planning and home follow-up intervention on elders hospitalized with common medical and surgical cardiac conditions. *Journal of Cardiovascular Nursing, 14,* 44–54.

Naylor, M. D., Bowles, K. H., & Brooten, D. (2000). Patient problems and advanced practice nurse interventions during transitional care. *Public Health Nursing, 17,* 94–102.

Oktay, J. S., & Volland, P. J. (1990). Post-hospital support program for the frail elderly and their caregivers: A quasi-experimental evaluation. *American Journal of Public Health, 80,* 39–46.

Penrod, J., & Dellasega, C. (1998). Caregivers' experiences in making placement decisions. *Western Journal of Nursing Research, 20,* 706–732.

Pohl, J. M., Collins, C., & Given, C. W. (1995). Beyond patient dependency: Family characteristics and access of elderly patients to home care services following hospital discharge. *Home Health Care Services Quarterly, 15,* 33–47.

Proctor, E., Morrow-Howell, N., Albaz, R., & Weir, C. (1992). Patient and family satisfaction with discharge plans. *Medical Care, 30,* 262–275.

Proctor, E. K., & Morrow-Howell, N. (1990). Complications in discharge planning with Medicare patients. *Health & Social Work, 15,* 45–54.

Proctor, E. K., Morrow-Howell, N., & Kaplan, S. J. (1996). Implementation of discharge plans for chronically ill elders discharged home. *Health & Social Work, 21,* 30–40.

Reiley, P., Iezzoni, L. I., Phillips, R., Davis, R. B., Tuchin, L. I., & Calkins, D. (1996). Discharge planning: Comparison of patients' and nurses' perceptions of patients following hospital discharge. *Image—the Journal of Nursing Scholarship, 28,* 143–147.

Reuben, D. B., Wolde-Tsadik, G., Pardamean, B., Hammond, B., Borok, G. M., Rubenstein, L. Z., & Beck, J. C. (1992). The use of targeting criteria in hospitalized HMO patients: Results from the demonstration phase of the Hospitalized Older Persons Evaluation (HOPE) Study. *Journal of the American Geriatrics Society, 40,* 482–488.

Rich, M. W., Beckham, V., Wittenberg, C., Leven, C. L., Freedland, K. E., & Carney, R. M. (1995). A multidisciplinary intervention to prevent the readmission of elderly patients with congestive heart failure. *New England Journal of Medicine, 333,* 1190–1195.

Riegel, B., Gates, D. M., Gocka, I., Medina, L., Odell, C., Rich, M., & Finken, J. S. (1996). Effectiveness of a program of early hospital discharge of cardiac surgery patients. *Journal of Cardiovascular Nursing, 11,* 63–75.

Rodgers, B. L. (1997). Family members' experiences with the nursing home placement of an older adult. *Applied Nursing Research, 10,* 57–63.

Rose, J. H., Bowman, K. F., & Kresevic, D. (2000). Nurse versus family caregiver perspectives on hospitalized older patients: An exploratory study of agreement at admission and discharge. *Health Communication, 12,* 63–80.

Ruane, T., & Brody, H. (1987). Understanding and teaching continuity of care. *Journal of Medical Education, 62,* 969–974.

Rubin, C. D., Sizemore, M. T., Loftis, P. A., Adams-Huet, B., & Anderson, R. J. (1992). The effect of geriatric evaluation and management on Medicare reimbursement in a large public hospital: A randomized clinical trial. *Journal of the American Geriatrics Society, 40,* 989–995.

Ryden, M. B., Snyder, M., Gross, C. R., Savik, K., Pearson, V., Krichbaum, K., & Mueller, C. (2000). Value-added outcomes: The use of advanced practice nurses in long-term care facilities. *Gerontologist, 40,* 654–662.

Saliba, D., Kington, R., Buchanan, J., Bell, R., Wang, M., Lee, M., Herbst, M., Lee, D., Sur, D., & Rubenstein, L. (2000). Appropriateness of the decision to transfer nursing facility residents to the hospital. *Journal of the American Geriatrics Society, 48,* 154–163.

Saltz, C. C., McVey, L. J., Becker, P. M., Feussner, J. R., & Cohen, H. J. (1988). Impact of a geriatric consultation team on discharge placement and repeat hospitalization. *Gerontologist, 28,* 344–350.

Satish, S., Winograd, C. H., Chavez, C., & Bloch, D. A. (1996). Geriatric targeting criteria as predictors of survival and health care utilization. *Journal of the American Geriatrics Society, 44,* 914–921.

Shaughnessy, P. W., & Kramer, A. M. (1990). The increased needs of patients in nursing homes and patients receiving home health care. *New England Journal of Medicine, 322,* 21–27.

Smith, D. M., Weinberger, M., Katz, B. P., & Moore, P. S. (1988). Postdischarge care and readmissions. *Medical Care, 26,* 699–708.

Stewart, C. J., Blaha, A. J., Weissfeld, L., & Yuan, W. (1995). Discharge planning from home health care and patient status post-discharge. *Public Health Nursing, 12,* 90–98.

Tappen, R. M., Muzic, J., & Kennedy, P. (2001). Elder care. Preoperative assessment and discharge planning for older adults undergoing ambulatory surgery. *AORN Journal, 73,* 464.

Tierney, A. J., Closs, S. J., Hunter, H. C., & Macmillan, M. S. (1993). Experiences of elderly patients concerning discharge from hospital. *Journal of Clinical Nursing, 2,* 179–185.

Weaver, F. M., Perloff, L., & Waters, T. (1998). Patients' and caregivers' transition from hospital to home: Needs and recommendations. *Home Health Care Services Quarterly, 17*(3), 27–48.

Weinberger, M., Oddone, E. Z., & Henderson, W. G. (1996). Does increased access to primary care reduce hospital readmissions? Veterans Affairs Cooperative Study Group on Primary Care and Hospital Readmission. *New England Journal of Medicine, 334,* 1441–1447.

Wilson, S. A. (1997). The transition to nursing home life: A comparison of planned and unplanned admissions. *Journal of Advanced Nursing, 26,* 864–871.

Wolock, I., Schlesinger, E., Dinerman, M., & Seaton, R. (1987). The posthospital needs and care of patients: Implications for discharge planning. *Social Work in Health Care, 12,* 61–76.

Chapter 6

Interventions for Family Members Caring for an Elder with Dementia

GAYLE J. ACTON AND MARY A. WINTER

ABSTRACT

This chapter reviews 73 published and unpublished research reports of interventions for family members caring for an elder with dementia by nurse researchers and researchers from other disciplines. Reports were identified through searches of MEDLINE, CINAHL, Social Science Index, PsycINFO, ERIC, Social Work Abstracts, American Association of Retired Persons database, CRISP index of the National Institutes of Health, Cochrane Center database, and Dissertation Abstracts using the following search terms: *caregiver, caregiving, dementia, Alzheimer's, intervention study, evaluation study, experimental,* and *quasi-experimental design.* Additional keywords were used to narrow or expand the search as necessary. All nursing research was included in the review and nonnursing research was included if published between 1991 and 2001. Studies were included if they used a design that included a treatment and control group or a one-group, pretest-posttest design (ex post facto designs were included if they used a comparison group). Key findings show that approximately 32% of the study outcomes (e.g., burden, depression, knowledge) were changed after intervention in the desired direction. In addition, several problematic issues were identified including small, diverse samples; lack of intervention specificity; diversity in the length, duration, and intensity of the intervention strategies; and problematic outcome measures.

Keywords: caregiver, dementia, cognitive impairment, Alzheimer's disease, intervention

The number of persons with chronic cognitive impairment is increasing because, as persons age, the incidence of dementia of the Alzheimer's type increases dramatically. A thorough discussion of Alzheimer's disease and its consequences can be found in chapter 2 in this volume by Burgener. Because of the long tenure of the disease, 2 to 20 years with an average of 8 years, the burden of caring for a loved one with dementia may become overwhelming, and family caregivers often express hopelessness and helplessness about their situations (Schulz & Beach, 1999; Schulz, O'Brien, Bookwala, & Fleissner, 1995). Researchers have been testing interventions to alleviate caregiver stress and burden since the late 1970s. This chapter will review nursing research (1988–2001) and research from other disciplines (1991–2001) testing interventions for family caregivers. Two questions are addressed in the review.

1. What family caregiver interventions have been tested, and what features are important for nurses to consider?
2. What are the important issues for researchers to address concerning caregiver intervention research?

METHOD

Search Strategy

An extensive and comprehensive search of the literature was undertaken to locate published and unpublished research related to intervention strategies designed to affect the consequences of caregiving. A computerized search of MEDLINE, CINAHL, Social Science Index, PsycINFO, ERIC, Social Work Abstracts, American Association of Retired Persons database, and Dissertation Abstracts was conducted. Keywords *caregiver, caregiving, dementia, Alzheimer's, intervention study, evaluation study,* and *experimental/quasi-experimental design* were used to initiate the searches. Additional keywords were used to narrow or expand the search as necessary. The CRISP index of the National Institutes of Health, Grants and Contracts Web site, was searched to obtain the abstracts of currently funded caregiving research. Manual searches of indexes of journals such as *The Journal of Gerontology, The Gerontologist,* and *Research in Aging* were completed to increase the likelihood of retrieving studies. After potential studies were located, the reference list of each article was examined to identify other research that might be included. To identify unpublished studies, dissertation abstracts, the Cochrane Center (a meta-analytic clearinghouse), and published abstracts from learned societies (e.g., Gerontological Society of America) were searched for researchers conducting caregiver intervention research. Researchers were contacted via e-mail, phone, or U.S. mail to inquire if they had any unpublished findings.

The following inclusion criteria were used to select studies: (a) a sample of family caregivers of adults with dementia; (b) a sample of care receivers who had cognitive impairment (studies were included if the researchers mentioned that the care receivers had cognitive impairment but failed to specify the percentage that were impaired; however, some studies included care receivers with and without dementia. Table 6.1 indicates if the researchers specified that less than 50% of the care receivers had dementia); (c) an education, support and education, counseling, respite, case management, or multicomponent intervention designed to lessen the negative impact of caregiving or improve the positive aspects of caregiving; and (d) a design that included a treatment and control group or a one-group, pretest-posttest design (ex post facto designs were included if they used a comparison group). Studies were excluded if they did not mention that caregivers were caring for family members with dementia. There were no age limits imposed on the sample selection.

Seventy-three studies are included in this review and there are approximately 34 pre-1991 studies not in this review (the list is available from the authors). Outcomes reviewed include dysphoric variables (e.g., burden, stress, anxiety), positive psychosocial variables (e.g., coping, life satisfaction, morale), perceived physical health, and rate of institutionalization. There may be other outcomes not included in this review (e.g., cost, physiologic responses). The reader is also referred to other meta-analyses of caregiver interventions (Acton & Kang, 2001; Bourgeois, Schultz, & Burgio, 1996; Knight, Lutzky, & Macofsky-Urban, 1993; Toseland & Rossiter, 1989).

RESULTS

What Family Caregiver Interventions Have Been Tested and What Features Are Important for Nurses to Consider?

The studies were grouped by intervention type (education, support and education, counseling, respite, case management, and multicomponent) and then examined for design, sample, intervention, and significant find-

TABLE 6.1   Interventions for Family Caregivers of Persons with Dementia

Study	Design/sample	Description of intervention	Significant findings
Intervention: Education			
Barusch & Spaid (1991)	Quasi-experimental T:95 (70 grp, 25 home; 59 individual, 36 family)	Didactic/relaxation training by professional 2 hr/wk × 6 wks.	Coping: Grp ↑, Ind ↑; Obj burden: Grp ↓, Ind ↓, Family ↓
Belmin, Hee, & Ollivet (1999)	Pre/posttest T:18; No ctrl grp	Practical info about dementia by professional/peer 3 hrs/wk × 3 wks.	↓ Burden
Bourgeois, Burgio, Schulz, Beach, & Palmer (1997)	Pre/posttest T:7; No ctrl grp	Individualized home session 60 mins × 11 + 3 hr workshop.	↑ Self-efficacy
Brodaty, Roberts, & Peters (1994)	Quasi-experimental T:28; C:23	Didactic session + group discussion by professional/peer leader 18 hrs over 4 mos.	↑ Knowledge
Buckwalter ♦, Gerdner, Kohout, Hall, Kelly, Richards, & Sime (1999)	Experimental T:95; C:80	Home visits + phone calls by nurses × 6 mos.	Depression, Tension, Anger: T < C
Burgener ♦, Bakas, Murray, Dunahee, & Tossey (1998)	Experimental T:11; T:12* T: 2*; C:12	Home didactic/behavioral session by professional for 90 mins × 1.	↑ Knowledge

TABLE 6.1 *(continued)*

	Intervention: Education		
Study	Design/sample	Description of intervention	Significant findings
Butt ♦ (1989)	Quasi-experimental T:2; C:2	Information session 2 hr/wk × 7 wks.	
Chang ♦ (1999)	Experimental T:34; C:31	Videos providing behavioral modeling viewed in-home + phone calls × 8 wks.	Depression: T<C; ↓ Emotion-focused coping
Chiverton ♦ & Caine (1989)	Quasi-experimental T:20; C:20	Didactic/group discussion session by nurse 2 hr × 3 mos.	↑ Knowledge
Coen, O'Boyle, Coakley, & Lawlor (1999)	Pre/posttest T:28; No ctrl grp	2 hr/wk × 8 wks by professional.	↑ Knowledge; ↑ Burden; ↓ Support
Corbeil, Quayhagen, & Quayhagen (1999)	Experimental T:28; C:31	Active cognitive stimulation training 1×/wk × 12 wks.	
Davis ♦ (1998)	Pre/posttest T:17; No ctrl grp	2 hr home problem-solving training × 1 + weekly phone calls by nurses × 12 wks.	↓ Depression; ↑ Life satisfaction
Gendron, Poitras, Dastoor, & Perodeau (1996)	Pre/posttest T:17; No ctrl grp	Coping skills training/discussion by professional 1 1/2 hrs/wk × 8 wks.	

(continued)

TABLE 6.1   *(continued)*

	Intervention: Education		
Study	Design/sample	Description of intervention	Significant findings
Heacock ♦ (Unpub)	Pre/posttest T:20; No ctrl grp	Skills training session: one day grp session + 2 individual sessions + 2 phone calls/11 wks.	
Magni, Zanetti, Bianchetti, Binetti, & Trabucchi (1995)	Pre/posttest T:22; No ctrl grp	Didactic session by professional 2 hr/wk × 8 wks.	↓ Stress; ↑ Knowledge
McCallion, Toseland, & Freeman (1999)	Experimental T:32; C:34	Individual/grp communication training 1 1/2 hrs × 4 + 1 hr × 3–8 wks.	
McCurry, Logsdon, Vitiello, & Teri (1998)	Experimental T:21; C:15	Group didactic sleep problems + grp pt care ed × 6 wks followed by individual ed × 4 wks.	Sleep quality: T>C
Quayhagen ♦ & Quayhagen (1989)	Quasi-experimental T:10; C:6	Cognitive stimulation program + monthly contact for 8 mos studied.	Depression, Burden, Negative affect: T<C
Ripich, Kercher, Wykle, Sloan, & Ziol (1998)	Pre/posttest T:8; T:20; No ctrl grp	Communication skills training by speech-language pathologist 2 hr/wk × 4.	

TABLE 6.1 *(continued)*

	Intervention: Education		
Study	Design/sample	Description of intervention	Significant findings
Ripich, Ziol, & Lee (1998)	Quasi-experimental T:19; C:18	Communication skills training by speech-language pathologist 2 hr/wk × 4.	Knowledge: T > C; Comm hassles: T < C
Robinson ♦ (1988)	Quasi-experimental T:11; C:9	Social skills training by nurse 2 hr × 4 during 8 wks studied.	↓ Sub burden; ↓ Burden
Robinson ♦ & Yates (1994)	Experimental T:6; C:12	Social skills + behavioral management training 1 1/2 hr × 6/12 wks.	Obj burden: T < C
Zanetti, Metitieri, Bianchetti, & Trabucchi (1998)	Quasi-experimental T:12; C:9	Didactic session 1 hr/wk × 6 wks.	↓ Stress; Knowledge: T > C

	Intervention: Support group and education		
Acton ♦ & Miller (1996)	Pre/posttest T:26; No ctrl grp	Individualized session for each group by nurse 1 hr bi-weekly × 1 yr.	
Brennan ♦, Moore, & Smyth (1995)	Experimental T:47; C:49	Home-installed computer.	Decision confidence, T > C

(continued)

TABLE 6.1 *(continued)*

	Intervention: Support group and education		
Study	Design/sample	Description of intervention	Significant findings
Cummings, Long, Peterson-Hazan, & Harrison (1998)	Pre/posttest T:13; No ctrl grp	90 mins/wk × 8 wks by professional. Concurrent pt sessions, some joint.	↓ Strain; ↑ Coping; ↑ Readiness; ↑ Competence
Demers & Lavoie (1996)	Quasi-experimental § T:73; C:80	Discussion/ learning session 2 1/2 hrs/ wk × 10 wks.	Depression, Burden: T > C
Farran ♦ & Keane-Hagarty (1994)	Quasi-experimental T:29; C:35	Didactic/support session by professional 2 hr/ wk × 8 wks.	↑ Burden; ↑ Distress
Gage & Kinney (1995)	Ex post facto T:103; C:102	No description given	Depression, Negative affect: T > C
Gendron, Poitras, Dastoor, & Perodeau (1996)	Pre/posttest T:18; No ctrl grp	Didactic/ discussion by professional 1 1/2 hrs/wk × 8 wks.	
Hebert, Leclerc, Bravo, Girouard, & Lefrancois (1994)	Experimental T:23; C:18	Education/support/ relaxation training by nurse 3 hrs/wk × 8 wks.	↑ Knowledge
Hosaka & Sugiyama (1999)	Pre/posttest T:20; No ctrl grp	Psycho-education/ discussion/ relaxation training 1 1/2 hrs/ wk × 5 wks.	↓ Depression; ↓ Anger

TABLE 6.1 *(continued)*

Intervention: Support group and education			
Study	Design/sample	Description of intervention	Significant findings
Ostwald ♦, Hepburn, Caron, Burns, & Mantell (1999)	Experimental T:53; C:31	Education/family support session by professional 2 hr/wk × 7 wks.	Burden, Stress: T < C
Schultz, Schultz, & Smyrnios (1994)	Quasi-experimental § T:268; C:22	Group session by professional/ peer 2 1/2 hrs/ wk × 6 wks + 2 1/2 hrs/mo × 3 mos.	State anxiety, Well-being: T < C
Strawn, Hester, & Brown (1998)	Pre/posttest T:14; No ctrl grp	Phone calls. M = 8.8 in 12 wks by graduate student in clinical psychology.	↓ Burden; ↓ Stress
Teri, Logsdon, Uomoto, & McCurry (1997)	Experimental T:19; C:20	Problem-solving/ education/ advice & support by geriatrician 1 hr/wk × 9 wks.	Depression: T < C
Toseland, Labrecque, Goebel, & Whitney (1992)	Quasi-experimental § T:42; C:47	Support/education/ discussion/ problem solving/stress reduction 2 hr/ wk × 8 wks.	Coping, Knowledge: T > C Burden: T < C
Intervention: Counseling			
Gallagher-Thompson & Steffen (1994)	Pre/posttest T:21; T:30	Therapy session 2×/wk × 4 wks + 1×/wk × 12–16 wks.	

(continued)

TABLE 6.1   *(continued)*

Intervention: Counseling			
Study	Design/sample	Description of intervention	Significant findings
Larsen ♦ (1998)	Pre/posttest T:5; no ctrl grp	Individualized counseling 1 1/2 hrs/wk × 8 wks.	
Perkins & Poyn-ton ♦ (1990)	Experimental T:6; C:6	Problem-solving session by pro-fessional nurse 1 1/4 hrs/wk × 10 wks.	Knowledge, Morale: T > C
Roberts ♦, Browne, Milne, Spooner, Gafni, Drum-mond-Young, LeGris, Watt, LeClair, Beaumont, & Roberts (1999)	Experimental T:38; C:39	Problem-solving therapy. Home visits (M = 8) + 40 total phone calls/6 mos.	
Intervention: Respite			
Adler, Ott, Jelin-ski, Morti-mer, & Christensen (1993)	Pre/posttest T:25, no ctrl grp	One-time admis-sion to geriat-ric ward for 2 wks: nursing and medical staff.	
Adler, Kuskow-ski, & Morti-mer (1995)	Ex post facto T:23; C:35	Admission to memory loss clinic for max of 4 wks dur-ing the yr stud-ied.	Burden: T > C

TABLE 6.1 *(continued)*

	Intervention: Respite		
Study	Design/sample	Description of intervention	Significant findings
Conlin ♦, Caranasos, & Davidson (1992)	Quasi-experimental T:7; C:8	Home care/institutional stay. M = 15.3 hrs/wk × 10 wks.	Stress: T < C
Deimling (1991)	Pre/posttest T:78; No ctrl grp	Min 4 mo total home/institutional stay during 2 yrs studied.	
Graham ♦ (1989)	Pre/posttest T:15	Stay in day care 2–5 days/wk × 3 wks.	
Guttman (1991)	Quasi-experimental T:63; C:55	Stay in day care 2–5 days/wk × 6 mos.	Stress: T < C
Homer & Gilleard (1994)	Pre/posttest § T:54; No ctrl grp	Hospital stay.	↓ Depression
Johnson ♦ & Maguire (1989)	Pre/posttest T:32: No ctrl grp	Stay in day care center 8 hrs/wk × 4 mos.	↓ Anxiety
Larkin & Hopcroft (1993)	Pre/posttest T:22; No ctrl grp	Hospital stay of 2 wks.	↓ Depression; ↓ Anxiety; ↓ Distress; ↓ Hostility
Rothman, Diehr, Hedrick, Erdly, & Nickinovich (1993)	Pre/posttest T:148; No ctrl grp	Day care in medical center facility during 1 yr studied.	
Rothman, Hedrick, Bulcroft, Erdly, & Nickinovich (1993)	Pre/posttest T:264; No ctrl grp	Day care in government-sponsored facility during 1 yr studied.	

(continued)

TABLE 6.1   *(continued)*

Intervention: Respite			
Study	Design/sample	Description of intervention	Significant findings
Skelly, McA-doo, & Osterg-ard (1993)	Ex post facto § T:16; C:14	Hospital stay coor-dinated by nurse during 2 yrs preceding the study.	
Strang ♦ & Neu-feld (1990)	Pre/posttest § T:10; No ctrl grp	Day care by pro-fessionals 5 1/2 hrs/day × 2 days/wk × 3 mos.	
Theis ♦, Moss, & Pearson (1994)	Pre/posttest § T:18; No ctrl grp	Referral/home re-spite/institu-tional respite managed by nurses; care provided by volunteers. Respite max: 4 hr home/wk or 14 days institu-tional during the yr studied.	
Wimo, Mattsson, Adolfsson, Er-iksson, & Nel-vig (1993)	Quasi-experimental T:55; C:44	Stay in day care during 1 yr studied.	Institutionalization: T<C
Zarit, Stephens, Townsend, & Greene (1998)	Quasi-experimental T:73; C:120	Stay in day care during 1 yr studied.	Depression, Role overload, Strain, Anger: T < C

TABLE 6.1 *(continued)*

Intervention: Case management			
Study	Design/sample	Description of intervention	Significant findings
Miller, New-comer, & Fox (1999)	Experimental T:4151; C:3944	Planning/ coordination/ monitoring by case mgr. Individual education by case mgr + group ed and support × 3 yrs.	
Newcomer, Yordi, DuNah, Fox, & Wilkinson (1999)	Experimental T:2728; C:2576	Planning/ coordination/ monitoring by case mgr. Individual education by case mgr + group support × 4 yrs.	
Pynoos & Ohta (1991)	Pre/posttest; T:12; No ctrl grp	Home visit by multidisciplinary team.	
Schwarz ♦ & Blixen (1997)	Quasi-experimental T:49; C:51	Care by home care professional/ aid M = 55.3 visits during 3 mos studied.	
Silverman, Musa, Martin, Lave, Adams, & Ricci (1995)	Quasi-experimental § T:42; C:26	Assessment/ planning/referral by professionals during 12 mos studied.	Strain, Burden: T < C

(continued)

TABLE 6.1 *(continued)*

Study	Design/sample	Description of intervention	Significant findings
Intervention: Case management			
Weinberger, Gold, Divine, Cowper, Hodgson, Schreiner, & George (1993)	Experimental T:166; C:61	Planning/referral of needed services by social worker in 1 visit + 1 phone call/7 days.	Outpatient doctor visits: T > C
Intervention: Multicomponent			
Archbold ♦, Stewart, Miller, Harvath, Greenlick, Van Buren, Kirschling, Valanis, Brody, Schook, & Hagan (1995)	Quasi-experimental T:11; C:11	Case mgt, phone advice and keep-in-touch system by nurse for 3–6 mos.	Care effectiveness: T > C
Drummond, Mohide, Tew, Streiner, Pringle, & Gilbert (1991)	Experimental T:22; C:20	Home visits × 6 mo., referral, consultation, and education. Home respite 4 hr wkly + support group meeting 2 hr monthly.	
Grunow ♦ (1991)	Quasi-experimental T:25; C:58	Home visit or phone call 1/ wk × 8 wks: support/education/referral.	↓ Burden; ↓ Distress; ↓ Negative coping

TABLE 6.1 *(continued)*

		Intervention: Multicomponent	
Study	Design/sample	Description of intervention	Significant findings
Harper, Manasse, James, & Newton (1993)	Pre/posttest T:45; No ctrl grp	Home care aid service + monthly cger mtgs × 3 mos.	↓ Psychological distress
Lo Giudice, Waltrowicz, Brown, Burrows, Ames, & Flicker (1999)	Experimental T:23, C:23	Advice/ counseling/ education, discharge planning by professional ×2	Psychosocial quality of life, T > C
Millan-Calenti, Gandoy-Crego, Antelo-Martelo, Lopez-Martinez, Riveiro-Lopez, & Mayan-Santos (2000)	Pre/posttest T:14; No ctrl grp	Home visits by volunteers for support/respite + home visit by professional every 2 wks for education, environmental safety, & grp psychotherapy during 1 yr.	↓ Anxiety state
Mittelman, Ferris, Shulman, Steinberg, Mackell, & Ambinder (1994)	Experimental T:39; C:42	Individual counseling × 2 + family education × 4 by counselor in 4 mos followed by support grp meeting 1/wk.	↑ Satisfaction with support; Institutionalization T<C

(continued)

TABLE 6.1 *(continued)*

	Intervention: Multicomponent		
Study	Design/sample	Description of intervention	Significant findings
Moniz-Cook, Agar, Gibson, Win, & Wang (1998)	Quasi-experimental T:5; C:4	Home-based info/counseling/memory aids by psychologist 6–12 hrs/4–14 wks.	
O'Connor, Pollitt, Brook, Reiss, & Roth (1991)	Quasi-experimental T:86; C:73	Advice/counseling/referral/respite/in-home help by professionals × 2 yrs.	
Riordan & Bennett (1998)	Quasi-experimental T:19; C:19	Home support service/information/advice by care assistants during 1 yr studied.	Institutionalization: T < C @ 1 yr
Teri, Logsdon, Uomoto, & McCurry (1997)	Experimental T:23; C:20	Behavior therapy/pleasant events topics by geriatrician 1 hr/wk × 9 wks.	Depression: T < C
Warrington & Eagles (1996)	Quasi-experimental T:33; C:27	T: Respite/case mgt/grp support by professional × 11 mo. C: Respite	Depression: T>C

Notes: (1) ♦ = nurse; (2) * = omitted in the present analysis; (3) ↓ = variable decreased after intervention; (4) ↑ = variable increased after interventions; (5) § = pts. < 50% with dementia; (6) significant findings represent researchers choice of significance level; (7) T vs. C outcomes listed when significant differences between the treatment and control groups were reported.

ings. These aspects are reported in Table 6.1. Each group of interventions was also evaluated for strengths and weaknesses in design, sample, intervention, and outcomes.

Education Interventions

For this review, education is defined as those interventions designed to provide specific information about the disease process, disruptive behaviors, and caregiving skills. The education interventions in this review were often delivered in a group setting by experts or professionals in the caregiving field. In some studies, time was allotted for the caregivers to practice or discuss the educational skills and materials.

In 23 studies, researchers tested an education intervention (Table 6.1); treatment group sample sizes ranged from 2 to 95. Researchers focused primarily on evaluating the effect of education on the negative consequences of caregiving (the most commonly measured outcomes were burden, depression, and stress). It is interesting to note that in only 9 of the 24 education interventions was a change in knowledge evaluated. Knowledge seems a logical outcome to assess post education; however, many researchers evaluated the effects of education on more global variables (e.g., burden and depression).

There was no consistent direction (increase or decrease) in most of the outcomes measured; some researchers found outcomes such as burden to be decreased after intervention (e.g., Ostwald, Hepburn, Caron, Burns, & Mantell, 1999; Robinson, 1988) while other research teams found burden to increase after intervention (e.g., Coen, O'Boyle, Coakley, & Lawlor, 1999; Farran & Keane-Hagarty, 1994). Similarly, depression, negative affect, stress, anxiety, coping, support, and distress were found to be increased in some studies and decreased in others. Of the 90 outcome variables measured, 32 (36%) were found to be statistically significant (in the desired direction).

In 10 of the 23 education interventions nurse researchers conducted the study focusing primarily on individualized, home-based programs delivered one on one over time periods ranging from 1 to 8 months; treatment group sample sizes ranged from 2 to 95. Due to this type of approach, the intervention intensity was greater than interventions delivered in the group-based format used by many researchers in other disciplines. Nurse researchers found five dysphoric outcomes (depression, tension, anger, burden, negative affect) to be significantly reduced by education interventions; depression was significantly reduced in four studies and burden was significantly reduced in three. Regarding positive outcomes, nurse researchers reported that knowledge, coping, and life satisfaction were significantly increased in 3 studies.

Support and Education Interventions

For this review, support and education interventions are defined as those strategies that use interactions among group members to share experiences and give mutual support. In addition, education is provided to group members either by peers or professionals. Support and education groups have long been the traditional mode of intervention for caregivers of adults with dementia. These types of groups are often established by the Alzheimer's Association or other local community group concerned about the stress of family caregiving. Groups may be conducted by lay persons with caregiving experience or by professionals with special training or skills. Typically, the support and education interventions in this review were delivered in a group setting with approximately half of the intervention session devoted to an educational topic and the last half of the session with time for supportive interactions among the members.

There are 14 studies classified as support and education interventions (Table 6.1); treatment group sample sizes ranged from 13 to 268. Of the 59 outcome variables measured, only 18 (31%) were found to be statistically significant (in the desired direction) in 12 of the 14 studies. Decreased burden and depression, and increased knowledge were the most common statistically significant outcomes.

There were four studies by nurse researchers in the support and education intervention category; treatment group sample sizes ranged from 26 to 53. Three of the studies were conducted in a group, community-based format and the fourth was a computerized intervention (see chapter 10 in this volume by Jones and Brennan for a thorough discussion of interventions with elders who use computers). Similar to the nursing studies in the education-only intervention category above, the nurse researchers tended to individualize the education content of the support and education interventions. Most of the nurse researchers used a stress-mediation theoretical model to frame their studies, as did many of the researchers from other disciplines. Few researchers, including nurses and those from other disciplines, specifically described the support component of the support and education intervention.

Only 3 of the 18 nursing research outcomes were significantly changed in the desired direction (burden, stress, and decision confidence). In contrast, Farran and Keane-Hagarty (1994) found burden and distress to be significantly increased after a support and education intervention. These researchers speculated that the caregivers in their study may have underreported the negative impact of caregiving on initial assessment and when trust among the intervention team and participants was developed during the study, subsequent assessments were more realistic. This explanation is plausible and may account for the low rate of statistical significance (in the desired direction) found in much of the caregiver intervention research.

Counseling Interventions

Counseling interventions facilitate change by helping caregivers to understand the behavioral symptoms exhibited by the care receiver and to understand their own reactions to the behavioral symptoms. In addition, counselors may individualize interventions based on needs and problems presented by caregivers. Counseling interventions may be delivered via group meetings but are often conducted during individual or family sessions.

Four studies were classified as counseling interventions (Table 6.1); treatment group sample sizes ranged from 5 to 38. Only two of the eight outcomes (25%) in one of the four research studies resulted in statistically significant changes in the desired direction (Perkins & Poynton, 1990).

There were three studies by nurse researchers; treatment group sample sizes ranged from 5 to 39. Larsen (1998) tested an individualized intervention and Roberts and colleagues (1999) offered individual counseling sessions in person or by phone. Only Perkins and Poynton (1990) found significant changes in outcome variables (increased knowledge and morale) after group counseling, although Roberts and colleagues found decreased psychological distress and improved psychological adjustment in a subgroup of subjects (those caregivers with poor logical analysis coping skills at baseline). Both Larsen (1998) and Roberts and colleagues (1999) used a model of problem solving to frame their interventions while Perkins and Poynton (1990) did not specify a guiding framework. The problem-solving model (most frequently used) followed by cognitive-behavioral therapy were the most common theoretical perspectives used by nurse and non-nurse researchers.

Respite Interventions

Respite care is defined as interventions designed to give caregivers a break from the responsibilities of caregiving. Respite care delivers short-term relief by providing care outside the home or in-home care for a temporary period of time. Care may be provided by community-based group respite programs or by individuals coming into the home to stay with the afflicted person while the caregiver is relieved from his or her duties.

Respite interventions were tested in 16 studies (Table 6.1); treatment group sample sizes ranged from 7 to 264. Eight studies focused on the effects of day care, five evaluated inpatient respite; three studies allowed research subjects to use either day care, in-home, or inpatient respite; and one study tested in-home respite. Most notable in the respite studies was the significant reduction in several negative outcomes (depression, stress, anxiety, role overload, strain, and anger). Of the negative aspects of caregiving measured, respite strategies were found to be successful in significantly reducing 33% of them.

Five nurse researchers tested the effect of respite interventions for caregivers; treatment group sample sizes ranged from 7 to 32. Three nurse researchers evaluated the effects of day care (Graham, 1989; Johnson & Maguire, 1989; Strang & Neufeld, 1990) while Conlin, Caranasos, and Davidson (1992) and Theis and colleagues (1994) tested the effect of either in-home or in-patient respite. A problematic issue in evaluating respite interventions is differences in the amount of respite used. For example, in the three nursing studies of day care respite, participants' respite use ranged from 1 to 5 days per week. In addition, the duration of the interventions ranged from 1 to 4 months. Significant outcomes in the nursing respite studies included a decrease in anxiety (Johnson & Maguire, 1989) and stress (Conlin et al., 1992). However, because the combination of use and duration varied considerably across studies, it is difficult to determine what amount of respite over what time period is optimal.

In a national survey of family caregivers, the National Family Caregivers Association (1999) reported that respite was the number one need expressed by family caregivers, thus it would seem reasonable that respite interventions would be successful in reducing the negative consequences of caregiving; however, this review does not support that conclusion. Most respite services are offered at specific times and locations which may not fit into caregivers' work schedules or life situations. Thus, family caregivers may not find prescribed respite helpful and may need more flexible respite options than are currently being tested by researchers.

Case Management Interventions

Case management is described as a means of linking caregivers with needed services. Case management typically entails assessment, planning, coordination, collaboration, and monitoring by a professional case manager (e.g., nurse, social worker). The family is visited in the home, an assessment is made, and services are provided based on individual need. There are six case management studies in this review (Table 6.1); treatment group sample sizes ranged from 12 to 4151. Only one study reported a significant reduction (in the desired direction) in a negative outcome (stress) (Silverman, Musa, Martin, Lave, Adams, & Ricci, 1995). One nurse research team (Schwarz & Blixen, 1997) tested a case management intervention and found no significant reductions in depression and strain and no significant increases in positive appraisal.

One explanation for the poor outcomes found in the case management interventions is offered by MaloneBeach, Zarit, and Spore (1992). These researchers note that many caregivers discontinue case management services because they find them difficult to use or inappropriate for their needs. Problems reported by caregivers include unreliable workers, rigid and complicated procedures for obtaining services, and lack of control over the services or delivery.

Multicomponent Interventions

As it is hard to pinpoint what types of interventions caregivers need in the differing stages of caregiving, comprehensive, multicomponent interventions (multiple strategies) are becoming more common (Bourgeois et al., 1996). An example of a multicomponent strategy is the Drummond and colleagues' (1991) study testing education, support groups, home visits, referral, consultation, and respite. Twelve studies reporting tests of multicomponent interventions are included in this review (Table 6.1); treatment group sample sizes ranged from 5 to 86. Few multicomponent studies were reported prior to 1991, thus this strategy represents a reconceptualization of caregiver intervention delivery.

Both positive and negative consequences of caregiving were measured as outcomes of the multicomponent interventions and most researchers found mixed results. However, one exception was the rate of institutionalization which was significantly reduced in two studies. In 8 of the 12 studies, researchers found significant changes in outcomes after intervention. Ten outcome variables (27%) were found to be significantly changed in the expected direction, and institutionalization rate was the only outcome to be significantly changed in more than one study.

Two nurse researchers tested multicomponent strategies; treatment group sample sizes ranged from 11 to 58. Each of the nurse-initiated interventions contained aspects of in-home services as did many of the multicomponent interventions tested by nonnurse researchers. The vast array of services offered by researchers testing multicomponent interventions presents a major problem when comparing these intervention strategies. The diversity inherent in multicomponent interventions introduces many extraneous variables (e.g., case management services are individualized and the level of service providers may range from volunteers to professionals) making a comprehensive synthesis of multicomponent interventions extremely difficult. Bourgeois and colleagues (1996) argue that researchers must evaluate each component of a multicomponent intervention. An example of appropriate intervention and outcome matching is found in Archbold and colleagues' (1995) research to help caregivers better care for their family members. These researchers chose one evaluation measure that closely corresponded to the focus of the intervention: care effectiveness. On evaluation, care effectiveness was significantly improved; however, more global indicators of change (depression and global strain) were not significantly improved.

DISCUSSION

What Are the Important Issues for Researchers to Address Concerning Caregiver Intervention Research?

Overall this review shows that only 32% of the interventions (all strategies combined) had significant effects in the desired direction on caregiver outcomes. These findings are disappointing and there may be several reasons for these results. Problematic areas noted in this review include small sample sizes; lack of sampling homogeneity; lack of intervention specificity; diversity in length, duration, and intensity of specific intervention strategies; poor matches between interventions and outcomes; lack of prescreening caregivers for levels of outcome variables; and lack of attention to matching caregiver needs to intervention strategies.

Due to the stressful and burdensome nature of caregiving, it is often very difficult to recruit family caregivers into research studies. Because of this difficulty, researchers routinely tolerate small sample sizes and a great deal of heterogeneity in their study subjects. For example, in this review it was not unusual to examine a study with a sample consisting of adult child and spouse caregivers of varying ages, in various caregiving situations (some caring for family members in the home, some caring for family members in institutions). This diversity certainly introduces many problems in delivering and evaluating interventions because the needs of adult child and spouse caregivers may differ drastically depending on their current circumstances. Similarly, the responses to interventions may be different depending on age-related developmental processes or current caregiving circumstances. Thus, outcomes of studies with diverse samples are bound to be difficult to evaluate unless the sample size is large, the intervention individualized, and appropriate outcomes for each type of caregiver are taken into account.

Intervention specificity is also problematic in caregiving intervention research. For example, case management and multicomponent interventions are difficult to specify and standardize. These interventions rely on coordination and collaboration among an array of services. Additionally, nurse researchers in this review relied heavily on individualized interventions guided by assessments of caregiver needs. Interventions based on needs dictate a lack of specificity (although guiding principles can be formulated). However, it is unclear whether standardized or individualized interventions produced better outcomes.

Another area of concern in the caregiver intervention literature is diversity in the length, intensity, and duration of the intervention strategies. For example in this review of respite studies, the time in respite ranged from 2 weeks to 1 year. Similarly, the actual amount of respite used ranged from 8 to 168 hours per week. Differences of this kind can also be found in other intervention strategies; most of the education interventions were delivered in group sessions of 1–3 hours per week for several weeks. However, Buckwalter and colleagues (1999) tested the effect of education delivered by home visits with follow up telephone calls over 6 months.

Thus, differences in length, intensity, and duration of the caregiver intervention strategies make comparisons and replication very difficult.

The lack of matching caregiver need to intervention strategy was also noted in this review. For example, teaching a caregiver with a family member in the early stages of dementia how to manage behaviors such as incontinence or wandering which occur in the later stages of the disease, may actually increase stress and anxiety regarding the inevitable decline of their loved one. Buckwalter and colleagues' (1999) investigation is an example of a successful study testing interventions linked to caregiver needs. The interventions in Buckwalter's study produced significant reductions in depression, tension, and anger.

Similarly, it was noted that few researchers mentioned recruiting subjects who were in need of the intervention. An exception was McCurry, Logsdon, Vitiello, and Teri (1998) who recruited caregivers having sleep difficulties for an educational intervention that included ways to get better sleep. This recruitment strategy resulted in significant increases in sleep quality among the treatment group; however, similar gains were not found for depression or burden.

Little attention to matching participants' preintervention state to postintervention outcomes was noted in this review. Few researchers prescreened participants on any variables planned for intervention evaluation. Thus, many researchers noted that because preintervention levels of the outcomes were low (or high), there was no room for improvement after intervention.

Another reason for the poor intervention effects may be that outcomes chosen by researchers were not sensitive to change following intervention. Burden, for example, is a measure of the global impact that caregiving has on the caregiver's life. It has been suggested that caregiver burden may not be alterable (Bourgeios et al., 1996), and Acton and Kang (2001) found that caregiver interventions had no statistically significant effect on caregiver burden. Instead, Toseland, Labrecque, Goebel, and Whitney (1992) suggest that "researchers may want to develop measures designed to assess the specific goals of a particular caregiver intervention program, rather than relying solely on global measures of change" (p. 389). An example of this is Ripich, Kercher, Wykle, Sloan, and Ziol's (1998) findings that knowledge was increased and communication hassles decreased after a communication skills intervention; however, more global variables such as depression, were not significantly changed.

The methods and procedures used by researchers in caregiver intervention studies are maturing; however, even though over half the researchers in this review used experimental and quasi-experimental designs, in reality social scientists have very little control over extraneous variables. For example, issues such as problems adult child caregivers may have with their own children or financial difficulties that can increase stress and burden for a spouse caregiver may override any gains made by the caregiver during intervention.

Suggestions for ways to improve caregiver intervention research are many, and they begin with increasing sample sizes and sample homogeneity. Study samples should be limited to adult child or spouse caregivers. Age limits and living arrangements should be specified to reduce sample diversity. Attention is also needed to determine whether standardized or individualized interventions produce the best outcomes in family caregivers. Theoretically, those interventions linked to caregiver needs should produce the best outcomes, but this idea must be tested and validated or refuted. Researchers must also evaluate the optimal length, duration, and intensity of specific intervention strategies. Ideally, interventions that are at least 1 hour in duration and occur over a period of weeks to months are preferable to one- or two-time interventions. Researchers must select outcomes that are likely to be changed by intervention. This review shows that global variables such as burden were less likely to change than intervention-specific variables such as knowledge. Another recommendation for improving family caregiver research is to prescreen caregivers for baseline levels of outcome variables and exclude persons with baseline measurements that leave little room for change after intervention.

It is essential to discover which interventions work under which conditions. Researchers must continue to search for the best ways to help family caregivers. As our nation ages and the numbers of persons with cognitive impairment increases, the nursing profession will be front-line providers and they must be armed with the best empirical evidence on which to base their nursing practice. Addressing the issues raised in this review may improve research and elevate the state of the science regarding interventions for family caregivers.

ACKNOWLEDGMENT

This review was funded by NIH Grant R15NR04459, NINR.

REFERENCES

Acton, G. J., & Kang, J. (2001). Interventions to reduce the burden of caregiving for an adult with dementia: A meta-analysis. *Research in Nursing & Health, 24,* 349–360.

Acton, G. J., & Miller, E. W. (1996). Affiliated-individuation in caregivers of adults with dementia. *Issues in Mental Health Nursing, 17*, 245–260.

Adler, G., Kuskowski, M. A., & Mortimer, J. (1995). Respite use in dementia patients. *Clinical Gerontologist, 15*(3), 17–30.

Adler, G., Ott, L., Jelinski, M., Mortimer, J., & Christensen, R. (1993). Institutional respite care: Benefits and risks for dementia patients and caregivers. *International Psychogeriatrics, 5*(1), 67–77.

Archbold, P. G., Stewart, B. J., Miller, L. L., Harvath, T. A., Greenlick, M. R., Van Buren, L., Kirschling, J. M., Valanis, B. G., Brody, K. K., Schook, J. E., & Hagan, J. M. (1995). The PREP system of nursing interventions: A pilot test with families caring for older members. *Research in Nursing & Health, 18*, 3–16.

Barusch, A. S., & Spaid, W. M. (1991). Reducing caregiver burden through short-term training: Evaluation findings from a caregiver support project. *Journal of Gerontological Social Work, 17*(1/2), 7–33.

Belmin, J., Hee, C., & Ollivet, C. (1999). Letters to the Editor. A health education program lessens the burden of family caregivers of demented patients. *Journal of the American Geriatrics Society, 47*, 1388–1389.

Bourgeois, M. S., Burgio, L. D., Schulz, R., Beach, S., & Palmer, B. (1997). Modifying repetitive verbalizations of community-dwelling patients with AD. *Gerontologist, 37*, 30–39.

Bourgeois, M. S., Schulz, R., & Burgio, L. (1996). Interventions for caregivers of patients with Alzheimer's disease: A review and analysis of content, process, and outcomes. *International Journal of Aging and Human Development, 43*, 35–92.

Brennan, P. F., Moore, S. M., & Smyth, K. A. (1995). The effects of a special computer network on caregivers of persons with Alzheimer's disease. *Nursing Research, 44*, 166–172.

Brodaty, H., Roberts, K., & Peters, K. (1994). Quasi-experimental evaluation of an educational model for dementia caregivers. *International Journal of Geriatric Psychiatry, 9*, 195–204.

Buckwalter, K. C., Gerdner, L., Kohout, F., Hall, G. R., Kelly, A., Richards, B., & Sime, M. (1999). A nursing intervention to decrease depression in family caregivers of persons with dementia. *Archives of Psychiatric Nursing, 13*, 80–88.

Burgener, S. C., Bakas, T., Murray, C., Dunahee, J. A., & Tossey, S. (1998). Effective caregiving approaches for patients with Alzheimer's disease. *Geriatric Nursing— American Journal of Care for the Aging, 19*, 121–126.

Butt, G. (1989). *A quasi randomized controlled study of the effects on caregiver burden of an educational intervention for primary caregivers of individuals with Alzheimer's disease.* Unpublished doctoral dissertation, McMaster University, Hamilton, Ontario, Canada.

Chang, B. L. (1999). Cognitive-behavioral intervention for homebound caregivers of persons with dementia. *Nursing Research, 48*, 173–182.

Chiverton, P., & Caine, E. D. (1989). Education to assist spouses in coping with Alzheimer's disease. A controlled trial. *Journal of the American Geriatrics Society, 37*, 593–598.

Coen, R. F., O'Boyle, C. A., Coakley, D., & Lawlor, B. A. (1999). Dementia care education and patient behaviour disturbance. *International Journal of Geriatric Psychiatry, 14,* 302–306.

Conlin, M. M., Caranasos, G. J., & Davidson, R. A. (1992). Reduction of caregiver stress by respite care: A pilot study. *Southern Medical Journal, 85,* 1096–1100.

Corbeil, R. R., Quayhagen, M. P., & Quayhagen, M. (1999). Intervention effects on dementia caregiving interaction. A stress-adaptation modeling approach. *Journal of Aging and Health, 11,* 79–95.

Cummings, S. M., Long, J. K., Peterson-Hazan, S., & Harrison, J. (1998). The efficacy of a group treatment model in helping spouses meet the emotional and practical challenges of early stage caregiving. *Clinical Gerontologist, 20*(1), 29–45.

Davis, L. L. (1998). Telephone-based interventions with family caregivers: A feasibility study. *Journal of Family Nursing, 4,* 255–270.

Deimling, G. T. (1991). Respite use and caregiver well-being in families caring for stable and declining AD patients. *Journal of Gerontological Social Work, 18,* 117–134.

Demers, A., & Lavoie, J. P. (1996). Effect of support groups on family caregivers to the frail elderly. *Canadian Journal on Aging, 15,* 129–144.

Drummond, M. F., Mohide, E. A., Tew, M., Streiner, D. L., Pringle, D. M., & Gilbert, J. R. (1991). Economic evaluation of a support program for caregivers of demented elderly. *International Journal of Technology Assessment in Health Care, 7,* 209–219.

Farran, C. J., & Keane-Hagarty, E. (1994). Multimodal intervention strategies for caregivers of persons with dementia. In E. Light, G. Niederehe, & B. D. Lebowitz (Eds.), *Stress effects on family caregivers of Alzheimer's patients. Research and interventions* (pp. 242–259). New York: Springer Publishing Co.

Gage, M. J., & Kinney, J. M. (1995). They aren't for everyone: The impact of support group participation on caregivers' well-being. *Clinical Gerontologist, 16*(2), 21–34.

Gallagher-Thompson, D., & Steffen, A. M. (1994). Comparative effects of cognitive-behavioral and brief psychodynamic psychotherapies for depressed family caregivers. *Journal of Consulting and Clinical Psychology, 62,* 543–549.

Gendron, C., Poitras, L., Dastoor, D. P., & Perodeau, G. (1996). Cognitive-behavioral group intervention for spousal caregivers: Findings and clinical considerations. *Clinical Gerontologist, 17*(1), 3–19.

Graham, R. W. (1989). Adult day care: How families of the dementia patient respond. *Journal of Gerontological Nursing, 15*(3), 27–31.

Grunow, J. A. L. (1991). *A home-based intervention program for family caregivers of dementia patients.* Unpublished doctoral dissertation, Rush University, Chicago, IL.

Guttman, R. A. (1991). Adult day care for Alzheimer's patients: Impact on family caregivers. In S. Bruchey (Ed.), *The elderly in America* (pp. 1–168). New York: Garland.

Harper, D. J., Manasse, P. R., James, O., & Newton, J. T. (1993). Intervening to reduce distress in caregivers of impaired elderly people: A preliminary evaluation. *International Journal of Geriatric Psychiatry, 8,* 139–145.

Heacock, P. (Unpublished). *Intervention for caregiver and dementia client dyads.*

Hebert, R., Leclerc, G., Bravo, G., Girouard, D., & Lefrancois, R. (1994). Efficacy of a support group programme for caregivers of demented patients in the community: A randomized controlled trial. *Archives of Gerontology and Geriatrics, 18,* 1–14.

Homer, A. C., & Gilleard, C. J. (1994). The effect of inpatient respite care on elderly patients and their carers. *Age & Aging, 23,* 274–276.

Hosaka, T., & Sugiyama, Y. (1999). A structured intervention for family caregivers of dementia patients: A pilot study. *Tokai Journal of Experimental and Clinical Medicine, 24*(1), 35–39.

Knight, B. G., Lutzky, S. M., & Macofsky-Urban, F. (1993). A meta-analytic review of interventions for caregiver distress: Recommendations for future research. *Gerontologist, 33,* 240–248.

Johnson, M., & Maguire, M. (1989). Give me a break: Benefits of a caregiver support service. *Journal of Gerontological Nursing, 15*(11), 22–26.

Larkin, J. P., & Hopcroft, B. M. (1993). In-hospital respite as a moderator of caregiver stress. *Health & Social Work, 18,* 132–138.

Larsen, L. S. (1998). Effectiveness of a counseling intervention to assist family caregivers of chronically ill relatives. *Journal of Psychosocial Nursing, 36*(8), 26–32.

Lawton, M. P., Brody, E. M., & Saperstein, A. R. (1989). A controlled study of respite service for caregivers of Alzheimer's patients. *Gerontologist, 29,* 8–16.

Lo Giudice, D., Waltrowicz, W., Brown, K., Burrows, C., Ames, D., & Flicker, L. (1999). Do memory clinics improve the quality of life of carers? A randomized pilot trial. *International Journal of Geriatric Psychiatry, 14,* 626–632.

Magni, E., Zanetti, O., Bianchetti, A., Binetti, G., & Trabucchi, M. (1995). Evaluation of an Italian educational programme for dementia caregivers: Results of a small-scale pilot study. *International Journal of Geriatric Psychiatry, 10,* 569–573.

MaloneBeach, E. E., Zarit, S. H., & Spore, D. S. (1992). Caregivers' perceptions of case-management and community-based services: Barriers to service use. *Journal of Applied Gerontology, 11,* 146–159.

McCallion, P., Toseland, R. W., & Freeman, K. (1999). An evaluation of a family visit education program. *Journal of American Geriatrics Society, 47,* 203–214.

McCurry, S. M., Logsdon, R. G., Vitiello, M. V., & Teri, L. (1998). Successful behavioral treatment for reported sleep problems in elderly caregivers of dementia patients: A controlled study. *Journal of Gerontology: Psychological Sciences, 53B,* P122–P129.

Millan-Calenti, J. C., Gandoy-Crego, M., Antelo-Martelo, M., Lopez-Martinez, M., Riveiro-Lopez, M. P., & Mayan-Santos, J. M. (2000). Helping the family carers of Alzheimer's patients: From theory . . . to practice. A preliminary study. *Archives of Gerontology and Geriatrics, 30,* 131–138.

Miller, R., Newcomer, R., & Fox, P. (1999). Effects of the Medicare Alzheimer's disease demonstration on nursing home entry. *Health Services Research, 34,* 691–714.

Mittelman, M., Ferris, S., Shulman, E., Steinberg, G., Mackell, J., & Ambinder, A. (1994). Efficacy of multicomponent individualized treatment to improve the well-being of Alzheimer's caregivers. In E. Light, G. Niederehe, & B. D. Lebowitz (Eds.), *Stress effects on family caregivers of Alzheimer's patients. Research and interventions* (pp. 156–184). New York: Springer Publishing.

Moniz-Cook, E., Agar, S., Gibson, G., Win, T., & Wang, M. (1998). A preliminary study of the effects of early intervention with people with dementia and their families in a memory clinic. *Aging & Mental Health, 2,* 199–211.

National Institute on Aging/National Institutes of Health (NIA/NIH). (1999). *Progress report Alzheimer's disease.* Silver Spring, MD: Alzheimer's Disease Education and Referral Center.

National Family Caregivers Association. (1999). *National report on the status of caregiving in America.* Kensington, MD: Author.

Newcomer, R., Yordi, C., DuNah, R., Fox, P., & Wilkinson, A. (1999). Effects of the Medicare Alzheimer's disease demonstration on caregiver burden and depression. *Health Services Research, 34,* 669–689.

O'Connor, D. W., Pollitt, P. A., Brook, C. P. B., Reiss, B. B., & Roth, M. (1991). Does early intervention reduce the number of elderly people with dementia admitted to institutions for long term care? *British Medical Journal, 302,* 871–875.

Ostwald, S. K., Hepburn, K. W., Caron, W., Burns, T., & Mantell, R. (1999). Reducing caregiver burden: A randomized psychoeducational intervention for caregivers of persons with dementia. *Gerontologist, 39,* 299–309.

Perkins, R. E., & Poynton, C. F. (1990). Group counselling for relatives of hospitalized presenile dementia patients: A controlled study. *British Journal of Clinical Psychology, 29,* 287–295.

Pynoos, J., & Ohta, R. J. (1991). In-home interventions for persons with Alzheimer's disease and their caregivers. *Physical & Occupational Therapy in Geriatrics, 3/4,* 83–92.

Quayhagen, M. P., & Quayhagen, M. (1989). Differential effects of family-based strategies on Alzheimer's disease. *Gerontologist, 29,* 150–155.

Riordan, J. M., & Bennett, A. V. (1998). An evaluation of an augmented domiciliary service to older people with dementia and their carers. *Aging & Mental Health, 2,* 137–143.

Ripich, D., Kercher, K., Wykle, M., Sloan, D. M., & Ziol, E. (1998). Effects of communication training on African American and white caregivers of persons with Alzheimer's disease. *Journal of Aging and Ethnicity, 1,* 163–178.

Ripich, D. N., Ziol, E., & Lee, M. M. (1998). Longitudinal effects of communication training on caregivers of persons with Alzheimer's disease. *Clinical Gerontologist, 19*(2), 37–55.

Roberts, J., Browne, G., Milne, C., Spooner, L., Gafni, A., Drummond-Young, M., LeGris, J., Watt, S., LeClair, K., Beaumont, L., & Roberts, J. (1999). Problem-solving counseling for caregivers of the cognitively impaired: Effective for whom? *Nursing Research, 48,* 162–172.

Robinson, K., & Yates, K. (1994). Effects of two caregiver-training programs on burden and attitude toward help. *Archives of Psychiatric Nursing, 8,* 312–319.

Robinson, K. M. (1988). A social skills training program for adult caregivers. *Advances in Nursing Science, 10*(2), 59–72.

Rothman, M. L., Diehr, P., Hedrick, S. C., Erdly, W. W., & Nickinovich, D. G. (1993). Effects of contract adult day health care on health outcomes and satisfaction with care. *Medical Care, 31*(9), SS75–SS83.

Rothman, M. L., Hedrick, S. C., Bulcroft, K. A., Erdly, W. W., & Nickinovich, D. G. (1993). Effects of VA adult day health care on health outcomes and satisfaction with care. *Medical Care, 31*(9), SS38–SS49.

Schultz, C. L., Schultz, N. C., & Smyrnios, K. X. (1994). Caring for family caregivers of dependent ageing persons: Process and outcome evaluation. *Australian Journal of Ageing, 13,* 193–196.

Schulz, R., & Beach, S. R. (1999). Caregiving as a risk factor for mortality. *Journal of the American Medical Association, 282,* 2215–2219.

Schulz, R., O'Brien, A. T., Bookwala, J., & Fleissner, K. (1995). Psychiatric and physical morbidity effects of dementia caregiving: Prevalence, correlates, and causes. *Gerontologist, 35,* 771–791.

Schwarz, K. A., & Blixen, C. E. (1997). Does home health care affect strain and depressive symptomatology for caregivers of impaired older adults? *Journal of Community Health Nursing, 14*(1), 39–48.

Silverman, M., Musa, D., Martin, D. C., Lave, J. R., Adams, J., & Ricci, E. M. (1995). Evaluation of outpatient geriatric assessment: A randomized multi-site trial. *Journal of the American Geriatric Society, 43,* 733–740.

Skelly, M. C., McAdoo, C. M., & Ostergard, S. M. (1993). Caregiver burden at McGuire Veterans Administration Medical Center. *Journal of Gerontological Social Work, 19*(3/4), 3–13.

Strang, V., & Neufeld, A. (1990). Adult day dare programs. A source for respite. *Journal of Gerontological Nursing, 16*(11), 16–20.

Strawn, B. D., Hester, S., & Brown, W. S. (1998). Telecare: A social support intervention for family caregivers of dementia victims. *Clinical Gerontologist, 18*(3), 66–69.

Teri, L., Logsdon, R. G., Uomoto, J., & McCurry, S. M. (1997). Behavioral treatment of depression in dementia patients: A controlled clinical trial. *Journal of Gerontology: Psychological Sciences, 52B,* P159–P166.

Theis, S. L., Moss, J. H., & Pearson, M. A. (1994). Respite for caregivers: An evaluation study. *Journal of Community Health Nursing, 11*(1), 31–44.

Toseland, R. Q., & Rossiter, C. (1989). Group interventions to support family caregivers: A review and analysis. *Gerontologist, 29,* 434–448.

Toseland, R. W., Labrecque, M. S., Goebel, S. T., & Whitney, M. H. (1992). An evaluation of a group program for spouses of frail elderly veterans. *Gerontologist, 32,* 382–390.

Warrington, J., & Eagles, J. M. (1996). A comparison of cognitively impaired attenders and their coresident carers at day hospitals and day centres in Aberdeen. *International Journal of Geriatric Psychiatry, 11,* 251–256.

Weinberger, M., Gold, D. T., Divine, G. W., Cowper, P. A., Hodgson, L. G., Schreiner, P. J., & George, L. K. (1993). Social service interventions for caregivers of patients with dementia: Impact on health care utilization and expenditures. *Journal of the American Geriatrics Society, 41,* 153–156.

Wimo, A., Mattsson, B., Adolfsson, R., Eriksson, T., & Nelvig, A. (1993). Dementia day care and its effects on symptoms and institutionalization—A controlled Swedish study. *Scandinavian Journal of Primary Health Care, 11,* 117–123.

Zanetti, O., Metitieri, T., Bianchetti, A., & Trabucchi, M. (1998). Effectiveness of an educational program for demented person's relatives. *Archives of Gerontology & Geriatrics,* (Suppl. 6), 531–538.

Zarit, S. H., Stephens, M. A. P., Townsend, A., & Greene, R. (1998). Stress reduction for family caregivers: Effects of adult day care use. *Journal of Gerontology: Social Sciences, 53B,* S267–S277.

Chapter 7

End-of-Life Care for Older Adults in ICUs

JUDITH GEDNEY BAGGS

ABSTRACT

This review was undertaken to present and critique the most recent (1990–2000) empirical evidence about end-of-life care for older adult patients in ICUs, their families, and care providers. The studies (including descriptive, correlational, longitudinal, and intervention) were found using a combination of these terms: (a) *intensive care (units)* or *critical care (units)*, and (b) *critical illness, critically ill patients, terminally ill, terminal care, life support care,* or *palliative care.* The computerized databases searched were CINAHL and MEDLINE. Only published studies of persons 44 years of age or older, written in English, and conducted in the U.S. or Canada were included. Research was not limited to studies conducted by or written by nurses. Excluded were articles focused on physiology, for example, studies of treatment for specific conditions, and articles focused on predictors of ICU outcomes.

Findings and Implications for Research

There is little research specifically focused on end-of-life care of older adults in ICUs. Most research has been retrospective, and most has involved either providers or patients and families but not both.

Research is needed in many areas. The mechanism by which age affects choice of care needs further exploration. The experience of patients, families, and providers and how those experiences change with interventions needs investigation. The influence of the ICU culture, variation in decisions made and reasons for that variation, the decision-making process, and variations in care, all require further attention. Four domains were identified for research needed to improve care for older adults at the end of life in intensive care: symptom relief, communication improvement, psychological support, and relationship improvement. No one has assessed whether the ICU is a good place for transition to palliation to occur, or whether it would be better to transfer patients to another type of unit.

Keywords: intensive or critical care [units], critical illness, terminal care, terminally ill, palliative care, life support care, adults, aged

Care that is provided at the end of life is a crucial part of health care. It may ease or make more difficult a passage that all of us will make. The quality of the care delivered also has an important impact on the surviving family and friends of the person who dies and on the health care providers who deliver the care.

A renewed desire to improve the care provided to the dying has been demonstrated over the past decade in new initiatives from the National Institutes of Health, from private foundations, and from local communities and institutions. The forces giving impetus to this movement are varied and include early and continuing research demonstrating problems with end-of-life care and the interest of private foundations and the government in funding improvements in end-of-life care. There has been increasing use of high technology to sustain life, with a growing recognition by both health care providers and the public that intensive, technological care is not always the best care for the dying. The media, television in particular, have highlighted coverage of this type of care.

In the ICU setting in particular there is a high level of technology used and interest in the treatment provided during the transition from life to death. Much of the recent interest in research on patients dying in the ICU has focused on the topic of decision making about limitation of treatment. Almost half of the research reports discovered for this review were about this decision.

As people age, the likelihood that they are close to the end of life increases. Excellence in end-of-life care for older adults is particularly important. The Intensive Care Unit (ICU) is the locale for end-of-life care for many patients, and many ICU patients are older. There is very little research specifically about end-of-life care for older adult patients in ICUs. For this review, studies of adult ICU patients were assumed to be studies that were about older patients because the average age for ICU patients is 65 (Baggs, 1999), and approximately 50% of ICU patients are 65 or older (Chelluri, Grenvik, & Silverman, 1995). In-hospital mortality for

ICU patients over 65 in most studies is about 30% (Chelluri et al., 1995). The studies that were focused on older adults are identified in the text, and mean age of research participants is provided for studies when it was relevant and available. Many authors have addressed the relevance of age to ICU care and to outcomes of that care. Most of that research points to the lack of a significant relationship between age and outcomes of care; age, however, appears to be important in determining what level and type of care will be given.

Aims

This review of the research literature was undertaken with the intention of presenting, critiquing, and synthesizing the most recent empirical evidence about end-of-life care for older patients in ICUs, their families, and care providers. The purpose was to use this review as a basis to suggest where research needs to be undertaken to help develop standards for measuring and improving that care.

METHOD

The research studies and review articles accessed for this chapter were found using a combination of the following search terms: (a) *intensive care [units]* or *critical care [units]*, and (b) *critical illness, critically ill patients, terminally ill, terminal care, life support care*, or *palliative care*. The computerized databases searched were CINAHL and MEDLINE. Limitations placed on the search included published studies of people 44 years of age or older. The lower age of 44 was chosen as an artifact of the computerized databases, where the age range for adults is 44 to 65. Omitting that range would have eliminated 60–64 year olds. It might also have eliminated studies of "adult" patients that actually included many older adult participants. Studies accessed were written in English, conducted in the U.S. or Canada, and published between 1990 and 2000. In addition to the database search, articles were located by reviewing reference lists of the articles found through the databases. Because so much health care research is interdisciplinary, and because research from other disciplines is applicable to and affects nursing, research was not limited to studies conducted by or written by nurses. Studies and research reviews by nurses are identified. Excluded were articles focused on physiology, for example, studies of treatment for specific conditions and articles focused on ICU outcome predictors. Many excluded studies were not relevant to most nursing care or nursing interventions. Eighty-five research studies (26 of them by nurse first authors) and 13 research reviews (6 of them by nurse first authors) are included.

The review is grouped by six major questions related to end-of-life care of older patients:

1. What is hospital end-of-life care like and what should it be?
2. What factors affect older patients dying in ICUs?
3. What is important to families of dying patients in acute care?
4. What is important to health care professionals caring for dying patients in ICUs?
5. What influences decision making at the end of life for ICU patients?
6. How can end-of-life care and decision making be improved?

Limitations

In most studies reviewed, a single ICU was studied or ICUs were treated as a homogeneous entity, when, in fact, numerous types of ICUs for the care of specific populations exist, including medical ICUs (MICUs), surgical ICUs (SICUs), and coronary care units (CCUs), among others. When specific types of ICUs were studied, the type is named. In some studies, acute hospital care and ICU care were combined or studies of acute care were included, as the acute care experience was closely enough related to ICU care to warrant its inclusion. Those instances are noted in the text.

WHAT IS HOSPITAL END-OF-LIFE CARE LIKE AND WHAT SHOULD IT BE?

What Is Hospital End-of-Life Care Like?

Several researchers have provided a perspective on what care currently is like in the United States and Canada for dying patients in acute care institutions (Table 7.1). The Study to Understand Prognoses and Preferences for Outcomes and Risks of Treatments (SUPPORT Principal Investigators, 1995) was designed to assess end-of-life care in seriously ill patients and to test an intervention to improve the process of end-of-life decision making. There was evidence of inadequate communication about patient wishes between patients and physicians. Other researchers who have studied deaths in hospitals or in ICUs have demonstrated inability of patients to participate when decisions to forgo life-sustaining treatment were made. There also is an increasing use of do-not-resuscitate (DNR) orders in ICUs (Tables 7.1 and 7.7).

What Should End-of-Life Care in Hospitals Be?

All published guidelines for management of limitation-of-treatment decisions and care of the dying patient have been based on expert opinion rather than on research data (American College of Chest Physicians, 1990; American Geriatrics Society Ethics Committee, 1995; American Thoracic Society, 1991; Council on Ethical and Judicial Affairs, 1991; Council on Scientific Affairs, 1996; Levetown, 1998; Luce, 1998; Rocker & Dunbar, 2000; Todres, Armstrong, Lally, & Cassem, 1998; Weissman, 2000).

A few studies had as a goal clarification of the lay or patient perspective on what end-of-life care should be, and from which standards of care could be developed. None of these studies were focused on older patients dying in the ICU, however, dying ICU patients of any age often do not have "capacity" and so are seldom available to be studied. Participants in these studies included healthy Americans anticipating future wishes, terminally or chronically ill patients, bereaved family members, and health care providers and volunteers who care for dying patients. Studies including the patient perspective are particularly valuable because they form the best basis for interventions to improve care based not on expert opinion but on what patients or members of the general public have identified as important for their care as they are dying.

In 1997, 385 American individuals participated in 36 focus groups in a study funded by The Robert Wood Johnson Foundation (American Health Decisions, 1997). Participants were selected to represent the American public and came from both genders and from varied income and education levels, age groups, and religious and ethnic backgrounds. The key findings were that Americans "fear reaching the end of their lives

TABLE 7.1   End-of-Life Care in the Hospital or ICU

Study author(s), date of publication	Methods	Key findings
Faber-Langendoen, 1996	Design: retrospective chart review of deceased patients in 4 acute care hospitals Measures/Variables: diagnosis, mental status, length of stay, timing of first decision to forgo treatment, range and sequence of treatments forgone Sample: 274 deaths (charts)-Mean age 63.8 years	• 229 (84%) deaths preceded by withholding or withdrawing potentially life-sustaining treatment • 75 (35%) were able to participate in first decision to forgo treatment
Prendergast, Claessens, & Luce, 1998	Design: prospective survey Measures/Variables: frequency of withdrawal of life support in medical-surgical ICUs Sample: 131 ICUs at 110 institutions in 38 US states; 6303 deaths Age of patients not reported	Life support was limited preceding 74% of deaths, with wide range of variation among ICUs Deaths occurred after (range): • failed CPR (4–79%) • DNR order (0–83%) • withholding life-support (0–67%) • withdrawing life-support (0–79%)
Prendergast & Luce, 1997	Design: prospective survey Measures/Variables: recommendations to limit life-sustaining treatment at 2 ICUs in San Francisco, CA, 1992–1993 Sample: ICU patients; mean age 52 years	• Results are compared with findings of Smedira et al. (1990) below • Recommendation to limit life support preceded 90% of patient deaths vs. only 51% in 1987–1988 • 3.4% of patients were competent to participate in treatment decisions vs. 4.3% in 1987–1988 sample • 4.5% of patients had advance directives vs. 0% in 1987–1988

TABLE 7.1 *(continued)*

Study author(s), date of publication	Methods	Key findings
Smedira et al., 1990	Design: Measures/Variables: decisions to withhold or withdraw life support from patients in 2 ICUs in San Francisco, CA, 1987–1988 Sample: 1719 ICU patients (aged 1 year or older), mean age of patients reported as 51 (in Prendergast & Luce, 1997)	• Life-support was withheld or withdrawn from 45% (89/115) of patients who died in the ICU • 4% (5/115) of patients made decision to limit care; the remainder were incompetent • 87% of families were involved
The SUPPORT Principal Investigators, 1995	Design: Phase I: prospective observation Phase II: randomized, controlled trial Measures/Variables: communication, frequency of aggressive treatment, characteristics of hospital death Sample: Phase I: 4804 patients, median age 65 years Phase II: control group (n = 2152), median age 64 years; intervention group (n = 2652), median age 66 years	Phase I: • 47% of physicians knew patients wishes to avoid CPR • 46% DNR orders written within 2 days of death • 38% of patients who died spent at least 10 days in ICU • family members reported moderate to severe pain in 50% of conscious patients who died in hospital Phase II: Intervention • failed to show improvements

Notes: CPR = cardiopulmonary resuscitation; DNR = do not resuscitate; ICUs = intensive care units; SUPPORT = Study to Understand Prognoses and Preferences for Outcomes and Risks of Treatments; US = United States hooked up to machines [and] prefer a natural death in familiar surroundings with loved ones" (p. 5). At the same time, participants feared that care providers might decide to provide or withdraw treatment based on financial considerations rather than on patient and family wishes, or that they might withdraw care before patients or family were ready for such an action.

Three groups of researchers have used data, including patient data, to identify crucial domains to assess end-of-life care. Singer, Martin, and Kelner (1999) conducted focus groups with 126 participants for whom death was likely to occur sooner than for the general public: dialysis patients, HIV-positive patients, and residents of a long-term care facility. From their study, five domains of quality end-of-life care were identified (Table 7.2).

Steinhauser, Clipp, and colleagues (2000) conducted focus group interviews with health care professionals, hospice volunteers, patients, and recently bereaved family members. From the focus groups they identified six components of a good death (Table 7.2). The data from the focus groups were analyzed and used to develop an instrument to measure factors considered important at the end of life (Steinhauser, Christakis, et al., 2000). The instrument was sent to a national sample representing the same populations as in the focus groups. The factors rated as important by all groups were pain and symptom management, preparation for death, achieving a sense of completion, treatment decisions, and being treated holistically (Steinhauser, Christakis, et al., 2000).

Emanuel, Alpert, Baldwin, and Emanuel (2000) interviewed 988 patients identified as having a prognosis of surviving 6 months or less; 650 were interviewed a second time. Eight factors were identified as representing measurable dimensions (Table 7.2).

Although there are some differences among the factors derived from each of these studies, there are also similarities. They may be combined into four factors (Table 7.2). The first is provision for relief of symptoms. Although Emanuel and colleagues (2000) found psychometric problems and did not name pain as a factor, the physical issue of pain and symptom management forms one clear factor in the other two studies. A second factor is support for communication for decision making, including avoiding prolonged dying. The third factor is psychological support involving maintenance of control, affirmation of the whole person, sense of purpose, spirituality, and acceptance. The fourth factor concerns importance of relationships with others, both families and providers. It involves relieving burden and strengthening relationships. These factors are important to keep in mind while reviewing the research about care for the dying older adult in ICUs.

TABLE 7.2   Research-Based Factors Important to End-of-Life Care

Four Factors	Singer, Martin, & Kelner (1999)	Steinhauser, Clipp, et al. (2000)	Emmanuel et al. (2000)
Symptom relief	• Adequate pain and symptom management	• Pain and symptom management	• Caregiving needs
Communication support	• Avoiding inappropriate prolongation of dying	• Clear decision making	
Psychological support	• Achieving a sense of control	• Preparation support • Completion • Affirm whole person	• Psychological distress • Spirituality and religiousness • Personal acceptance • Sense of purpose
Relationship improvement	• Relieving burden • Strengthening relationships with loved ones	• Contributing to others	• Patient–clinician relationship • Social connectedness • Clinician communication

WHAT FACTORS AFFECT OLDER PATIENTS DYING IN THE ICU?

Four reviews of research on older adult ICU patients were found, all written by nurses, although none of them focused on dying patients. Their authors highlighted physiology (Stanley, 1992) and adverse psychological responses (Foreman, 1992) of older adult ICU patients that should be considered in care provision. Tullmann and Dracup (2000) reviewed factors leading to increased risk for older patients in ICUs based on their physiology, cognition, and psychosocial issues such as ageism and likelihood of lessened social support. They noted that aspects of illness, treatments, and the ICU environment might generate risk. Based on these factors, the authors proposed that the liberalization of family visiting would be an important way to improve care for older adult ICU patients that would be particularly applicable if the patients are dying.

What Is the ICU Patient Experience?

The fourth research review on older adult ICU patients focused on patient experiences. Most of the studies were conducted using questionnaires or interviews with patients recently discharged from the ICU (Stein-Parbury & McKinley, 2000). Recall of the ICU experience was variable. Negative experiences reported included discomfort, impaired cognitive function, difficult sleeping, and anxiety. Positive experiences included a sense of safety and security.

For their descriptions of the experience of critically ill older patients' experience, three studies are noteworthy (Table 7.3). The researchers described how ICU patients experience nurses' caring, the symptom burden of dying patients, and the experience of being unable to communicate their preferences in speech (Burfitt, Greiner, Miers, Kinney, & Branyon, 1993; Desbiens, Mueller-Rizner, Connors, Wenger, & Lynn, 1999; Happ, 2000).

How Do Older Patients Differ or Not Differ from Other ICU Patients?

Chelluri and colleagues (1995) reviewed the research literature on outcomes of ICU care for older adults. They found that age alone was not a predictor of critical illness mortality or quality of life of survivors. Their recommendation was to consider therapeutic trials of intensive care before deciding whether limitation of life-supporting treatment for the older patient is appropriate. This finding of lack of outcome prediction based on age has been supported in studies of various groups of older adults, including the "oldest old" ($\geq$ 85 years; Table 7.4). The works by Kleinpell and Ferrans (1998) and Elpern and colleagues (1992) are the only ones by nurses. Older adults had a lower cost of care than younger patients, and age did not predict desire for ICU care or preferences for treatment at the end of life (Cicirelli, MacLean, & Cox, 2000). Despite low predictive

TABLE 7.3   Critically Ill Elderly Patients' ICU Experiences

Author(s), date	Methods	Selected findings
Burfitt, Greiner, Miers, Kinney, & Branyon (1993)	Design: phenomenology, Spiegelberg technique Objective: description of ICU patients' perceptions and meanings of caring by professional nurses Sample: adults (n = 13) aged 23–80 (mean = 61)	Patients experienced caring as vigilance, including attentiveness, nurturing, and skilled practice; mutuality, a sense of reciprocal process; and healing, including life-saving behaviors, acts freeing patients from anxiety and worry, and a holistic approach to care
Desbiens, Mueller-Rizner, Connors, Wenger, & Lynn, for the SUPPORT Investigators (1999)	Design: statistical analysis of Phase I SUPPORT study data (see Table 1) Measures/Variables: symptom burden and associated factors Sample: adults (n = 1582), median age 62.5 years, able to respond to a symptom questionnaire	67% of symptoms in the following categories were moderately severe at least half of the time: pain, dyspnea, anxiety, depression, nausea. 76% of patients reported fatigue. Greater symptom burden associated with: male gender, more comorbidities, more dependence in ADLs prior to illness, and poorer QoL. There was no association between symptom burden and age.
Happ (2000)	Design: grounded theory Objective: describe communication processes in critically ill voiceless older adult patients Sample: adults (n = 16) aged 64–87 (mean = 75.4); ICU nurses (n = 9) were also included in the study, as were family members (n = 4) and physicians (n = 3)	The experience of voicelessness, where patients are unable to communicate their preferences in speech, was explored. Nurses and family members responded by trying to serve as interpreters of patients' wishes.

ADLs = activities of daily living; ICU = intensive care unit; QoL = quality of life.

TABLE 7.4   Differentiating Elderly from Other ICU Patients

Author(s), date	Methods	Selected findings
Boyd, Teres, Rapoport, & Lemeshow (1996)	Design: secondary data analysis Measures/Variables: evaluate use of DNR orders in ICUs and age, controlling for illness severity Sample: adults aged 18–≥ 85 years	• Elders had more frequent orders to limit treatment than younger patients; 11.4% overall, increasing to 32.6% for elders over 85 years
Chelluri, Pinsky, Donahoe, & Grenvik (1993)	Design: prospective comparison of outcomes in patients 65–74 vs. ≥ 75 years Measures/Variables: long-term morbidity and mortality of critically-ill elders in ICUs Sample: adults aged ≥ 65 years (n = 97)	• Severity of illness was a greater predictor of mortality than age • No significant differences between groups on LOS, hospital charges, mortality, or QoL
Chelluri, Pinsky, & Grenvik (1992)	Design: retrospective chart review and follow-up telephone interview Measures/Variables: short and long-term outcomes for critically ill elders ≥ 85 years Sample: elders aged ≥ 85 (n = 34)	• 62% (21/34) survived to discharge from the hospital • 59% (10/17 able to be contacted) were still alive at follow-up of 18 ± 10 months (range = 1–32 months)
Cicirelli, MacLean, & Cox (2000)	Design: survey Measures/Variables: psychosocial and demographic characteristics, end-of-life decision preferences, responses to scenarios Sample: community dwelling elders aged 60–90 (n = 200)	• Age did not predict end-of-life treatment preferences • Significant influences were religiosity, value for preserving life, quality of life, fear of death, and locus of control • Safeguarding autonomy was very important
Elpern, Patterson, Gloskey, & Bone (1992)	Design: survey Measures/Variables: preferences for ICU care Sample: adults mean age 58 years (n = 84)	• Age did not predict desire to return to ICU

TABLE 7.4 *(continued)*

Author(s), date	Methods	Selected findings
Ely, Evans, & Haponik (1999)	Design: prospective cohort study Measures/Variables: mechanical ventilation and age Sample: adults ≥ 75 ($n = 63$) vs. ≤ 75 ($n = 237$)	• Elderly patients receiving mechanical ventilation had a lower cost of ICU care compared to younger patients
Hall & Rocker (2000)	Design: retrospective chart review Measures/Variables: use of technology, medications, and physician practice in end-of-life care of ICU patients Sample: adults in Canadian ICUs	• Elders had more frequent orders to limit treatment than younger patients
Hamel et al. (1996)	Design: prospective cohort Measures/Variables: age, resource use, severity of illness, life-support preference Sample: seriously ill adults ($n = 4301$), SUPPORT data (Phase I)	• Elders had fewer invasive procedures than younger patients • Hospital costs were lower for patients aged ≥ 80 years
Hamel, Davis, et al. (1999)	Design: secondary analysis of SUPPORT data Measures/Variables: age and short-term survival, controlling for baseline patient characteristics and aggressiveness of care Sample: seriously-ill adults ($n = 9105$), mean age 63	• Acute physiology and prognosis correlated more highly with increased mortality than age alone
Hamel, Teno, et al. (1999)	Design: prospective cohort Measures/Variables: age and decisions to withhold life-sustaining treatments Sample: SUPPORT study data; seriously-ill adults ($n = 9105$), mean age 63	• Elders had more frequent decisions to limit treatment than younger patients

(continued)

TABLE 7.4   *(continued)*

Author(s), date	Methods	Selected findings
Hanson & Danis (1991)	Design: retrospective chart review Measures/Variables: ICU and CPR utilization rates for elderly patients Sample: terminal admissions (n = 524) of adults aged 35–74 years vs. ≥ 75 years	• Elders admitted to ICU less often than younger patients • Nursing home residence, advanced malignancy, severe chronic illness, and older age independently predicted withholding ICU care
Jayes, Zimmerman, Wagner, Draper, & Knaus (1993)	Design: prospective inception cohort Measures/Variables: patient demographics and DNR orders in ICUs Sample: consecutive ICU admissions (n = 17,440) from 1988–1990	• Elders had more frequent orders to limit treatment than younger patients
Kass, Castriotta, & Malakoff (1992)	Design: cohort study Measures/Variables: age, previous functional status, severity of acute illness, acute (ICU) and long-term survival of elderly (≥ 85) Sample: elders aged ≥ 85 years (n = 105)	• Age and preadmission functional status not associated with increased ICU mortality • Severity of illness was associated with higher ICU mortality
Kleinpell & Ferrans (1998)	Design: retrospective chart review Measures/Variables: severity of illness demographics, survival of critically ill elders Sample: adults aged 45 and older (n = 275)	• Predictors of ICU nonsurvival were severity of illness, intubation, increased ICU LOS • Age was not a predictor of nonsurvival
Koch, Rodeffer, & Wears (1994)	Design: retrospective chart review Measures/Variables: terminal care management changes over time Sample: consecutive ICU admissions (n = 237) of adults (mean age 63 years) with terminal care decisions	• Elders had more frequent orders to limit treatment than younger patients

TABLE 7.4 *(continued)*

Author(s), date	Methods	Selected findings
Stillman, Braitman, & Grant (1998)	Design: vignette response comparison Measures/Variables: therapeutic aggressiveness Sample: internal medicine residents ($n = 46$) and practicing internists ($n = 41$)	• Elders with mental or physical impairment associated with age had more frequent orders to limit treatment
Wenger et al. (1995)	Design: secondary data analysis Measures/Variables: patient and hospital characteristics of DNR patients Sample: Medicare patients ($n = 14,008$), by diagnosis, with DNR orders (11.6%)	• Elders had more frequent orders to limit treatment than younger patients
Wu, Rubin, & Rosen (1990)	Design: retrospective chart review Measures/Variables: advanced age, severity of illness, mortality Sample: adults aged 55–65 years ($n = 135$) compared to adults aged ≥ 75 ($n = 130$)	• Older age did not predict mortality controlling for severity of illness, admitting diagnosis, and presence of underlying malignancy
Yu, Ash, Levinsky, & Moskowitz (2000)	Design: retrospective review of Medicare data Measures/Variables: age, ICU admissions, mortality Sample: > 65 years ($n = 89,667$)	• ICU use decreased with age, particularly for those > 85 years. The majority of the elderly survived at least 90 days.

DNR = do-not-resuscitate; ICU = intensive care unit; LOS = length of stay; QoL = quality of life; SUPPORT = Study to Understand Prognoses and Preferences for Outcomes and Risks of Treatments.

power of age and despite patient preferences of older adults that are similar to those of younger patients, limitations in treatment for critically ill older adults have been demonstrated (Table 7.4). Thus, while age by itself does not predict outcome of ICU care, the care given to older adults is generally less aggressive than care given to younger patients.

WHAT IS IMPORTANT TO FAMILIES OF DYING PATIENTS IN ACUTE CARE?

Family members of patients who have died in acute care hospitals and ICUs have been studied to gather their impressions of the process and the care delivered as well as their suggestions for improving care of the dying (Table 7.5). Families reported that in their last three days of life patients commonly suffered from pain, dyspnea, and fatigue, and most would have preferred comfort care, but nonetheless they received life-sustaining technical care. Factors leading to family satisfaction or dissatisfaction with care have been described (Table 7.5). Pierce was the only nurse researcher in this group.

In general, although family members are the appropriate persons to ask about their responses to, and satisfaction with, care, their interpretations of patient responses should be recognized as interpretations. For example, a family member's description of a patient's pain or other symptoms may be a misinterpretation or may reflect the family member's anxiety rather than the patient's pain. The data are important and they may be all researchers are able to obtain, particularly in retrospect after a patient death, but they are proxy, not primary, data.

WHAT IS IMPORTANT TO HEALTH CARE PROFESSIONALS CARING FOR DYING PATIENTS IN ICUS?

None of the studies that were found on care of dying ICU patients were specific to older adults (Table 7.6). All of the studies were about nursing care rather than care by other providers, and all but one (Asch, Shea, Jedrziewski, & Bosk, 1997) were conducted by nurses.

ICU nurses from Alberta, Canada, reported confusion about the meaning of DNR orders (Thibault-Prevost, Jensen, & Hodgins, 2000). The

TABLE 7.5   **Family Issues for Dying Patients in Acute Care Hospitals**

Author(s), date	Methods	Selected findings
Baker et al. (2000)	Design: randomized, controlled trial Measures/Variables: factors associated with family satisfaction with end-of-life care Sample: SUPPORT data Family members of seriously ill hospitalized adults ($n = 767$) who died	• 16% of families were dissatisfied with patient comfort • 30% were dissatisfied with communication and decision making
Jacobson et al. (1997)	Design: focus group interviews Objectives: explore family experiences of death of patient in hospital Sample: 46/81 "emergency contacts" or last address of deceased patients	• Most important issues to family members were: support and sensitivity from medical staff, access to the patient, communication, pain management, and advance directives
Johnson et al. (1998)	Design: descriptive survey Measures/Variables: family needs assessment Sample: Canadian next of kin ($n = 99$) and secondary family members ($n = 16$)	• Family satisfaction was increased with consistency of ICU providers (both nurses and physicians)
S. P. Keenan, Mawdsley, Plotkin, Webster, & Priestap (2000)	Design: survey Measures/Variables: family satisfaction after withdrawal of life support Sample: Canadian next of kin ($n = 29$)	• Family satisfaction increased with explanation of process of withdrawal, when death proceeded as expected, when patient appeared comfortable
Lynn et al. (1997)	Design: prospective cohort study Measures/Variables: surrogate decision makers perspectives on dying patients' experiences Sample: SUPPORT study data 73% of family members of deceased patients ($n = 3357$)	• 55% of patients were conscious in the last 3 days of life • Pain, dyspnea, and fatigue were commonly reported • Family members believed 70% of patients would have preferred comfort care, but 15% of these received life-sustaining care

(continued)

TABLE 7.5   *(continued)*

Author(s), date	Methods	Selected findings
Pierce (1999)	Design: qualitative interviews Variables: describe family members' suggestions for improvement of end-of-life care Sample: family members of decedents ($n = 29$)	• Most important issues to family members were: facilitate patient and family interaction, facilitate caregiver and patient/family interaction, create conducive caregiving setting, demonstrate respect for dying person's personhood

ICU = intensive care unit; SUPPORT = Study to Understand Prognoses and Preferences for Outcomes and Risks of Treatments.

major issue in most other studies of nurses and DNR patients in the ICU is how care differs before and after the DNR order is written or between patients with and without DNR orders. Tittle, Moody, and Becker (1992a, 1992b) found an increase in use of nursing resources after the DNR order. The resource they measured was focused on technology and did not include psychosocial care such as patient and family support. In intervention studies that involved an interdisciplinary team and moving DNR patients out of the ICU, Campbell and Field (1991) and Campbell and Thill-Baharozian (1994) showed that nursing intensity could be decreased. Again, the measure of nursing intensity was primarily a measure of technological support.

In several more recent studies a broader conceptualization of nursing resource use was applied and resource use diminished or was predicted to diminish after a DNR order (Keenan & Kish, 2000; Sherman & Branum, 1995). Nurses believed physical care should be less intense in DNR patients whereas psychosocial care should remain the same. This finding, that nurses expect different levels of the two types of care, helps to explain the seemingly contradictory findings of more and less treatment after the DNR order. There have been two types of study: One type is focused on technical care and the other type takes a broader view of nursing care. Findings differ depending on whether the study is focused narrowly on technical care or broadly on all kinds of care potentially needed. Nurses have approved of diminished levels of physical or medical care for patients with a DNR order, but have endorsed continued high levels of psychosocial supports.

TABLE 7.6   Studies of ICU Professionals' Care for Dying Patients

Author(s), date	Methods	Selected findings
Asch, Shea, Jedrziewski, & Bosk (1997)	Design: content analysis of mailed survey Measures/Variables: critical care nurses' views of euthanasia Sample: Random sample of U.S. critical care nurses ($n = 468$)	• Themes: importance of concerns of patients and families, and nurses' personal and professional; need improved physician behavior; need more clarity in end-of-life care; and importance of clinical, social, legal, and religious issues
Campbell & Field (1991)	Design: prospective descriptive study Measures/Variables: interdisciplinary terminal care team focused on physical, psychological, and spiritual needs of dying ICU patients and families Sample: mean age 68 ($n = 131$)	• Technological nursing care can be decreased by moving DNR patients out of ICU
Campbell & Thill-Baharozian (1994)	Design: prospective descriptive study Measures/Variables: DNR patient care requirements and outcomes Sample: mean age 63 ($n = 100$)	• Technological nursing care can be decreased by moving DNR patients out of ICU
C. H. Keenan & Kish (2000)	Design: descriptive study Measures/Variables: effect of DNR order on care of cancer patients in SICU Sample: Patients ($n = 23$) mean age 59	• ICU patients with cancer who had a DNR order received fewer medical interventions but had a constant level of supportive nursing care
Kirchhoff & Beckstrand (2000)	Design: mailed survey Measures/Variables: critical care nurses' perceptions of obstacles and helps to providing end-of-life care Sample: ICU nurses ($n = 199$)	• Obstacles: families' not understanding life-support, not accepting poor prognosis, requesting more technology than the patient desires, anger • Helps: agreement among health care team, dying with dignity, families' acceptance of prognoses

(continued)

TABLE 7.6 *(continued)*

Author(s), date	Methods	Selected findings
Kirchhoff et al. (2000)	Design: focus groups Objectives: ICU nurses' perceptions of end-of-life care for dying patients Sample: ICU nurses ($n = 21$)	• "Good" end-of-life care ensures patients' dignity and pain control, family involvement, clear prognosis, continuity of care providers
McClement & Degner (1995)	Design: exploratory interview Objectives: identify expert nursing behaviors in care of adults dying in ICUs Sample: ICU nurses ($n = 10$)	• Six critical nursing behaviors: responding after death, responding to the family and colleagues, responding to anger, facilitating transition to palliation, comfort
Sherman & Branum (1995)	Design: descriptive, cross-sectional Measures/Variables: ICU nurses' perceptions of appropriate care for patients with and without DNR Sample: ICU nurses ($n = 87$)	• ICU nurses believed physical care should be less intense in DNR patients but psychosocial care should remain the same
Thibault-Prevost, Jensen, & Hodgins (2000)	Design: survey Measures/Variables: nurses' perceptions of DNR decisions in ICU Sample: ICU nurses ($n = 405$)	• The meaning of DNR orders was confusing/ambiguous and rationale for DNR orders was poorly articulated
Tittle, Moody, & Becker (1992a; 1992b)	Design: prospective descriptive study Measures/Variables: ICU resource allocation before and after DNR Sample: 62 ICU patients with DNR (convenience sample; mean age 74), 62 ICU patients without DNR (random sample; mean age 68)	• Technology and nursing resource use (e.g., frequency of vital signs) and LOS increased after DNR • Aggressive treatment (e.g., mechanical ventilation) often continued after DNR

DNR = do not resuscitate; ICU = intensive care unit; LOS = length of stay; SICU = surgical intensive care unit; SUPPORT = Study to Understand Prognoses and Preferences for Outcomes and Risks of Treatments; US = United States.

In other studies of nurses caring for dying ICU patients, researchers have investigated a variety of topics: nurses' experiences with end-of-life care, how nurses define expert care in this realm, and what nurses perceive as helpful or not for such patients. Asch, Shea, Jedrziewski, and Bosk (1997) assessed critical care nurses' views on euthanasia. The comments nurses provided, however, were more general, about "critical care nurses' views of hospital care at the end of life" (p. 1661). The authors concluded that nurses were frustrated at their limited role in end-of-life care management and were confused about appropriate care. Some worked in ICU environments that did not foster excellence in end-of-life care. Three studies of ICU nurses' perceptions of good and poor end-of-life care were found (Kirchhoff & Beckstrand, 2000; Kirchhoff et al., 2000; McClement & Degner, 1995). In most cases, interactions between nurses and families could be facilitated by nurses' attending to patient and family needs.

WHAT INFLUENCES DECISION MAKING AT THE END OF LIFE FOR ICU PATIENTS?

Reviews of the End-of-Life Decision-Making Literature

Two reviews of end-of-life decision making about adult ICU patients in general were found. Cook (1997) reviewed the research on DNR orders and other treatment directives about life support in ICUs. She noted that ICU decisions are distinguished from decisions in other health care areas by greater urgency and uncertainty, a continually changing environment, and higher costs. From the studies reviewed she highlighted disagreements among health care professionals about decisions they would make, weak correlations between provider and patient choices, and the importance of the providers' manner of presenting information about choices. She concluded that there is a need for qualitative research to study behavior, perceptions, and values in end-of-life decision making. Covinsky and colleagues (2000) reviewed the SUPPORT data and found that providers and families were often unaware of what patients wanted, and care delivered was inconsistent with patient wishes.

Three reviews specific to end-of-life treatment decision making in critically ill older patients were located. Clarke, Goldstein, and Raffin

(1994) highlighted four ethical dilemmas identified in the literature that are key for older patients: ICU care and whether age restrictions are appropriate; outcomes of CPR in older adult versus younger patients, where the research findings from different studies are contradictory; appropriate use of DNR orders; and a search for ways to improve patient and provider communication about end-of-life decisions. Their conclusion was that "elderly people in the United States often receive treatment through an enormous array of medical technology when they become critically ill. Some, or all, such interventions may be unwanted, and patients have the right to be informed" (p. 99).

Schecter (1994) reviewed literature on life support decisions for geriatric surgical patients, where the most rapidly growing group is octogenarians. His focus was how to improve decision making about limiting treatment to older adults. He concluded with his principles for good decision making: patients deserve a diagnosis, prognosis is usually uncertain, consider potential risks and benefits, respect patient autonomy, be cautious, communicate, try to understand the patient's values, and achieve consensus. Prendergast (1997), after a similar review not focused on older adults, concluded that a fiduciary model, committing the physician to patient interests but maintaining the physician's role in defining those interests, is better than decision making based on futility. Most recently Baggs and Mick (2000), who are nurses, reviewed the literature on ethical issues for older ICU patients near the end of life. They concluded that collaborative decision making involving health care professionals, patients, and families has the potential to improve the decision making.

What Is the Epidemiology of Limitation-of-Treatment Decisions for ICU Patients?

In a series of studies, the increasing use of DNR orders in ICUs and lack of patient participation in decision making has been described, primarily by physician authors (Table 7.7). None of the studies focused solely on older adults. Smedira and colleagues (1990, Table 7.1) demonstrated that 45% of ICU patients had life-supporting treatments withdrawn or withheld before death. Few patients but many families were involved in decision making. Daly and colleagues (1996, Table 7.7), in the sole nurse-led study in this group, compared patients in a special care unit for the chronically critically ill with other ICU patients and found no difference in frequency

TABLE 7.7   Epidemiology of Treatment-Limitation Decisions in ICU Patients

Study author(s), date of publication	Methods	Selected findings
Daly et al. (1996)	Design: randomized, prospective study Measures/Variables: frequency of DNR orders in chronically critically ill, patient characteristics, cost, practice differences in two types of unit Sample: ICU patients ($n = 75$) vs. special care patients ($n = 145$) mean age 64	• 43% of patients had DNR orders in both settings
Jayes et al. (1993)	See Table 7.4.	• Rates of DNR in ICU patients increased over time
Koch et al. (1994)	See Table 7.4.	• Rates of DNR in ICU patients increased over time
McLean, Tarshis, Mazer, & Szalai (2000)	Design: retrospective chart review Measures/Variables: ICU deaths, 1988 vs. 1993, 2 Canadian hospitals Sample: 439 charts of deceased patients Males mean age 55 years, females mean age 62 years	• Withdrawal of life support in ICU increased (43% to 66% in Hospital A; 46% to 80% at Hospital B) over time
Prendergast & Luce (1997)	See Table 7.1.	• Limitation of life support increased from 51% during 1987–88 to 90% during 1992–93
Smedira et al. (1990)	See Table 7.1.	• 45% of patients dying in ICU had life-support treatments withheld or withdrawn before death • 4% of patients were involved in the decision to limit treatment • 87% of families were involved in the decision to limit treatment

DNR = do not resuscitate; ICU = intensive care unit.

of DNR orders. Prendergast and Luce (1997, Table 7.1) studied patients in the same units studied earlier by Smedira and colleagues. They compared patients who died in 1992–93 versus 1987–88. They reported an increase in limitation of life support, little patient participation in decision making, and minimal use of advance directives. In similar studies comparing ICU treatment withdrawal over periods in both the U.S. and Canada from the 1980s through the 1990s (Table 7.7), others have found increasing rates of DNR orders (Jayes et al., 1993; Koch et al., 1994; McLean, Tarshis, Mazer, & Szalai, 2000; Prendergast et al., 1998).

What Is the Process for Limitation of Treatments in ICUs?

The process of forgoing life-supporting treatment in acute care or ICU patients was described in a number of research studies from 1990 to 2000, primarily by physician researchers (Table 7.8). None of the studies focused solely on older patients. Faber-Langendoen and Bartels (1992) studied patients who died in acute care hospitals and noted that "it is often not until a patient is unable to interact with others that the wisdom of further aggressive therapy is questioned" (p. 574). The researchers concluded that this decision making is not one discrete event but occurs over several days and involves multiple decisions. This is supported by the work of others (Lee, Swinburne, Fedullo, & Wahl, 1994). In another U.S. study, a distinct sequence of withdrawal of forms of life support was identified (Asch, Faber-Langendoen, Shea, & Christakis, 1999). Canadian findings about limitation of treatment are similar (Heyland, Lavery, Tranmer, Shortt, & Taylor, 2000; S. P. Keenan et al., 1997; 1998; McLean et al., 2000; Wood & Martin, 1995).

Wide variability in limiting treatment has been found, in both factors influencing decisions and decisions made (Cook et al., 1995; Jayes, Zimmerman, Wagner, & Knaus, 1996; Prendergast et al., 1998; Walter et al., 1998; Wenger et al.). In one study of level of care at the end of life in the hospital, patients designated to receive comfort care received less aggressive care, but there was no standard treatment (Goodlin, Winzelberg, Teno, Whedon, & Lynn, 1998).

Four studies described below were undertaken for different reasons, considered different aspects of decision making, and used different methods. Yet they are linked by the researchers' attempts to discover and describe aspects of limitation-of-treatment decision making. Jezewski,

TABLE 7.8   Process for Limitation of ICU Treatments

Author(s), date	Methods	Selected findings
Asch, Faber-Langendoen, Shea, & Christakis (1999)	Design: retrospective chart review Measures/Variables: order of withdrawal of life-sustaining treatments Sample: 211 consecutive dying patients, adults mean age 66 years	• Rank order of withdrawal (earliest to latest): blood products, hemodialysis, vasopressors, mechanical ventilation, total parenteral nutrition, antibiotics, intravenous fluids, tube feedings
Cook, Giacomini, Johnson, & Willms, for the Canadian Critical Care Trials Group (1999)	Design: qualitative, naturalistic inquiry; participant observation and interviews Objectives: explore why advanced life support is withheld, provided, continued, or withdrawn in ICU Sample: 25 ICU rounds, 11 family meetings, interviews with ICU care providers ($n = 26$)	• Life-support technologies, presumed to treat illness and prevent death, may also be used to orchestrate the dying process
Cook, et al., for the Canadian Critical Care Trials Group (1995)	Design: cross-sectional survey Measures/Variables: health care workers' attitudes about withdrawing life support Sample: ICU care providers ($n = 1314$) in 37 Canadian university-affiliated hospitals	• Factors used by health care providers for limitation of treatment decisions were found to be extremely variable
Faber-Langendoen (1996)	See Table 7.1.	• The DNR order was found to be the first step in making treatment limitation decisions
Faber-Langendoen & Bartels (1992)	Design: retrospective chart review Measures/Variables: patient demographics, range and sequence of treatments withheld or withdrawn Sample: deceased patients ($n = 70$). Acute care non-ICU and pediatric patients were included	• 27% of patients participated in decision making • Often, aggressive therapy was not addressed until patients were unable to interact with others

(*continued*)

TABLE 7.8   *(continued)*

Author(s), date	Methods	Selected findings
Goodlin, Winzelberg, Teno, Whedon, & Lynn (1998)	Design: retrospective chart review Measures/Variables: symptoms and treatments in last 2 days of life in hospitalized adults Sample: deceased patients (n = 104), mean age 68.9 years	• 46% had pain • 51% had dyspnea and restlessness or agitation • 12% had CPR • 27% received ventilator support • 18% were restrained • 48% had order or note specifying comfort measures only • Patients receiving comfort care received less aggressive care
Heyland, Lavery, Tranmer, Shortt, & Taylor (2000)	Design: cross sectional analysis of Canadian death records, 1997 Measures/Variables: Place of death Sample: deaths (n = 201, 892) in Canada during 1997	• 73% of deaths occurred in hospital, 18.6% of these were in ICUs • In 1950, 45% of Canadians died in hospital
Jayes, Zimmerman, Wagner, & Knaus (1996)	Design: prospective inception cohort Measures/Variables: frequency of DNR; terminal care guidelines and qualitative observations, 9 ICUs Sample: 42 US ICUs, consecutive ICU admissions (n = 17,440)	• Treatment limitation practices were found to be variable
Jezewski, Scherer, Miller, & Battista (1993)	Design: grounded theory Objectives: ICU nurses' perspectives of patients'/families' DNR decisions Sample: ICU nurses (n = 22)	• Core category: gaining consent for DNR orders • Intervening conditions: meaning of DNR, importance of time and timing, nurse's role, conflicts

TABLE 7.8   *(continued)*

Author(s), date	Methods	Selected findings
Kaufman (1998)	Design: ethnography Objectives: to study dying elderly patients in ICUs Sample: 80 ICU patients over age 50 observed, 3 case studies	• See text
S. P. Keenan et al. (1997)	Design: retrospective cohort study Measures/Variables: patients who died in Canadian ICU after limiting life support Sample: ICU deaths ($n = 419$), adults mean age 62.7	• 70% of patients died after limitation of treatment
S. P. Keenan et al., for the Southwestern Ontario Critical Care Research Network (1998)	Design: prospective cohort study, retrospective chart review Measures/Variables: withdrawing and withholding life support in teaching and community hospital ICUs Sample: community ($n = 160$) vs. teaching hospital deaths ($n = 292$)	• 71% of community hospital deaths and 68% of teaching hospital deaths followed limitation of life-supporting treatments
Lee, Swinburne, Fedullo, & Wahl (1994)	Design: retrospective case series Measures/Variables: process and outcome of withdrawing and withholding life support in community hospital MICU Sample: mean age 71 years ($n = 28$)	• Treatment limitation discussions occurred over an average of 5 days
McLean et al. (2000)	See Table 7.7.	• Treatment limitation decisions were reported as 66% and 80% at 2 different tertiary care ICUs

(continued)

TABLE 7.8   *(continued)*

Author(s), date	Methods	Selected findings
Prendergast et al. (1998)	See Table 7.1.	• Wide variation in practice of end-of-life treatment limitations, see also Table 1 findings
Prendergast & Luce (1997)	See Table 7.1.	• End-of-life decision-making is not one discrete event but occurs over several days and involves multiple decisions
Simmonds (1996)	Design: grounded theory Objectives: nurse/physician experiences working with dying ICU patients Sample: nurses ($n = 7$), house staff ($n = 6$), and attending physicians ($n = 8$)	• All believed over treatment of ICU patients was common • None wanted life-prolonging, technical treatment for selves or family when they were dying • Physicians reported it was easier to continue aggressive treatment than to have discussions with families about limiting treatment
Smedira et al. (1990)	See Table 7.1.	• End-of-life decision-making is not one discrete event but occurs over several days and involves multiple decisions
Walter et al., for the Canadian Critical Care Trials Group (1998)	Design: cross-sectional survey Measures/Variables: ICU health care workers confidence in decisions to limit life support Sample: Canadian ICU workers; ICU intensivists ($n = 149$), house staff ($n = 142$), and nurses ($n = 1070$)	• Providers chose a level of care for patients described in a scenario. In less extreme scenarios, responses were variable, and providers were confident

TABLE 7.8   *(continued)*

Author(s), date	Methods	Selected findings
Wenger et al. (1995)	See Table 7.4.	• Treatment limitation practices were found to be variable
Wilson (1997)	Design: retrospective chart review and caregiver interview Measures/Variables: inpatient end-of-life care, Alberta Canada Sample: deceased patients mean age 70.9 ($n = 137$), caregivers ($n = 60$)	• Impending, certain death was heralded by irreversible unconsciousness (93% of cases); in all cases, DNR orders were written after unconsciousness occurred
Wood & Martin (1995)	Design: prospective observational study Measures/Variables: rationale and procedures for limiting life-sustaining treatments for Canadian ICU patients Sample: ICU deaths ($n = 110$); mean age 66.5	• The DNR order was found to be the first step in making treatment limitation decisions; 64.5% died after treatment was limited

CPR = cardiopulmonary resuscitation; DNR = do not resuscitate; ICU = intensive care unit; LOS = length of stay; MICU = medical intensive care unit; US = United States.

Scherer, Miller, and Battista (1993), a group of nurse researchers, studied critical care nurses who described their experiences with the process of gaining consent for DNR orders. They described the role of the nurse as ascertaining whether the time is right to approach patients and families, establishing a trusting relationship, providing information, supporting family decision making, and brokering interactions of families and patients with physicians or among family members. They concluded by noting the absence of similar studies from the perspectives of others involved in this process. A later study by Simmonds (1996), a nurse researcher, involved interviews with ICU care providers about their experiences working with dying patients.

Cook, Giacomini, Johnson, Willms, and the Canadian Critical Care Trials Group (1999) conducted a qualitative descriptive investigation of the purposes of life-support technologies. They found that decisions about technology are part of a process to "synchronize understanding and expectations" (p. 1109) between family members and clinicians. Orchestration by technology was described as a way to modify the "aesthetic, ethical, and social experiences" of those involved in patient care: significant others, family, and clinicians.

Kaufman (1998) conducted an ethnographic study of older dying patients in a community hospital ICU. Hers is the only one of these qualitative studies focused on older adults. The findings from this study, therefore, are particularly relevant to the topic at hand, end-of-life care for older patients in ICUs. Kaufman observed 80 ICU patients over 50, 31 of whom died. She noted the current interest in dying, including an emphasis on the abstract concept of "death with dignity." She found that in the reality of technology of critical care, "death with dignity" is irrelevant. More important were ambivalence about what decisions to make as the patient became more ill and ambiguity about "goals as death approaches" (p. 716). She noted that older adults who die in the ICU represent patients whom physicians and families hoped to treat successfully and hesitated to define as dying. Kaufman identified the sources of problems with older adults who die in the ICU as: the commitment of the ICU setting to full therapeutic treatment, the power of medicine "as cultural knowledge," the commitment to action in treatment, and the "incommensurability of lay and medical worlds." Kaufman concluded that biomedicine has become the framework for understanding death and dying, that physicians orchestrate dying, and that they often do not acknowledge that the patient is dying until the end is near. Discussion of treatment limitation, then, becomes their way of allowing the dying process to begin. This process is only allowed "when outcomes of specific treatments are repeatedly negative and the patient has an obviously downward course" (p. 721). She observed that family members are unprepared for the type of decisions they are asked to make, do not understand terminology such as "code status," and face choices that arise from biomedicine, not from the families' world of experience. The family cannot provide the immediate, simple answers that care providers seek. Technical information does not alter the ambivalence and ambiguity of the lay person. Kaufman's recommendations were that only through a reconsideration of medicine's dominant role, a reshaping of institutional practices and values, and an acknowledgement that the life-to-death transition is highly variable will we begin to improve this process.

It is clear from these studies that decision making about the end of life is complex and difficult for everyone involved, and that control rests primarily with care providers. Discussion of limitation-of-treatment decision making occurs primarily when patients no longer have the capacity to participate.

How Are Health Care Providers Involved in End-of-Life Decision Making in ICUs?

Several researchers have investigated the factors that influence ICU care providers' end-of-life decision making (Table 7.9) (Cook et al., 1995; Society of Critical Care Medicine [SCCM] Ethics Committee, 1992). Despite evidence that age by itself is not a good predictor of outcome, it is used by ICU physicians to make decisions about limitation of life-sustaining treatment.

Differences in decision making by discipline and practice locale have been studied (Eliasson, Howard, Torrington, Dillard, & Phillips, 1997; SCCM Ethics Committee, 1992; Walter et al., 1998). Physicians were more willing than nurses to limit treatment, and those in academic practice were more willing to limit than those in private practice. ICU nurses' involvement in end-of-life decision making seldom has been described (Hiltunen et al., 1995; Kennard et al., 1996; Thibault-Prevost et al., 2000). This is an area in need of further exploration.

Solomon and colleagues (1993) surveyed acute care hospital nurses and physicians who worked "with critically and terminally ill adults" (p. 15). Few thought staff had found out what patients wanted, that patients understood the information, or that patients got the help they needed in decision making. The researchers concluded that more interdisciplinary discussion is needed. The lack of satisfaction reported by providers in this study may be explained in part by the work of Asch, Hansen-Flaschen, and Lanken (1995). They found that many ICU physicians made life-sustaining treatment decisions without the knowledge or consent of patient or family. Although such decisions may be comfortable for the attending physician, they may be dissatisfying for other members of the health care team.

How Are Families Involved in End-of-Life Decision Making in ICUs?

None of the studies of families involved in end-of-life decision making in the ICU were focused on older patients; all used some form of qualitative

TABLE 7.9   Health Care Providers' Involvement in End-of-Life Decision Making in ICUs

Author(s), date	Methods	Selected findings
Asch, Hansen-Flaschen, & Lanken (1995)	Design: survey Measures/Variables: futility, limiting life-support treatments, decision making, concurrence of patients/surrogates Sample: US ICU physicians (n = 879)	• 34% of ICU physicians continued life-sustaining treatments despite family/patients wish to stop • 82–83% of physicians stopped treatment unilaterally because treatment was "futile"
Cook et al. (1995)	See Table 7.8.	• Important factors in limitation decisions: chance of survival, premorbid cognitive function, age
Eliasson, Howard, Torrington, Dillard, & Phillips (1997)	Design: opinion survey Measures/Variables: DNR decisions, nurse/physician agreement/disagreement Sample: 368 medical ICU admissions; mean age 61	• Academic physicians more likely to limit life-sustaining treatments than private practice physicians
Hiltunen et al. (1995)	See Table 7.1. The SUPPORT Principal Investigators (1995) Report of study nurses' roles end-of-life decision making	• Staff nurses underestimate patients' value of their health, but were accurate in estimating patients' rating of health
Kennard et al. (1996)	Design: Survey. See Table 7.1. The SUPPORT Principal Investigators (1995) Measures/Variables: nurses' roles in decision-making for patients at end of life Sample: 696 nurses; 50% ICU nurses	• Nurses found to be actively involved in end-of-life decision-making process of dying patients

(continued)

TABLE 7.9 *(continued)*

Author(s), date	Methods	Selected findings
Society of Critical Care Medicine Ethics Committee (1992)	Design: survey/questionnaire Measures/Variables: critical care professionals' attitudes about forgoing life-sustaining treatments in critically-ill patients Sample: SCCM conference registrants ($n = 600$); 84% physicians, 11% nurses, 5% other critical care professionals	• 96% would withhold or withdraw • Influential factors: patient's QoL, likelihood of survival, comorbidity • For 43%, age not a consideration, for 40% it was important, for 12% very important • Age more important to physicians • Physicians more willing to limit
Solomon et al. (1993)	Design: survey Measures/Variables: nurse/physician views on life-sustaining treatments Sample: physicians ($n = 687$) and nurses ($n = 759$) from 5 US acute care hospitals	• 1/3 of respondents satisfied with patient participation in end-of-life decision making • Physicians most satisfied, nurses least; house officers about as satisfied as nurses • Respondents were troubled by over- rather than under-treatment
Thibault-Prevost et al. (2000)	See Table 7.6.	• ICU nurses believe patients, families, and nurses should be involved in DNR decisions, but that physicians are responsible
Walter et al. (1998)	See Table 7.8.	• Academic practice physicians are more likely to limit life-sustaining treatments than private practice

DNR = do not resuscitate; ICU = intensive care unit; QoL = quality of life; SCCM = Society of Critical Care Medicine; SUPPORT = Study to Understand Prognoses and Preferences for Outcomes and Risks of Treatments; US = United States.

analysis; and all but one (Miller, Coe, & Hyers, 1992) were nursing studies (Table 7.10). This last analysis, written by two physicians and a PhD, assessed the situation much more simplistically than Kaufman's (1998) work described above.

Four qualitative studies by nurse researchers involved interviews of families who had made, or who were in the process of making, limitation-of-treatment decisions. Two studies were retrospective (Jacob, 1998; Tilden, Tolle, Garland, & Nelson, 1995). Two were conducted with family decision makers during the decision-making process (Reckling, 1997; Swigart, Lidz, Butterworth, & Arnold, 1996). The quality of family-to-provider interactions stands out in all these studies as crucial to the decision-making process, to satisfaction with the process, and to the ability of families to live comfortably with the decisions made.

HOW CAN END-OF-LIFE CARE AND DECISION MAKING BE IMPROVED

Methodological Articles

Three methodological articles were found that were designed to assist care providers trying to improve care and researchers studying end-of-life care and decision making. None of them were focused on older adults or ICUs, but they could be helpful conceptually. Donaldson and Field (1998) and Morrison, Siu, Leipzig, Cassel, and Meier (2000) wrote about measuring quality of care at the end of life. Heyland, Tranmer, and Feldman-Stewart (2000) proposed an "organizing framework" for end-of-life decision making. In a preliminary study to assess whether the identified analytic steps (information exchange, deliberation, and decision making) could be measured in seriously ill patients, they found that they could measure some identified aspects. In general, the patients had considered end-of-life issues, few had held discussions with their physicians, few had advance directives, and most were willing to discuss the topic with physicians and wanted to be involved in decision making.

Intervention Studies

In a review of studies of clinical interventions at the end of life, the interventions were found not to be research based and, for the most part,

TABLE 7.10   Family Involvement in End-of-Life Decision Making in ICUs

Author(s), date	Methods	Selected findings
Jacob (1998)	Design: grounded theory analysis of interview Objectives: describe and explain family members' experiences of end-of-life decision making Sample: family members ($n =$ 17) involved in limitation decisions for ICU patient who died in ICU within preceding year	• Decision-making was burdensome but they wanted to be involved • Decision-making was easier with a sense of patient's wishes • Patient's history and future life were important • Families were comforted by a feeling of working harmoniously with providers • Quality of interaction between care providers and family facilitated the family's acceptance
Kaufman (1998)	See Table 7.8.	• See text
Miller, Coe, & Hyers (1992)	Design: conversational analysis of audiotaped family meetings Objectives: examine decision-making process about limiting life support Sample: physicians and family members of 15 critically ill patients; 7 patients able to participate	• "Patient's wishes" central theme • Physicians gave direct, clear information on the patient's situation in lay language and described possible treatment options in unbiased manner • Physicians narrowed treatment options to those they judged best • Families often, but not always, agreed
Reckling (1997)	Design: participant observation, interview, case study Objectives: explore activities related to withholding or withdrawing ICU treatments; patients without capacity Sample: critical informants (family members and health care professionals) for ICU patients ($n = 10$)	• Physicians always raised the question about limiting treatment with families in this study • Participants' roles in advocating or resisting treatment limitation decisions was explored

TABLE 7.10   *(continued)*

Author(s), date	Methods	Selected findings
Swigart, Lidz, Butterworth, & Arnold (1996)	Design: Grounded theory analysis of interviews Objectives: describe family decision making about life support in ICUs Sample: family members ($n = 30$) of critically ill patients ($n = 16$)	• Processes: understanding the critical illness, reviewing the patient's life, and maintaining family roles and relationships
Tilden, Tolle, Garland, & Nelson (1995)	Design: content analysis of interviews Objectives: exploration of physician and nurse behaviors that supported or increased burden of family decision making about ICU patients Sample: family members ($n = 32$) of ICU patients without advance directives who died 2–6 months earlier	• Helpful provider behaviors: encouraging advance planning, timely communication, clarification of families' roles, facilitating family consensus, accommodation of family grief • Burdensome behaviors: putting off discussions about limitation, delaying withdrawal, asking for one family member to make decisions, withdrawing from the family, presenting death as failure

ICU = intensive care unit.

were focused on numbers of advance directives completed (Hanson, Tulsky, & Danis, 1997). In the SUPPORT study (1995, Table 7.1) nurse facilitators were hired to improve patient to family to physician communication about end-of-life wishes. None of the outcome variables studied were changed by this intervention. No nurses were involved in the original formulation for this study, which may have been one reason for the lack of success of a nurse intervention.

The possibility that advance directives are associated with treatment differences at the end of life has been investigated using SUPPORT and other data (Table 7.11). Only modest, if any, effects in limiting treatment have been found (Goodman, Tarnoff, & Slotman, 1998; Teno et al., 1994;

TABLE 7.11   Improving End-of-Life Care and Decision Making in ICUs: Intervention Studies

Author(s), date	Methods	Selected findings
Dowdy, Robertson, & Bander (1998)	Design: prospective, controlled study Measures/Variables: effect of proactive ethics consultation on patient care communication and decision making about ICU patients Sample: ICU patients ($n = 99$) on continuous mechanical ventilation > 4 days; mean age 63.2 years	• Ethics consultation resulted in more frequent communications, more decisions to limit life supports, and decreased ICU LOS
Goodman, Tarnoff, & Slotman (1998)	Design: retrospective chart review Measures/Variables: effect of advance directives on treatment of elderly, critically ill patients Sample: 401 records; adults aged ≥ 65	• Advance directives were rarely present (5%) and had no effect on level of care delivered
Holloran, Starkey, Burke, Steele, & Forse (1995)	Design: descriptive Measures/Variables: effect of case-based medical ethics educational program	• SICU LOS decreased by 46% between 1990 and 1994 • Ethics discussions occurred earlier and more frequently when the program was in place
Lilly et al. (2000)	Design: prospective, change-of-practice intervention Measures/Variables: use of a communication process (interdisciplinary team meeting intervention) to consider use of advanced support technology Sample: before intervention cases ($n = 134$), postintervention cases ($n = 396$); adults mean age 60 (preintervention), 58 (postintervention)	• Intervention was a proactive, interdisciplinary, "intensive communication" for MICU patients with predicted LOS > 5 days, high predicted mortality, or likely irreversible loss of functional status • ICU care providers met with patients/families within 72 hours of admission • Intervention facilitated earlier access to palliative care

(continued)

TABLE 7.11 *(continued)*

Author(s), date	Methods	Selected findings
Schneiderman, Gilmer, & Teetzel (2000)	Design: prospective, randomized, controlled study Measures/Variables: ethics consultation: intervention and benefits; ICU LOS and treatments to patients who fail to survive to hospital discharge Sample: ICU patients ($n = 74$) with "values based conflicts"	• Ethics consultation was associated with decreased ICU LOS and fewer treatments for patients who died
Teno et al. (1994)	See Table 7.1. The SUPPORT Principal Investigators (1995). This report refers to SUPPORT Phase I data only	• There was no association between advance directives and resuscitation decisions or resource use
Teno et al. (2000)	See Table 7.1. The SUPPORT Principal Investigators (1995).	• Patients were more likely to receive care consistent with preferences when they discussed those preferences with physicians

ICU = intensive care unit; LOS = length of stay; MICU = medical intensive care unit; SICU = surgical intensive care unit; SUPPORT = Study to Understand Prognoses and Preferences for Outcomes and Risks of Treatments.

Teno et al., 2000). This minimal influence may be because some patients have advance directives that they have neither shared nor discussed with their physicians. It is clear from the studies reviewed that physicians take a major role in the decision making.

Three interventions for ICUs have been described, each quite different from the others. Each could be helpful in improvement of end-of-life care decision (Table 7.11). In the sole nurse-developed intervention, Holloran, Starkey, Burke, Steele, and Forse (1995) developed an interdisciplinary, case-based educational program for surgical residents during their SICU rotation. Two groups have studied the impact of proactive ethics consultation (Dowdy, Robertson, & Bander, 1998; Schneiderman, Gilmer, & Teetzel, 2000). The third intervention involved patients, families, and care providers (Lilly et al., 2000) in a family meeting to review the medical situation, discuss the patients' wishes, and agree on a care plan and criteria for judging success or failure of the plan with time frames for assessment. Further meetings were held based on these time frames. All these interventions were interdisciplinary, but outcomes measured were limited primarily to patient length of stay and mortality.

RESULTS AND DISCUSSION

What Are the Implications of the Studies Reviewed for Research?

There are few studies of the end-of-life experiences of older patients in ICUs, and 50% of ICU patients are 65 or older (Chelluri et al. 1995). In addition, most deaths occur in persons who are aged, and many deaths occur in ICUs. In light of the large number of the aged who may die in ICUs, this lack of research represents a critical gap in the literature. Attention is needed to older adults in ICUs at the end of life, to assure that samples are representative of the populations studied. Age should be a variable in studies of adult ICU patients, and researchers should analyze data considering whether age is a differentiating variable.

Both qualitative and quantitative research studies are needed to assess end-of-life treatment focusing on older patients at the end of life in ICUs. The mechanism by which age functions to affect care chosen needs further exploration, particularly in light of the absence of an independent effect of age on patient outcome. The influence of age could be on patient choice (although most studies suggest this is unlikely), on family choice, or on provider decision making.

The experience of patients, families, and providers should be explored and how those experiences change with interventions. The influence of the culture of the ICU, variation in decisions made and reasons for that variation, the process of decision making, and variation in treatment, all require further attention.

Based on research conducted with lay persons, patients, families, and care providers (see Table 7.2), four domains were identified for research needed to improve care for older adults at the end of life in intensive care. Each of these domains needs further work. One domain would involve assessments of the best ways to relieve symptoms, such as pain, dyspnea, fatigue, and anxiety. This research should, whenever possible, involve primary data collection from patients. A second domain would involve assessment of ways to improve communication, to transmit information clearly and in an understandable way to patients and families to support decision making. Timeliness and timing of communications should be studied. Also included in this domain would be further assessment of the appropriate ways to access and honor advance directives, including both signed documents and verbal communications with other care providers, family, and friends. Although the emphasis in this review was not on physiology, there are physiological changes with aging, among them sensory and cognitive changes, that may influence both patients and close family members in ways that would affect communication.

A third domain to be studied would be psychological support, assisting patients to achieve a sense of control, to accept and prepare for death with a sense of purpose. A fourth domain would involve assessing ways to improve interactions and relationships among providers, among patients and family members, and between these two groups. A study of the effect of promoting family visiting, touching, and participation in care would be one possibility. The quality of interactions (respectful, empathic, and holistic), should be measured, and the importance of those qualities considered. Ways should be sought to improve understanding of patient's wishes when patients are aware but voiceless, and to interpret those wishes.

Crossing this domain of relationships and the domain of decision making is study of what it means to share decision making with patients and families and with various members of the health care team. If decision making is collaborative or shared, where should control lie, and are physicians willing to give up some of the control they currently have? Improving this process probably will require framing it differently so that the knowledge of clinicians and lay persons is valued more equally and the discussions are held on a different and more level playing field. Moving the discussions to an earlier point in the process, through recognition that discussion should begin before death is inevitable, is also supported by the research findings.

Baggs and Schmitt (2000), both nurses, reviewed end-of-life decision studies in adult ICUs and found that most research has been retrospective, few researchers have considered nurses' involvement in decision making, and most have concerned either providers, or patients and families, but not both. Thus, prospective research that considers involvement of patients, families, and all relevant providers is needed. It is important to assess why so few patients are involved in end-of-life decision making. It may be that earlier discussions could be held, in the ICU or before ICU admission, or at any opportunity when the patient is able to participate. Research about why this does not appear to happen is needed.

There are other questions not yet studied. For example, no one has assessed whether the ICU is a good place for this transition to palliation to occur or whether it would be better for patients to be transferred to some other type of unit at some point in this transition. If so, what type of unit should that be? It may be that only in the ICU can many of these patients receive the intense nursing care needed. Transfer would also affect continuity of care, which has been identified by families as important to their assessment of the quality of care.

Intervention research is needed to assess how care and decision making might be improved. The current intervention research has focused on the outcomes of length of stay and mortality, which do not begin to support understanding of how patients, families, and providers experience the effects of these interventions. Testing of interventions is encouraging for the development of the field of research and treatment for patients dying in ICUs.

Development of interventions will require attention to types of ICUs where care is delivered, types of hospitals in which they are located, and individual unit characteristics. Very little attention has been paid to the effect of differences in unit culture on end-of-life care. This also raises the issue of different types of ICU, an issue ignored in most studies, which are either based in one type of unit or aggregate data from multiple types of units. Are cultural differences based on the institution or on the hospital? Are MICUs generally different from SICUs and other types of units? Is the unit culture a function of institution, type of ICU, or a more individualized feature such as the leadership style of the manager?

Nurses are struggling with how to deliver high-quality care to dying patients and indicate a wish to be more involved as decisions are made about limiting treatments. They have opinions about how this might occur. Researchers could assess ways to empower nurses to implement their interventions and examine outcomes of patients, families, and other providers.

What Are the Implications of the Studies Reviewed for Practice?

The same domains, increasing comfort, improving decision making, offering psychological support, and improving interactions and communication also should be attended to in order to improve practice. Sensitivity to the patient-family perspective is essential, including sensitivity to the physical, sensory, and cognitive changes associated with aging. Proactive interventions that make changes systematic rather than reliance on multiple, individual judgments appear to offer hope for the future. Finding ways to improve family access to patients, and to maintain continuity and high-quality care is a challenge. The best chances for improved care for older adults in ICUs at the end of life appear to rest in collaborative, interdisciplinary, holistic efforts to bring comfort to patients and families and to improve communications and interactions among all participants in that care.

ACKNOWLEDGMENT

I appreciate the assistance of Craig R. Sellers, MS, RN, CS-ANP, ACRN, doctoral student, with literature identification, access, and development of aspects of this chapter, particularly the tables.

REFERENCES

American College of Chest Physicians/Society of Critical Care Medicine Consensus Panel. (1990). Ethical and moral guidelines for the initiation, continuation, and withdrawal of intensive care. *Chest, 97,* 949–958.
American Geriatrics Society Ethics Committee. (1995). The care of dying patients: A position statement from the American Geriatrics Society. *Journal of the American Geriatrics Society, 43,* 577–578.
American Health Decisions. (1997). *The quest to die with dignity: An analysis of Americans' values, opinions and attitudes concerning end-of-life care.* Atlanta, GA: Author.
American Thoracic Society. (1991). Withholding and withdrawing life-sustaining therapy. *Annals of Internal Medicine, 115,* 478–485.
Asch, D. A., Faber-Langendoen, K., Shea, J. A., & Christakis, N. A. (1999). The sequence of withdrawing life-sustaining treatment from patients. *American Journal of Medicine, 107,* 153–156.
Asch, D. A., Hansen-Flaschen, J., & Lanken, P. N. (1995). Decisions to limit or continue life-sustaining treatment by critical care physicians in the United States: Conflicts between physicians' practices and patients' wishes. *American Journal of Respiratory & Critical Care Medicine, 151*(2, Pt. 1), 288–292.
Asch, D. A., Shea, J. A., Jedrziewski, M. K., & Bosk, C. L. (1997). The limits of suffering: Critical care nurses' views of hospital care at the end of life. *Social Science & Medicine, 45,* 1661–1668.
Baggs, J. G. (1999). Women in the intensive care unit. *American Journal of Critical Care, 8,* 207–209.

Baggs, J. G., & Mick, D. J. (2000). Collaboration: A tool addressing ethical issues for elderly patients near the end of life in intensive care units. *Journal of Gerontological Nursing, 26*(9), 41–47.

Baggs, J. G., & Schmitt, M. H. (2000). End-of-life decisions in adult intensive care: Current research base and directions for the future. *Nursing Outlook, 48,* 158–164.

Baker, R., Wu, A. W., Teno, J. M., Kreling, B., Damiano, A. M., Rubin, H. R., Roach, M. J., Wenger, N. S., Phillips, R. S., Desbiens, N. A., Connors, A. F., Jr., Knaus, W., & Lynn, J. (2000). Family satisfaction with end-of-life care in seriously ill hospitalized adults. *Journal of the American Geriatrics Society, 48*(Suppl.), S61–S69.

Boyd, K., Teres, D., Rapoport, J., & Lemeshow, S. (1996). The relationship between age and the use of DNR orders in critical care patients: Evidence for age discrimination. *Archives of Internal Medicine, 156,* 1821–1826.

Burfitt, S. N., Greiner, D. S., Miers, L. J., Kinney, M. R., & Branyon, M. E. (1993). Professional nurse caring as perceived by critically ill patients: A phenomenologic study. *American Journal of Critical Care, 2,* 489–499.

Campbell, M. L., & Field, B. E. (1991). Management of the patient with do not resuscitate status: Compassion and cost containment. *Heart & Lung, 20,* 345–348.

Campbell, M. L., & Thill-Baharozian, M. (1994). Impact of the DNR therapeutic plan on patient care requirements. *American Journal of Critical Care, 3,* 202–207.

Chelluri, L., Grenvik, A., & Silverman, M. (1995). Intensive care for critically ill elderly: Mortality, costs, and quality of life. Review of the literature. *Archives of Internal Medicine, 155,* 1013–1022.

Chelluri, L., Pinsky, M. R., Donahoe, M. P., & Grenvik, A. (1993). Long-term outcome of critically ill elderly patients requiring intensive care. *Journal of the American Medical Association, 269,* 3119–3123.

Chelluri, L., Pinsky, M. R., & Grenvik, A. (1992). Outcome of intensive care of the "oldest-old" critically ill patients. *Critical Care Medicine, 20,* 757–761.

Cicirelli, V. G., Cox, L. S., & MacLean, A. P. (2000). Hastening death: A comparison of two end-of-life decisions. *Death Studies, 24,* 401–419.

Clarke, D. E., Goldstein, M. K., & Raffin, T. A. (1994). Ethical dilemmas in the critically ill elderly. *Clinics in Geriatric Medicine, 10,* 91–101.

Cook, D. J. (1997). Health professional decision-making in the ICU: A review of the evidence. *New Horizons, 5,* 15–19.

Cook, D. J., Giacomini, M., Johnson, N., & Willms, D., for the Canadian Critical Care Trials Group. (1999). Life support in the intensive care unit: A qualitative investigation of technological purposes. *Canadian Medical Association Journal, 161,* 1109–1113.

Cook, D. J., Guyatt, G. H., Jaeschke, R., Reeve, J., Spanier, A., King, D., Molloy, D. W., Willan, A., & Streiner, D. L., for the Canadian Critical Care Trials Group. (1995). Determinants in Canadian health care workers of the decision to withdraw life support from the critically ill. *Journal of the American Medical Association, 273,* 703–708.

Council on Ethical and Judicial Affairs of the American Medical Association. (1991). Guidelines for the appropriate use of do-not-resuscitate orders. *Journal of the American Medical Association, 265,* 1868–1871.

Council on Scientific Affairs of the American Medical Association. (1996). Good care of the dying patient. *Journal of the American Medical Association, 275,* 474–478.

Covinsky, K. E., Fuller, J. D., Yaffe, K., Johnston, C. B., Hamel, M. B., Lynn, J., Teno, J. M., & Phillips, R. S. (2000). Communication and decision-making in seriously ill patients: Findings of the SUPPORT project. *Journal of the American Geriatrics Society, 48*(Suppl.), S187–S193.

Daly, B. J., Gorecki, J., Sadowski, A., Rudy, E. B., Montenegro, H. D., Song, R., & Dyer, M. A. (1996). Do-not-resuscitate practices in the chronically critically ill. *Heart & Lung, 25,* 310–317.

Desbiens, N. A., Mueller-Rizner, N., Connors, A. F., Jr., Wenger, N. S., & Lynn, J. for the SUPPORT Investigators. (1999). The symptom of burden of seriously ill hospitalized patients. *Journal of Pain & Symptom Management, 17,* 248–255.

Donaldson, M. S., & Field, M. J. (1998). Measuring quality of care at the end of life. *Archives of Internal Medicine, 158,* 121–128.

Dowdy, M. D., Robertson, C., & Bander, J. A. (1998). A study of proactive ethics consultation for critically and terminally ill patients with extended lengths of stay. *Critical Care Medicine, 26,* 252–259.

Eliasson, A. H., Howard, R. S., Torrington, K. G., Dillard, T. A., & Phillips, Y. Y. (1997). Do-not-resuscitate decisions in the medical ICU: Comparing physician and nurse opinions. *Chest, 111,* 1106–1111.

Elpern, E. H., Patterson, P. A., Gloskey, D., & Bone, R. C. (1992). Patients' preferences for intensive care. *Critical Care Medicine, 20,* 43–47.

Ely, E. W., Evans, G. W., & Haponik, E. F. (1999). Mechanical ventilation in a cohort of elderly patients admitted to an intensive care unit. *Annals of Internal Medicine, 131,* 96–104.

Emanuel, L. L., Alpert, H. R., Baldwin, D. C., Jr., & Emanuel, E. J. (2000). What terminally ill patients care about: Toward a validated construct of patients' perspectives. *Journal of Palliative Medicine, 3,* 419–431.

Faber-Langendoen, K. (1996). A multi-institutional study of care given to patients dying in hospitals: Ethical and practice implications. *Archives of Internal Medicine, 156,* 2130–2136.

Faber-Langendoen, K., & Bartels, D. M. (1992). Process of forgoing life-sustaining treatment in a university hospital: An empirical study. *Critical Care Medicine, 20,* 570–577.

Foreman, M. D. (1992). Adverse psychologic responses of the elderly to critical illness. *AACN Clinical Issues in Critical Care Nursing, 3,* 64–72.

Goodlin, S. J., Winzelberg, G. S., Teno, J. M., Whedon, M., & Lynn, J. (1998). Death in the hospital. *Archives of Internal Medicine, 158,* 1570–1572.

Goodman, M. D., Tarnoff, M., & Slotman, G. J. (1998). Effect of advance directives on the management of elderly critically ill patients. *Critical Care Medicine, 26,* 701–704.

Hall, R. I., & Rocker, G. M. (2000). End-of-life care in the ICU: Treatments provided when life support was or was not withdrawn. *Chest, 118,* 1424–1430.

Hamel, M. B., Davis, R. B., Teno, J. M., Knaus, W. A., Lynn, J., Harrell, F., Jr., Galanos, A. N., Wu, A. W., & Phillips, R. S. for the SUPPORT Investigators.

(1999). Older age, aggressiveness of care, and survival for seriously ill, hospitalized adults. *Annals of Internal Medicine, 131,* 721–728.

Hamel, M. B., Phillips, R. S., Teno, J. M., Lynn, J., Galanos, A. N., Davis, R. B., Connors, A. F., Jr., Oye, R. K., Desbiens, N., Reding, D. J., & Goldman, L. for the SUPPORT Investigators. (1996). Seriously ill hospitalized adults: Do we spend less on older patients? *Journal of the American Geriatrics Society, 44,* 1043–1048.

Hamel, M. B., Teno, J. M., Goldman, L., Lynn, J., Davis, R. B., Galanos, A. N., Desbiens, N., Connors, A. F., Jr., Wenger, N., & Phillips, R. S. for the SUPPORT Investigators. (1999). Patient age and decisions to withhold life-sustaining treatments from seriously ill, hospitalized adults. *Annals of Internal Medicine, 130,* 116–125.

Hanson, L. C., & Danis, M. (1991). Use of life-sustaining care for the elderly. *Journal of the American Geriatrics Society, 39,* 772–777.

Hanson, L. C., Tulsky, J. A., & Danis, M. (1997). Can clinical interventions change care at the end of life? *Annals of Internal Medicine, 126,* 381–388.

Happ, M. B. (2000). Interpretation of nonvocal behavior and the meaning of voicelessness in critical care. *Social Science & Medicine, 50,* 1247–1255.

Heyland, D. K., Lavery, J. V., Tranmer, J. E., Shortt, S. E. D., & Taylor, S. (2000). Dying in Canada: Is it an institutionalized, technologically supported experience? *Journal of Palliative Care, 16*(Suppl.), S10–S16.

Heyland, D. K., Tranmer, J., & Feldman-Stewart, D. (2000). End-of-life decision making in the seriously ill hospitalized patient: An organizing framework and results of a preliminary study. *Journal of Palliative Care, 16*(Suppl.), S31–S39.

Hiltunen, E. F., Puopolo, A. L., Marks, G. K., Marsden, C., Kennard, M. J., Follen, M. A., & Phillips, R. S. (1995). The nurse's role in end-of-life treatment discussions: Preliminary report from the SUPPORT project. *Journal of Cardiovascular Nursing, 9*(3), 68–77.

Holloran, S. D., Starkey, G. W., Burke, P. A., Steele, G., Jr., & Forse, R. A. (1995). An educational intervention in the surgical intensive care unit to improve ethical decisions. *Surgery, 118,* 294–298.

Jacob, D. A. (1998). Family members' experiences with decision making for incompetent patients in the ICU: A qualitative study. *American Journal of Critical Care, 7,* 30–36.

Jacobson, J. A., Francis, L. P., Battin, M. P., Green, G. J., Grammes, C., VanRiper, J., & Gully, J. (1997). Dialogue to action: Lessons learned from some family members of deceased patients at an interactive program in seven Utah hospitals. *Journal of Clinical Ethics, 8,* 359–371.

Jayes, R. L., Zimmerman, J. E., Wagner, D. P., Draper, E. A., & Knaus, W. A. (1993). Do-not-resuscitate orders in intensive care units: Current practices and recent changes. *Journal of the American Medical Association, 270,* 2213–2217.

Jayes, R. L., Zimmerman, J. E., Wagner, D. P., & Knaus, W. A. (1996). Variations in the use of do-not-resuscitate orders in ICUs: Findings from a national study. *Chest, 110,* 1332–1339.

Jezewski, M. A., Scherer, Y., Miller, C., & Battista, E. (1993). Consenting to DNR: Critical care nurses' interactions with patients and family members. *American Journal of Critical Care, 2,* 302–309.

Johnson, D., Wilson, M., Cavanaugh, B., Bryden, C., Gudmundson, D., & Moodley, O. (1998). Measuring the ability to meet family needs in an intensive care unit. *Critical Care Medicine, 26,* 266–271.

Kass, J. E., Castriotta, R. J., & Malakoff, F. (1992). Intensive care unit outcome in the very elderly. *Critical Care Medicine, 20,* 1666–1671.

Kaufman, S. R. (1998). Intensive care, old age, and the problem of death in America. *Gerontologist, 38,* 715–725.

Keenan, C. H., & Kish, S. K. (2000). The influence of do-not-resuscitate orders on care provided for patients in the surgical intensive care unit of a cancer center. *Critical Care Nursing Clinics of North America, 12,* 385–390.

Keenan, S. P., Busche, K. D., Chen, L. M., Esmail, R., Inman, K. J., & Sibbald, W. J. for the Southwestern Ontario Critical Care Research Network. (1998). Withdrawal and withholding of life support in the intensive care unit: A comparison of teaching and community hospitals. *Critical Care Medicine, 26,* 245–251.

Keenan, S. P., Busche, K. D., Chen, L. M., McCarthy, L., Inman, K. J., & Sibbald, W. J. (1997). A retrospective review of a large cohort of patients undergoing the process of withholding or withdrawal of life support. *Critical Care Medicine, 25,* 1324–1331.

Keenan, S. P., Mawdsley, C., Plotkin, D., Webster, G. K., & Priestap, F. (2000). Withdrawal of life support: How the family feels, and why. *Journal of Palliative Care, 16*(Suppl.), S40–S44.

Kennard, M. J., Speroff, T., Puopolo, A. L., Follen, M. A., Mallatratt, L., Phillips, R., Desbiens, N., Califf, R. M., & Connors, A. F., Jr. (1996). Participation of nurses in decision making for seriously ill adults. *Clinical Nursing Research, 5,* 199–219.

Kirchhoff, K. T., & Beckstrand, R. L. (2000). Critical care nurses' perceptions of obstacles and helpful behaviors in providing end-of-life care to dying patients. *American Journal of Critical Care, 9,* 96–105.

Kirchhoff, K. T., Spuhler, V., Walker, L., Hutton, A., Cole, B. V., & Clemmer, T. (2000). Intensive care nurses' experiences with end-of-life care. *American Journal of Critical Care, 9,* 36–42.

Kleinpell, R. M., & Ferrans, C. E. (1998). Factors influencing intensive care unit survival for critically ill elderly patients. *Heart & Lung, 27,* 337–343.

Koch, K. A., Rodeffer, H. D., & Wears, R. L. (1994). Changing patterns of terminal care management in an intensive care unit. *Critical Care Medicine, 22,* 233–243.

Lee, D. K. P., Swinburne, A. J., Fedullo, A. J., & Wahl, G. W. (1994). Withdrawing care: Experience in a medical intensive care unit. *Journal of the American Medical Association, 271,* 1358–1361.

Levetown, M. (1998). Palliative care in the intensive care unit. *New Horizons, 6,* 383–397.

Lilly, C. M., DeMeo, D. L., Sonna, L. A., Haley, K. J., Massaro, A. F., Wallace, R. F., & Cody, S. (2000). An intensive communication intervention for the critically ill. *American Journal of Medicine, 109,* 469–475.

Luce, J. M. (1998). Withholding and withdrawal of life-sustaining therapy. In J. B. Hall, G. A. Schmidt, & L. D. H. Wood (Eds.), *Principles of critical care* (2nd ed., pp. 249–255). New York: McGraw-Hill.

Lynn, J., Teno, J. M., Phillips, R. S., Wu, A. W., Desbiens, N., Harrold, J., Claessens, M. T., Wenger, N., Kreling, B., & Connors, A. F., Jr. for the SUPPORT Investigators. (1997). Perceptions by family members of the dying experience of older and seriously ill patients. *Annals of Internal Medicine, 126,* 97–106.

McClement, S. E., & Degner, L. F. (1995). Expert nursing behaviors in care of the dying adult in the intensive care unit. *Heart & Lung, 24,* 408–419.

McLean, R. F., Tarshis, J., Mazer, C. D., & Szalai, J. P. (2000). Death in two Canadian intensive care units: Institutional difference and changes over time. *Critical Care Medicine, 28,* 100–103.

Miller, D. K., Coe, R. M., & Hyers, T. M. (1992). Achieving consensus on withdrawing or withholding care for critically ill patients. *Journal of General Internal Medicine, 7,* 475–480.

Morrison, R. S., Siu, A. L., Leipzig, R. M., Cassel, C. K., & Meier, D. E. (2000). The hard task of improving the quality of care at the end of life. *Archives of Internal Medicine, 160,* 743–747.

Pierce, S. F. (1999). Improving end-of-life care: Gathering suggestions from family members. *Nursing Forum, 34*(2), 5–14.

Prendergast, T. J. (1997). Resolving conflicts surrounding end-of-life care. *New Horizons, 5,* 62–71.

Prendergast, T. J., Claessens, M. T., & Luce, J. M. (1998). A national survey of end-of-life care for critically ill patients. *American Journal of Respiratory & Critical Care Medicine, 158,* 1163–1167.

Prendergast, T. J., & Luce, J. M. (1997). Increasing incidence of withholding and withdrawal of life support from the critically ill. *American Journal of Respiratory & Critical Care Medicine, 155,* 15–20.

Reckling, J. B. (1997). Who plays what role in decisions about withholding and withdrawing life-sustaining treatment? *Journal of Clinical Ethics, 8,* 39–45.

Rocker, G., & Dunbar, S. (2000). Withholding or withdrawal of life support: The Canadian Critical Care Society Position Paper. *Journal of Palliative Care, 16*(Suppl.), S53–S62.

Schecter, W. P. (1994). Withdrawing and withholding life support in geriatric surgical patients: Ethical considerations. *Surgical Clinics of North America, 74,* 245–259.

Schneiderman, L. J., Gilmer, T., & Teetzel, H. D. (2000). Impact of ethics consultations in the intensive care setting: A randomized, controlled trial. *Critical Care Medicine, 28,* 3920–3924.

Sherman, D. A., & Branum, K. (1995). Critical care nurses' perceptions of appropriate care of the patient with orders not to resuscitate. *Heart & Lung, 24,* 321–329.

Simmonds, A. (1996). Decision-making by default: Experiences of physicians and nurses with dying patients in intensive care. *Humane Health Care International, 12,* 168–172.

Singer, P. A., Martin, D. K., & Kelner, M. (1999). Quality end-of-life care: Patients' perspectives. *Journal of the American Medical Association, 281,* 163–168.

Smedira, N. G., Evans, B. H., Grais, L. S., Cohen, N. H., Lo, B., Cook, M., Schecter, W. P., Fink, C., Epstein-Jaffe, E., May, C., & Luce, J. M. (1990). Withholding and withdrawal of life support from the critically ill. *New England Journal of Medicine, 322,* 309–315.

Society of Critical Care Medicine Ethics Committee. (1992). Attitudes of critical care medicine professionals concerning forgoing life-sustaining treatments. *Critical Care Medicine, 20,* 320–326.

Solomon, M. Z., O'Donnell, L., Jennings, B., Guilfoy, V., Wolf, S. M., Nolan, K., Jackson, R., Koch-Weser, D., & Donnelley, S. (1993). Decisions near the end of life: Professional views on life-sustaining treatments. *American Journal of Public Health, 83,* 14–23.

Stanley, M. (1992). Elderly patients in critical care: An overview. *AACN Clinical Issues in Critical Care Nursing, 3,* 120–126.

Stein-Parbury, J., & McKinley, S. (2000). Patients' experiences of being in an intensive care unit: A select literature review. *American Journal of Critical Care, 9,* 20–27.

Steinhauser, K. E., Christakis, N. A., Clipp, E. C., McNeilly, M., McIntrye, L., & Tulsky, J. A. (2000). Factors considered important at the end of life by patients, family, physicians, and other care providers. *Journal of the American Medical Association, 284,* 2476–2482.

Steinhauser, K. E., Clipp, E. C., McNeilly, M., Christakis, N. A., McIntyre, L. M., & Tulsky. J. A. (2000). In search of a good death: Observations of patients, families, and providers. *Annals of Internal Medicine, 132,* 825–832.

Stillman, A. E., Braitman, L. E., & Grant, R. J. (1998). Are critically ill older patients treated differently than similarly ill younger patients? *Western Journal of Medicine, 169,* 162–165.

SUPPORT Principal Investigators. (1995). A controlled trial to improve care for seriously ill hospitalized patients: The study to understand prognoses and preferences for outcomes and risks of treatments (SUPPORT). *Journal of the American Medical Association, 274,* 1591–1598.

Swigart, V., Lidz, C., Butterworth, V., & Arnold, R. (1996). Letting go: Family willingness to forgo life support. *Heart & Lung, 25,* 483–494.

Teno, J. M., Fisher, E., Hamel, M. B., Wu, A. W., Murphy, D. J., Wenger, N. S., Lynn, J., & Harrell, F. E., Jr. (2000). Decision-making and outcomes of prolonged ICU stays in seriously ill patients. *Journal of the American Geriatrics Society, 48*(Suppl.), S70–S74.

Teno, J. M., Lynn, J., Phillips, R. S., Murphy, D., Younger, S. J., Bellamy, P., Connors, A. F., Jr., Desbiens, N. A., Fulkerson, W., & Knaus, W. A. (1994). Do formal advance directives affect resuscitation decisions and the use of resources for seriously ill patients? *Journal of Clinical Ethics, 5,* 23–30.

Thibault-Prevost, J., Jensen, L. A., & Hodgins, M. (2000). Critical care nurses' perceptions of DNR status. *Journal of Nursing Scholarship, 32,* 259–265.

Tilden, V. P., Tolle, S. W., Garland, M. J., & Nelson, C. A. (1995). Decisions about life-sustaining treatment: Impact of physicians' behaviors on the family. *Archives of Internal Medicine, 155,* 633–638.

Tittle, M. B., Moody, L., & Becker, M. P. (1992a). Nursing care requirements of patients with DNR orders in intensive care units. *Heart & Lung, 21,* 235–242.

Tittle, M. B., Moody, L., & Becker, M. P. (1992b). Severity of illness and resource allocation in DNR patients in ICU. *Nursing Economics, 10,* 210–216.

Todres, I. D., Armstrong, A., Lally, P., & Cassem, E. H. (1998). Negotiating end-of-life issues. *New Horizons, 6,* 374–382.

Tullmann, D. F., & Dracup, K. (2000). Creating a healing environment for elders. *AACN Clinical Issues: Advanced Practice in Acute and Critical Care, 11,* 34–50.

Walter, S. D., Cook, D. J., Guyatt, G. H., Spanier, A., Jaeschke, R., Todd, T. R. J., & Streiner, D. L. for the Canadian Critical Care Trials Group. (1998). Confidence in life-support decisions in the intensive care unit: A survey of healthcare workers. *Critical Care Medicine, 26,* 44–49.

Weissman, D. E. (2000). New end-of-life guidelines. *Journal of Palliative Medicine, 3,* 149–150.

Wenger, N. S., Pearson, M. L., Desmond, K. A., Harrison, E. R., Rubenstein, L. V., Rogers, W. H., & Kahn, K. L. (1995). Epidemiology of do-not-resuscitate orders: Disparity by age, diagnosis, gender, race, and functional impairment. *Archives of Internal Medicine, 155,* 2056–2062.

Wilson, D. (1997). A report of an investigation of end-of-life care practices in health care facilities and the influences on those practices. *Journal of Palliative Care, 13*(4), 34–40.

Wood, G. G., & Martin, E. (1995). Withholding and withdrawing life-sustaining therapy in a Canadian intensive care unit. *Canadian Journal of Anaesthesia, 42,* 186–191.

Wu, A. W., Rubin, H. R., & Rosen, M. J. (1990). Are elderly people less responsive to intensive care? *Journal of the American Geriatrics Society, 38,* 621–627.

Yu, W., Ash, A. S., Levinsky, N. G., & Moskowitz, M. A. (2000). Intensive care unit use and mortality in the elderly. *Journal of General Inernal Medicine, 15,* 97–102.

Chapter 8

Nursing Homes and Assisted Living Facilities As Places for Dying

JULIANA C. CARTWRIGHT

ABSTRACT

This chapter reviews the state of knowledge about nursing homes and assisted living facilities as places for dying. Reviewed are 25 published and unpublished research reports by nurse researchers and researchers from other disciplines that address the following questions: (a) What is known about how communication and shared decision-making about end-of-life care preferences occur? (b) How are symptoms assessed and managed at end-of-life? and (c) What are facility characteristics that influence end-of-life care services delivery? Reports were identified through searches of the following databases: MEDLINE, CINAHL, Health Star, PsychLit, Ageline, Ebsco, and PubMed. The following terms guided the search: *advance directives, geriatric assessment or nursing, health services for the aged, hospice, residential facilities, palliative care, symptom management*, and *terminal care*. Reports were included if published between 1990 and 2000, if relevant to nursing research on end-of-life care, if conducted on samples age 65 or older and living in nursing home or residential care settings, and if published in English. The studies reviewed were primarily descriptive. The findings indicate that little is known about end-of-life care in these settings, and that family and staff perspectives differ on the nature and quality of the services provided. Both external and internal factors influence the ability of facilities to provide end-of-life care. Recommendations are provided for further research related to nursing homes and assisted living facilities as places for dying.

Keywords: elderly, end of life, palliative care, assisted living, nursing homes, symptoms, facility characteristics, communication

Little is known about end-of-life (EOL) care in nursing homes (NHs) or assisted living facilities (ALFs). Yet combined, these settings provide residential and care services for almost 3 million elders (Hawes, Rose, & Phillips, 1999; Strahan, 1997). The purpose of this chapter is to review the existing research literature on NHs and ALFs as places for dying. The questions focusing this review were:

1. What is known about how communication and shared decision-making about end-of-life care preferences occur?
2. How are symptoms assessed and managed at end-of-life?
3. What are facility characteristics that influence end-of-life care services delivery?

For the purposes of this paper, EOL refers to the time frame during which death is considered to be likely "within a few days to several months" (Field & Cassel, 1997, p. 27). EOL care represents palliative care at the end of life as defined by the Last Acts Task Force (1997, paragraph #1): "comprehensive management of physical, psychological, social, spiritual, and existential needs of patients."

HOW AND WHERE OLDER PEOPLE DIE

By 2020, 2 1/2 million deaths, primarily related to chronic diseases, will occur annually among older people (Brock & Foley, 1998). The three leading causes of death in the United States—heart disease, cancer, and stroke—have been described by the Institute of Medicine as "slow killers" (Field & Cassel, 1997). Increasingly, death involves living with progressive, terminal illness: periods of ordinary daily life interrupted by crises related to illness exacerbations that may, or may not, be reversible. Concurrent with these morbidity trends are changes in housing and long-term care services. Kane (1995) reported that distinctions are blurring between home and institutional services and settings. Factors contributing to these changes include elders' desires to avoid NH placement and to age in place in homelike settings, the increased availability of community-based care services, and policy maker concerns regarding the potential increase in expenses related to caring for older people (Kane, 1995; Wilson, 1995).

Nursing Homes

An estimated 1.5 million elders age 65 and older reside in NHs (Strahan, 1995). Half are permanent residents; 66% are projected to die in the facility (Mezey, Miller, & Linton-Nelson, 1999). However, the federal Omnibus

Budget Reconciliation Act of 1987 (OBRA '87) emphasized rehabilitation, restoration, and improvement in function for NH residents, not provision of EOL care. Federal and state surveillance regulations, including required resident assessment, treatment, and documentation protocols, reflect this focus (Engle, 1998; Keay, 1999).

Assisted Living Facilities

ALFs are among the fastest-growing housing options in long-term care (Allen, 1999). The term *assisted living* has over 30 definitions (Hawes, Rose, & Phillips, 1999), which may explain the broad estimate that between 800,000 and 1.5 million elders reside in ALFs (Allen, 1999). Some other terms describing this option include *residential care facilities*, *adult congregate housing*, and *board and care homes* (Hawes et al., 1999). The following characteristics are commonly associated with ALFs: (a) a congregate residential setting that includes 24-hour staffing; (b) a range of scheduled personal care and health monitoring services, including the capacity to accommodate unscheduled needs; (c) physical and social environments that maximize residents' autonomy, privacy, dignity, and choice; and (d) accommodations that minimize the need to move (National Center for Assisted Living, 2001). ALFs are state regulated, but regulations vary greatly in terms of staffing ratios and qualifications, and the nature of services required or permitted (Allen, 1999; Hawes et al., 1999; Mollica, 1998). Debate exists whether federal oversight of the industry is needed, and how best to balance resident choice and privacy along with safety and costs (Sheehy, 2000). ALFs are attractive to policy makers as a potentially less costly substitute for placement of up to 25% of nursing home residents (Manard & Cameron, 1997). Medicaid waivers for placement in ALFs have been approved in 35 states for residents who otherwise meet level-of-care criteria for NH placement (Mollica, 1998).

NHs and ALFs have markedly different philosophies and regulatory requirements guiding delivery of services. However, both are places where elders are likely to live during their final years and months. The nature of EOL care services in these settings, and factors that influence EOL care delivery, are important for nurses to understand because these are settings where nursing services can affect the EOL experience of elders.

METHOD

To identify data-based reports addressing EOL care in NHs or ALFs, electronic searches spanning 1990 through 2001 were conducted in the following databases: MEDLINE, CINAHL, Health Star, PsychLit, Ageline, Ebsco, and PubMed. The following MESH terms guided the searches: *advance directives, palliative care, terminal care, hospice, symptom management, residential facilities, geriatric assessment or nursing,* and *health services for the aged.* Additionally, the term *end of life* was searched in titles and abstracts. Searches were limited to reports specified as *age 65 and over.* When these strategies identified a large proportion of articles related to *advance care planning* (ACP), the term *advance directives* was deleted from the search strategy. This process eliminated 10 of 140 previously identified articles. Because ALFs are a relatively new phenomenon, the Agency on Aging website was searched for reports specific to EOL care in these types of facilities. Papers were also located through bibliographic lists and a manual review of the *Program Abstracts of the 53rd Annual Scientific Meeting of the Gerontological Society of America, 2000.*

An initial review of report abstracts eliminated nonprimary studies from the search results. Criteria for primary study reports to be included in this review were: (a) published in English, (b) addressed EOL care concepts suggested by the three questions framing this review, and (c) reported results that either focused on, or clearly delineated, analyses for NHs or ALFs as places for dying. Additional criteria were used in reviewing the extensive literature related to ACP: studies were included only if they addressed communication by residents or their families and staff related to treatment decision making. Excluded from the review of literature on ACP were studies that focused on the impact of the 1990 Patient Self Determination Act on documentation of advance directives, or studies that explored residents' preferences regarding ACP. The resultant sample of 25 papers includes 22 studies of NHs, 1 study of ALFs, and 2 studies that examined EOL care in both settings. The reader is referred to the excellent discussion by Moss (2001) for additional information on conceptual and methodological concerns related to death, dying, and bereavement in nursing homes. Additionally, a recent review by Rubenstein (2001) provides an in-depth exploration of the culture of death and dying in nursing homes.

RESULTS

The results of this review are organized by study question and by facility setting into three tables that summarize methodologies and relevant findings. All investigators used nonexperimental designs, with the exception of Kovach, Wilson, and Noonan, (1996). Sources of data for the studies included residents ($n = 6$), family members ($n = 5$), staff and administrators ($n = 12$), and document reviews, primarily using medical records ($n = 9$). Sample sizes ranged from a single NH resident case study (Kayser-Jones, 2000) to 16,945 NHs (Petrisek & Mor, 1999). Most of the studies provided either no information about sample ethnicity, or sampled white populations. Seventeen papers reported on facilities in the United States, 2 on NHs in the United Kingdom, two on NHs in Canada, and one on NHs in Australia. Additionally, Katz, Komaromy, and Sidell (1999) and Komaromy, Sidell, and Katz (2000) reported on research that examined both NHs and community residential care facilities in the U.K.

Teno, McNiff, and Lynn (2001) have suggested a framework for measuring EOL care as a component of institutional accountability based on three domains: (a) communication and shared decision making, (b) symptom assessment and treatment planning, and (c) characteristics of the health care system. This framework was the basis for identifying the three questions addressed in this review. For the purposes of this report, communication and shared decision making represent the tenet that patients and families have the right to understand and participate in decisions related to current and future prognosis and treatment options. Symptom assessment and treatment planning refer to recognition and management of physical, emotional, and spiritual symptoms that occur during the dying experience. Characteristics of the health care system refer to factors associated with comprehensive and coordinated care at EOL in a facility.

What Is Known About How Communication and Shared Decision Making About EOL Care Preferences Occur in NHs?

Four studies provide evidence that residents may have limited involvement in discussions about EOL care preferences (Table 8.1). Bradley, Walker, Blechner, and Wetle (1997), Levin and colleagues (1999), Lurie, Pheley, Miles, and Bannick-Mohrland (1992), and Palkner and Nettles-Carlson (1995) reported that fewer than 50% of residents, even when deemed alert and oriented by staff, participate in decision-making discussions about future treatment preferences. Further, how clearly residents understand EOL care options, or are comfortable with previously documented decisions, are questions raised by the findings of Lurie and colleagues (1992), and Palker and Nettles-Carlson (1995). Bradley and colleagues (1997),

TABLE 8.1   What Is Known Regarding How Communication and Decision Making About End-of-Life Care Preferences Occur?

Study	Method	Selected findings relevant to communication and decision making
	Nursing homes	
Bradley, Walker, Blechner, & Wetle (1997) Nonnurse	Design: Descriptive. Data collection: Chart reviews; interviews. Sample: $N = 600$ resident charts. 2 cohorts randomly selected pre- and post- Patient Self-Determination Act (1990 and 1994), 50 each from 6 NHs. $N = 19$ staff were purposely selected by role. Residents: M age = 83; 40% alert & oriented, and 50% independent in ADLs on admission.	• Someone other than the resident received information on future medical treatment options in 48% of admissions of oriented residents. • Likelihood of not receiving information was associated with < high school education (Odds ratio = 0.73, $p < .058$). • Reasons why staff excluded residents from information processes: (a) belief that the resident was cognitively impaired, (b) emotional distress of resident on admission, (c) perceived delegation of authority by resident to someone else for ACP.
Forbes, Bern-Klug, & Gessert (2000) Nurse	Design: Descriptive. Data collection: Focus groups. Sample: $N = 28$ family members of residents with severe dementia. Convenience sample from 4 NHs representing ethnically, socially, & economically diverse residents.	• Families reported lack of discussion about death and dying by staff, and lack of opportunities for consistent communication with a specific care provider. • Families wanted to make treatment decisions that preserve their own peace of mind: "knowing I did everything I could." • Families did not recognize dying trajectories.

TABLE 8.1   *(continued)*

Study	Method	Selected findings relevant to communication and decision making
	Nursing homes	
Kayser-Jones (1995) Nurse	Design: Case study. Data collection: Participant observation, interviews, event analysis. Sample: $N = 2$ dying elders, their families & staff. Theoretical framework: Decision-making theory.	• Families & staff brought different perspectives on the resident's situation to their decision-making processes. • Nurses were in a position to learn family perspectives, & to advocate these perspectives to the MD. • How MDs framed & presented the problem & treatment options influenced family decision-making processes.
Levin, Wenger, Ouslander, Zellman, Schnelle, Hirsch, & Reuben (1999) Nonnurse	Design: Descriptive. Data Collection: Chart review and interviews with residents and family members. Sample: $N = 413$ NH residents & 363 family members (83% response rate). Convenience sample from NHs in the West and New England. M age $= 84$; M length of stay in NH $= 2.7$ years.	• 29% of residents reported having discussions about life-sustaining treatments. • For 14 of 154 residents with DNR orders in chart, neither the resident nor family recalled any discussions about ACP. • Likelihood of resident-physician discussions decreased with age (Odds ratio $= 0.93$/year, 95% CI, .89–.97), decreased with a diagnosis of cognitive impairment (Odds ratio $= 0.41$, 95% CI, .17–.98), but increased with number of medical diagnoses (Odds ratio $= 1.22$ per diagnosis, 95% CI, 1.05–1.42).

(continued)

TABLE 8.1 *(continued)*

Study	Method	Selected findings relevant to communication and decision making
	Nursing homes	
Lurie, Pheley, Miles, & Bannick-Mohrland (1992) Nonnurse	Design: Descriptive. Data collection: In-person surveys. Sample: $N = 131$ residents, randomly sampled (87% response rate). M age = 71.2 (SD 14.7).	• 15% of residents ($n = 19$) recalled discussing ACP with an MD; of these, 11% ($n = 2$) had reservations about their directives. • 79% ($n = 15$) of discussions were provider initiated. • Residents aged 80 and older were less likely to have talked with a MD ($p < .05$) or family ($p < .01$).
Wilson & Daley (1999) Nurse	Design: Descriptive. Data Collection: Interviews within 4 weeks of NH death. Sample: $N = 11$ family members.	• Families desired assistance from the staff in treatment decision-making and in understanding the dying process. • Families needed to ask questions, receive answers, and talk about their concerns with staff.
Palker & Nettles-Carlson (1995) Nurse	Design: Descriptive. Data Collection: Chart review and interviews. Sample: $N = 77$ resident charts, 17 interviews (16%). Convenience sample. M age = 77.3.	• 13 interviewees (76%) could not correctly describe an advance directive (AD). • Only 7 interviewees (41%) could recall having discussions about ADs. • Unclear or conflicting directives were noted in some records (number unspecified).

TABLE 8.1 *(continued)*

Study	Method	Selected findings relevant to communication and decision making
	Assisted living facilities	
Mitty (2000) Nurse	Design: Descriptive. Data Collection: Mail Survey. Sample: $N = 107$ ALFs of 300 selected through a stratified national sampling plan (30% response rate). Facilities represented 7936 residents; 52% of the facilities were for-profit.	• 75% of ALFs provided educational info to residents through one-to-one conversations, brochures, or group meetings. • Barriers to AD completion: perceived physician responsibility (75%), resident disinterest (63%), decisionally impaired residents (61%), family disinterest (50%), regulations do not require (53%), no available proxy (60%).

Levin and colleagues (1999), and Lurie and colleagues (1992) identified the following variables that may be associated with whether or not residents are involved in discussions and decision making around EOL care: (a) resident age, level of education, cognitive status, and number of medical conditions; (b) staff perceptions that the admission process is emotionally distressful to residents; (c) staff beliefs that the resident has delegated responsibility for communication and decision making about EOL care to someone else, and (d) staff willingness to initiate discussions about EOL care and decisions.

That family members may feel alone or lacking sufficient knowledge when making decisions about EOL care for their resident is suggested by the findings of Forbes, Bern-Klug, and Gessert (2000), and Wilson and Daley (1999). Forbes and colleagues used a journey as a metaphor for EOL decision making by families of elders with dementia: "a long, arduous, and unwelcomed journey . . . in unfamiliar territory filled with unrecognizable landmarks" (2000, p. 256). Kayser-Jones (1995) reported that families consider their biographical knowledge of the resident while physicians emphasize medical futility in framing decision making situations. These studies provide evidence that families expect staff to initiate discussions about EOL issues. Additionally, the findings suggest that families desire (a) clearly stated information communicated by the same staff over time, (b) assistance in interpreting information about their loved one's clinical status and treatment options, (c) help in communicating their concerns to others, and (d) acknowledgment of their concerns regarding EOL care options and their loved one's dying.

LIMITATIONS

Although these studies included efforts to sample both rural and urban regions throughout the U.S., and included some relatively large sample sizes (N = 413 residents and 363 family members; Levin et al., 1999), most used small, convenience samples for data collection. Minimally addressed were specific cultural, ethnic, and religious variations that might influence communication and decision-making preferences, the impact of specific medical diagnoses or functional limitations on communication and decision making, and preferred conditions for information exchange and decision making from the perspectives of residents and families. Reports about EOL care preference discussions focused primarily on one component of EOL care: medical interventions (e.g., antibiotics for pneumonia, resuscitation, life support equipment).

What Is Known About How Communication About EOL Care Preferences and Shared Decision Making Occur in ALFs?

No research was located that specifically addressed communication and decision making regarding EOL care in ALFs. Mitty (2000) reported that state regulations vary regarding requirements for documenting EOL care preferences by residents, and that 53% of surveyed ALF administrators indicated that their facility is exempt from any requirements to inform residents about EOL care options (Table 8.1). These findings, coupled with the ALF industry philosophy emphasizing resident autonomy and privacy, suggest that communication and decision making about EOL care preferences in ALFs may be quite different than in NHs, and may be quite different across states and facilities.

LIMITATIONS

This single study by Mitty (2000) is the only located report on communication and decision making at EOL in ALFs. While the investigator is commended for this important, beginning effort, the findings are limited by its singular perspective (administrators) and low response rate (30%).

How Are Symptoms Assessed and Managed at EOL in NHs?

Studies located on symptom assessment and management were predominantly descriptive in nature, and based on resident, family, and staff reports (Table 8.2). Reports by Baer and Hanson (2000), Clare and DeBellis (1997), Engle, Fox-Hill, and Graney (1998), Hanson and Henderson (2000), and Kayser-Jones (2000) indicated that residents dying in NHs experience significant physical, emotional, and spiritual symptoms; that systematic, evidence-based strategies for recognizing common symptoms at EOL are absent; and that staff often lack knowledge about how best to assess and manage symptoms. In the only study located that specifically examined ethnic differences between dying residents, Engle and colleagues (1998) reported that Black residents expressed more unrelieved pain than White residents. Two reports suggested that families perceive EOL care and symptom management in NHs to be less positive than in hospitals or through hospice services (Baer & Hanson, 2000; Hanson et al., 1997). Noted by Hanson and Henderson (2000) were the desires of some NH staff to provide emotional and spiritual support to dying residents.

Building on the reports identified above are the findings of Kovach, Wilson, and Noonan (1996), who studied the effects of a hospice-oriented intervention on NH residents with end-stage dementia. Their findings indicated that staff education, environmental modifications, and care supervision by expert nurse case managers can reduce residents' levels of discomfort at EOL, and may decrease iatrogenic infections. Further, the knowledge and skills acquired by staff may positively influence the care they provide to residents who are not imminently dying.

LIMITATIONS

Limitations to these studies include findings based primarily on self-report, relatively small sample sizes, lack of use of standardized instruments for symptom assessment, and, with the exception of Engles, Fox-Hill, and Graney (1998), the absence of attention to cultural or ethnic variations in sampling strategies and analyses. Both conceptual and operational definitions for symptoms and management strategies were frequently missing in

TABLE 8.2   How Symptoms Are Assessed and Managed at End of Life

Study	Method	Selected findings related to symptom assessment and management
	Nursing homes	
Baer & Hanson (2000) Nonnurse	Design: Descriptive. Data Collection: Mail survey. Sample: $N = 292$ families of decedent NH hospice enrollees in North Carolina (73% of total).	• Family ratings of symptoms during final 3 months: 70% had severe to moderate pain; 56% had severe to moderate dyspnea; 61% had additional uncomfortable symptoms; 47% had moderate to severe depression; 50% had moderate to severe anxiety; 35% had loneliness. • Quality of physical symptom care: 64%"good to excellent" in NHs pre-hospice; 93% with hospice ($p < .001$). Quality of emotional and spiritual care: 64% "good to excellent" in NHs pre-hospice; 90% with hospice ($p < .001$). • NHs provided a home-like environment; hospice provided professional knowledge and skills regarding palliative care including anticipation of potential problems.

TABLE 8.2 *(continued)*

Study	Method	Selected findings related to symptom assessment and management
	Nursing homes	

Study	Method	Selected findings related to symptom assessment and management
Clare & De-Bellis (1997) Nurse	Design: Descriptive. Data Collection: Mail survey. Sample: $N = 71$ directors of NHs in urban and rural South Australia (47% response). Respondents represented 44% of 6908 NH beds in the region. Non-profit & for-profit NHs were represented.	• Identified needs of dying residents: psychological support (100%), full assistance with hygiene (97%), urinary incontinence management (88%), pain management (87%), help with eating and drinking (86%), pain consultation (68%), bowel management (80%), behavior management (72%); nursing care every 2 hours (76%), wound care (69%). • 3% of facilities used a specific instrument to assess pain in cognitively impaired residents.
Engle, Fox-Hill, & Graney (1998) Nurse	Design: Descriptive. Data Collection: Repeated interviews. Sample: $N = 13$ residents in 2 NHs. M age = 73 yr. 6 women; 8 black, 5 white residents. Purposive sampling.	• Black residents reported having unrelieved, moderate-to-severe pain and difficulty obtaining pain medications. • White residents rarely reported pain, and reported adequate pain relief. • Some residents perceived comfort, including pain relief, in religious activities (e.g., prayer, hymns) and services.

(continued)

TABLE 8.2 *(continued)*

Study	Method	Selected findings related to symptom assessment and management
	Nursing homes	
Hanson, Danis, & Garrett (1997) Nonnurse	Design: Descriptive. Data Collection: Phone interviews. Sample: N = 461 relatives of decedents over age 65 (80% response rate). 28% of decedents died in NHs.	• Positive comments about care management at EOL were less frequent for NHs (51%) than hospitals (69%). • Positive comments about care management in NHs: staff like extended family; tried hard. • Negative comments about care management in NHs: poorly trained staff, insufficient staff, poor quality of care, remote physicians.
Hanson & Henderson (2000) Nurse	Design: Descriptive. Data Collection: Focus group discussions. Sample: N = 77 staff from 2 NHs. Convenience sample of nurses (RN & LPN), aides, and physicians from 178 possible staff.	• Signs of pending death were nonspecific, recurrent, & difficult to interpret, making difficult early initiation of palliative care. • Participants disagreed about the frequency of pain at end-of-life in NHs, and how to identify signs of pain at end-of-life. • Most NH deaths were perceived as 'good deaths.' A good death included physical symptom management, and emotional & spiritual preparation. • 'Bad deaths' occurred with prolonged pain, physical disfigurement, and loss of personal dignity.

TABLE 8.2   *(continued)*

Study	Method	Selected findings related to symptom assessment and management
	Nursing homes	
		• Dying in a NH was reported as a lonely and isolating situation. • Staffs reported they became surrogate family to some dying residents. They engaged in spiritual care such as prayer with residents.
Kayser-Jones (2000) Nurse	Design: Case Study. Data Collection: Observations, interviews and event analysis. Sample: $N = 1$ woman, aged 101, with arthritis & mild cognitive impairment.	• Unable to use utensils, but not routinely assisted with meals or fluids. • Restrained in wheelchair throughout day despite 3 stage-2 decubitus ulcers on buttocks. • Resident expressed embarrassment at eating limitations; fatigue and emotional distress about wheelchair restraint 10 days before dying.

(continued)

TABLE 8.2   *(continued)*

Study	Method	Selected findings related to symptom assessment and management
	Nursing homes	
Kovach, Wilson, & Noonan (1996) Nurse	Design: pretest-posttest experimental design. Data Collection: SPMSQ for cognitive impairment; BEHAVE-AD scale for behavioral symptoms; DS-DAT for discomfort; chart review for physical problems. Sample: $N = 62$ severely, cognitively impaired residents in 3 facilities. The intervention included (a) a day-long staff class on hospice concepts, dementia, therapeutic activities, behavioral treatments, family & spiritual care; (b) classes for RNs on recognizing & treating common physical conditions; (c) a home-like setting that clustered 6 to 8 bed areas; and (d) case manager nurses with formal classes in hospice & case management.	• T group had less discomfort posttest ($t = 3,88, p < .001$). • T group had fewer iatrogenic infections ($n = 4$ versus $n = 15$). • No significant differences between groups posttest on physical complications or behavioral symptoms. • T group staff reported improved job satisfaction, sense of empathy & caring. (Significance or magnitude not mentioned.) • T group family members noted little or no difference in residents. (Significance or magnitude not mentioned.)
	Assisted living facilities	
Mitty (2000) Nurse	See Table 8.1.	• In the prior 12 months, palliative or comfort care services were reported for 171 residents (2% of total ALF population). • Prior 12 month in-facility services for all residents:

TABLE 8.2 *(continued)*

Study	Method	Selected findings related to symptom assessment and management
	Assisted living facilities	
		• Controlled substances administration = 60 residents (< 1% of total) • Oxygen therapy = 81 residents (1% of total)
	Nursing homes and assisted living facilities combined	
Katz, Komaromy, & Sidell (1999) Nurse	Design: Descriptive. Data Collection: Interviews and case study observations. Sample: $N = 100$ interviews with administrators randomly sampled from 412 responses to a prior survey in the UK. $N = 12$ facilities purposively sampled and observed.	• Dying trajectories were unpredictable, making difficult the recognition of a dying resident. • Physical pain was identified as a concern, but not other symptoms associated with dying (e.g., weakness, constipation, psychological distress). • Pain management was complicated by poor medical care, lack of staff knowledge about analgesics, & negative staff attitudes to narcotics.
Komaromy, Sidell, & Katz (2000) Nurse	Design: Descriptive. Data Collection: Mail surveys. Sample: $N = 412$ NHs & residential care homes (41% response rate) representing 10,035 residents (2% of total U.K. residential home population).	• Use of pastoral services varied greatly, & often depended on family or resident request for these services.

the reports. The general term, *EOL care*, was frequently used in describing findings, making difficult the ability to ascertain specific symptom assessment and management activities.

How Are Symptoms Assessed and Managed at EOL in ALFs?

Mitty (2000) provides the only study located that addressed symptom assessment and management at EOL in U.S. ALFs (Table 8.2). Management interventions commonly associated with EOL care, such as comfort care and controlled substance administration, were reported for the overall population of ALF residents, not specifically for dying residents.

How Are Symptoms Assessed and Managed at EOL in NHs and ALFs?

Katz, Komaromy, and Sidell (1999), and Komaromy, Sidell, and Katz (2000) combined survey, interview, and observational methodologies in exploring EOL care management in NHs and residential care facilities in the U.K. (Table 8.2). Overall, results were similar to those reported in U.S. NHs by Clare and DeBellis (1997), and Hanson and Henderson (2000). As with the reports on U.S. facilities, these findings indicated that staff had difficulty recognizing dying trajectories, and that staff focused on pain control as the primary symptom concern for dying residents (Katz et al., 1999; Komaromy et al., 2000).

LIMITATIONS

The findings of the U.K. studies were not specifically described for NHs or residential care facilities. This makes difficult interpretation of the results for one setting or the other, versus both settings.

What Are Facility Characteristics That Influence EOL Care Services Delivery in NHs?

Staff in U.S. facilities identified that regulatory requirements adversely affected EOL care, particularly federal emphasis on restorative and rehabilitative care that mandates the nature of resident assessments, and implementation of specific care protocols (Hanson & Henderson, 2000; Wilson & Daley, 1999). Also adversely affecting EOL care management were the high acuity levels of residents admitted from hospitals, negative family and public perceptions of NHs, and inadequate reimbursement rates with concurrent insufficient staffing to provide needed care (Hanson & Henderson, 2000; Wilson & Daley, 1999; Clare & DeBellis, 1997).

Investigators from Australia, Canada, and the U.K. reported that NH staff perceived they were inadequately educated to provide EOL care (Clare & DeBellis; Gibbs, 1995; Patterson, Molloy, Jubelius, Guyatt, & Bedard, 1997). In contrast, Eseck, Kraybill, and Hansberry (1999) reported that U.S. survey respondents rated their EOL care skills as high. However, Eseck and colleagues also found that, in focus groups, U.S. staff identified the following as problematic for nurses and aides: staff communication, hospice services collaboration, symptom management, time constraints, and emotional attachments to residents. Barriers to meeting EOL care educational needs included lack of awareness of learning resources (Gibbs, 1995), as well as lost salary and inconvenient times or locations for classes (Patterson et al., 1997). Further, Froggatt (2000) reported that the ability of staff to implement new knowledge was adversely influenced by organizational characteristics such as centralized decision making and lack of administrative support.

Three studies reported on factors associated with use of the hospice benefit in NHs. Castle (1998), and Petrisek and Mor (1999) identified that intense market competition, Medicare prospective payment reimbursements, and for-profit ownership status of NHs and hospices were associated with more NH use of hospice services. Jones, Nackerud, and Boyle (1997) found that administrators were less likely to use hospice if they perceived hospice staff as "taking over," as poor communicators, or as not valuing the NH staff. Additionally, concerns that the hospice benefit adversely affected facility reimbursements adversely influenced administrator decisions not to use this service (Jones et al., 1997).

LIMITATIONS

Limitations to the above-described studies include emphasis on self-report, and absence of data collection methods that use standardized measures for assessing staff knowledge or actual EOL care services delivery. While Castle (1998), and Petrisek and Mor (1999) delineated how variables were operationalized, some studies had limited or incomplete information about staffing ratios or patterns.

What Are Facility Characteristics That Influence EOL Care Services Delivery in ALFs?

Mitty (2000) reported that facilities were permitted, rather than mandated, to provide more nursing intensive services, resulting in within-state variations regarding facilities' willingness or ability to permit residents to die in their setting (Table 8.3). Administrators identified the following barriers to EOL care delivery in ALFs: lack of RNs and other care staffs, insufficient Medicare reimbursements, and attitudes of some staff and physicians that the facility was not an appropriate site for EOL care. Deemed essential for "good" EOL care to occur in ALFs were the presence of hospice, family support, and additional, privately purchased care services (Mitty, 2000).

What Are Facility Characteristics That Influence EOL Care Services Delivery in NHs and ALFs?

Komaromy and colleagues (2000) found similar facility challenges to providing EOL care as were reported separately in the NH literature: overextended staff, ambivalent attitudes towards use of external agency nurses in providing EOL care, and lack of staff and administrative education about palliative and hospice care (Table 8.3). Komaromy and colleagues noted that poor wages might contribute to recruitment and retention of staff. Budgetary restrictions also adversely affected some facilities' abilities to purchase special equipment for use in EOL care (e.g., delivery devices for continuous infusion of subcutaneous analgesics).

LIMITATIONS

As noted earlier in this chapter, limitations to this study by Komaromy and colleagues (2000) include lack of specificity in reporting results for NHs versus residential care facilities. While many of the findings appear similar to concerns identified in the U.S., applicability of these findings to other nations may be limited by the different regulatory climates existing among countries.

TABLE 8.3   Facility Characteristics That Influence End-of-Life Care Services Delivery

Study	Methods	Selected findings related to facility characteristics
	Nursing homes	
Castle (1998) Nonnurse	Design: Descriptive. Data collection: Medicare & Medicaid Automated Certification Survey for facility characteristics, & Area Resource File for market attributes. Sample: $N = 14,646$ national NHs.	• NHs were less likely to have hospice programs if the following community characteristics were present: (a) prospective payment reimbursement for Medicaid (Odds ratio = 0.82, CI, 0.72–0.92, $p < .001$), (b) less market competition (Odds ratio = 0.55, CI, 0.36–0.85, $p < .001$), and (c) higher levels of hospital inpatient services (Odds ratio = 0.97, CI, 0.95–0.98, $p < .01$). • NHs were more likely to have hospice programs if the following community characteristic was present: higher levels of hospital outpatient services (Odds ratio = 1.03, CI, 1.02–1.04, $p < .001$). • NHs were less likely to have pain management programs if the following community characteristics were present: (a) less market competition (Odds ratio = 0.77, CI, 0.58–1.00, $p < .05$), and (b) a moratorium on the building of new NH beds (Odds ratio = 0.84, CI, 0.76–0.93, $p < .01$).

(continued)

TABLE 8.3 *(continued)*

Study	Methods	Selected findings related to facility characteristics
	Nursing homes	
Clare & De Bellis (1997)	See Table 8.2	• Reimbursements did not reflect actual hours of care services. • 97% identified the need for increased staff knowledge about palliative care.
Ersek, Kraybill, & Hansberry (1999) Nurse	Design: Descriptive. Data collection: Surveys and focus groups. Sample: $N = 88$ RNs and LPNs (response rate = 42%) & 136 CNAs (response rate = 28%). Convenience sample.	• RNs, LPNs and CNAs self-identified few learning needs on the survey. • In RN and LPN focus groups, problems identified were: communication, symptom management, insufficient time for EOL care, and emotional attachment to residents. • In CNA focus groups, CNAs lacked basic knowledge about EOL care, and experienced distress about some care decisions. 'On-the-job' was the training method for EOL care.
Froggatt (2000) Nurse	Design: Responsive evaluation. Data collection: surveys, observations, interviews. Sample: $N = 4$ NHs and 43 staff from 54 NHs that participated in an EOL education project in the UK. Project provided EOL care courses for all types and levels of facility staff	• After completion of EOL courses, respondents reported their care improved in the following areas: communication with residents, families, and other providers; and pain control. • New knowledge of EOL care was difficult to implement without facility support or a critical mass of educated staff. • Facilities with centralized decision-making processes were less likely to support implementation of new knowledge.

TABLE 8.3 *(continued)*

Study	Methods	Selected findings related to facility characteristics
	Nursing homes	
Gibbs (1995) Nurse	Design: Descriptive. Data Collection: Semi-structured interviews about pain management Sample: $N = 24$ nurses randomly selected from government elder care wards and private NHs in the UK (response rate = 100%).	• The majority of nurses desired more education on palliative & pain care. • NH respondents were less familiar than acute care nurse respondents with pain assessment scales, had less contact with palliative & pain specialists, & reported more restrictions regarding pain control by physicians. • NH respondents identified fewer opportunities for additional education regarding palliative & pain care management.
Hanson & Henderson (2000)	See Table 8.2	• Negatively influencing EOL care delivery: lack of facility resources, intensity of regulations & paperwork, public negative perceptions of NHs, and federal regulatory assumption that NH residents will receive rehabilitation versus palliative care.

(continued)

TABLE 8.3 *(continued)*

Study	Methods	Selected findings related to facility characteristics
	Nursing homes	

Jones, Nackerud, & Boyle (1997) Nonnurse	Design: Descriptive. Data Collection: Mail survey & interviews. Sample: $N = 20$ NH administrators (response rate $= 87\%$) for survey. $N = 4$ administrators for interviews. Purposive sampling for interviews.	• Hospice services were less requested if pain control was not an identified problem.
		• Administrator attitudes that decreased use of hospice:
		  • Hospice staff perceived as 'taking over,' as poor communicators, as making difficult the coordination of services, and as not recognizing valuable care and knowledge of NH staff.
		  • Hospices perceived as reluctant to accept 'money loser' patients. Hospice services perceived as a money loser to facility.

Patterson, Molloy, Jubelius, Guyatt, & Bedard (1997) Nurse	Design: Descriptive. Data Collection: Mail survey. Sample: $N = 225$ RNs, LPNs, and aides in 3 NHs in Canada. (Response rate $= 54\%$). Convenience sample.	• EOL care learning needs included stress management for staff, palliative care team roles, physiologic impact of illness, pain assessment and management, and management of psychological needs of residents and families. • Barriers to attending courses included loss of pay and inconvenient course time or location.

TABLE 8.3 *(continued)*

Study	Methods	Selected findings related to facility characteristics
	Nursing homes	

Petrisek & Mor (1999) Nonnurse	Design: Descriptive. Data collection: 3 HCFA files: The On-line Survey & Certification of Automated Records, the Provider of Service File, and the Area Resource File. Sample: $N = 16,945$ national NHs surveyed between 6/95 & 4/97. Theoretical framework: Contingency theory.	• Relative risk of NH having at least 1 patient with Medicare hospice benefit was greater under the following facility conditions:
		  • For-profit, chain-affiliated, lacking full-time MD coverage, presence of other types of special care units in NHs.
		• Relative risk of NH having at least 1 patient with Medicare hospice benefit was greater under the following community conditions:
		  • More competitive NH market
		  • More for-profit, freestanding, & larger hospices in area
		  • Urban region > rural region

Wilson & Daley (1998) Nurse	Design: Descriptive. Data Collection: Focus groups. Sample: $N = 155$ staff and administrators across 11 proprietary and nonprofit NHs. Separate groups for staff and administrators. Purposive sampling for proprietary and nonprofit NHs.	• Staff attachment to residents facilitated quality terminal care. Attachment was defined as a "strong emotional bond and connectedness between staff & resident over time" (p. 25).

(continued)

TABLE 8.3 *(continued)*

Study	Methods	Selected findings related to facility characteristics

Nursing homes

		• Individual staff factors positively influencing attachment: *Presence* (being and staying with the resident), *communication* (talking openly with the resident & family about dying), & *knowledge* (of comfort measures, especially pain management). • Facility factors that negatively influenced EOL care: multiple time demands, lack of private rooms for the dying, & lack of pastoral support for residents, families, staff. • External factors that negatively influenced EOL care: acuity of new admits, unrealistic family expectations, negative image of NHs, regulatory requirements, & inadequate reimbursements to increase staff ratios.

Assisted living facilities

| Mitty (2000) | See Table 8.1 | • Identified concerns about EOL care in ALFS: RNs not available around the clock and every day (70%), legal liability for dying residents (62%), EOL care exceeds services stipulated in facility-resident contract (79%), "skilled nursing care" not permitted by state rules (88%), staff attitudes (46%), physician attitude (41%), insufficient reimbursement by Medicaid for hospice-like care (61%). |

TABLE 8.3 *(continued)*

Study	Methods	Selected findings related to facility characteristics
	Assisted living facilities	
		• 76% of facilities supported & used hospice services. • Factors needed for 'good' EOL care in ALFS: hospice, privately purchased additional care services, and family support.
	Nursing homes and assisted living facilities	
Komaromy, Sidell, & Katz (2000)	See Table 8.2	• Staffs were poorly paid, & responsible for a range of tasks including housekeeping & cooking besides direct care. • On-the-job training was the most common method for staff to learn how to provide EOL care. 5% of facilities employed staff with formal training in palliative care. • External (policy) and internal (facility budgets) factors influenced the availability of some equipment associated with terminal care. • External agency nurses who were following residents were sometimes perceived as negatively affecting quality of care within the home. • 8% of directors understood palliative care & its relevance to terminally ill residents. • 34% of directors stated they were familiar with the philosophy of hospice, but most perceived hospice as relevant only for a resident with cancer.

DISCUSSION

The majority of reports reviewed represent factor-isolating and factor-relating studies, which are appropriate for the limited body of existing knowledge (Dickoff, James, & Wiedenbach, 1968). These studies reflect efforts to identify key variables that influence NHs and ALFs as places for dying, and beginning efforts to describe relationships among the variables.

Methodological Issues

The studies reviewed were mostly atheoretical in nature. Theoretical or conceptual frameworks are needed to build a unified, comprehensive, and prescriptive body of knowledge on NHs and ALFs as places for dying. Sampling strategies relied predominately on small, convenience samples, and studies varied in the level of detail used to describe the samples. The findings represent predominantly the White, Anglo-Saxon experience of EOL care in NHs and ALFs. Ethnic, cultural, and religious diversity were minimally represented in the samples or discussed in the analyses. Self-report was the most common method for data collection.

State of Knowledge: NHs

Strengths to providing EOL care in NHs appear to be centered in the potential for a sustained, caring relationship between staff and residents, and staff and families. Several studies indicated that residents, families, and staff recognize the contribution that these types of relationships can make in providing EOL care management. However, there exists a large discrepancy between family and staff perceptions of the nature and quality of EOL care management. Families indicated that NH staffs have less knowledge and skill in EOL care than do hospital or hospice staffs. The poor quality of care was perceived as both general in nature and specific to symptoms at EOL, such as pain control and spiritual needs. Associated factors include (a) poor communication by staff with residents, families, and staff from other agencies; (b) lack of standardized tools or protocols for monitoring commonly occurring symptoms at EOL; (c) lack of recognition of issues other than pain control as part of EOL care; (d) limited staff access to educational offerings on EOL care; and (e) reimbursement mechanisms that do not reward EOL care services.

Staff members perceived that the federal regulatory emphasis on rehabilitation inhibits their abilities to provide EOL care. Dying trajectories were difficult to recognize, raising the question of whether new or additional frameworks for care in NHs are needed. Potential frameworks are the Mixed Model of Eventually Fatal Illness proposed by Fields and Cassel (1997), and Kolcaba's Model of Comfort Care (1995). These frameworks emphasize care that is supportive of individuals across a range of treatment goals including rehabilitation and palliation.

The reports on NH use of hospice services suggest confusion by NH staff about the clinical benefits to residents as well as fiscal implications of hospice services for facilities. Questions are raised by the findings that hospice staff may be perceived as intrusive by NH staff, and by the association of hospice use with proprietary, chain-affiliated status, and a highly competitive NH market.

State of Knowledge: ALFs

ALFs are at the opposite end of the spectrum of regulatory controls from NHs. While the extreme paucity of literature on ALFs as places for dying limits the conclusions that can be made, the EOL-specific findings reported by Mitty (2000) support other findings of extensive variation in the levels of care and nature of services generally provided in these facilities (Allen, 1999; Hawes et al., 1999; Mollica, 1998; Phillips et al., 2000). The findings from studies conducted in the U.K. suggest that ALFs may experience challenges for EOL care similar to NHs—challenges which may be compounded by the less stringent educational requirements for facility staff.

Directions for Future Research

Now programs of research are needed that lead to the long-term goal of prescribing the conditions required for "good deaths" to occur in NHs and ALFs. Studies that address the significance and magnitude of the effects of variables identified in this review will strengthen the preliminary, descriptive findings. Besides research that focuses on the three domains of institutional accountability suggested by Teno and colleagues (2001), studies that identify indicators of "good deaths" in these settings, and appropriate ethnic, cultural, and religious variations, could facilitate the design and testing of specific interventions.

The studies reviewed suggest that positive, long-term relationships can occur among residents, families, and staff members in NHs. ALFs also have the potential for similar, long-term relationships. How can these relationships be enhanced to improve EOL communication and decision making, along with supportive physical, emotional, and spiritual care for residents and their families?

Studies should be conducted that test the use of EOL symptom assessment tools and protocols in NHs and ALFs, particularly when used by ALF staff members who may be unlicensed and have limited formal education in caregiving. Studies are needed that (a) address early recognition of residents most likely to benefit from targeted, EOL care services, (b) analyze the impact of standardized assessment tools on resident and family satisfaction with symptom management, and (c) examine the impact of fiscal and regulatory policies on symptom assessment and management.

The findings of Kovach and colleagues (1996) support the need for larger replication studies with sample sizes sufficient to permit analysis of the various components of the intervention, and how each component contributes to specific care outcomes. Similar intervention research is appropriate with dying residents who do not have end-stage dementia.

ALF regulations vary considerably across states. Thus, single-state studies are desirable that focus on ALFs as places for dying from the perspectives of the key stakeholders: residents, family members, and care providers. State specific replications of the multimethod, in-depth descriptive studies conducted by Katz and colleagues (1999), and Komaromy and colleagues (2000) in the U.K. are appropriate to develop basic knowledge about EOL experiences and care in ALFs that operate in common regulatory environments in the U.S.

Within-state studies are also needed that compare NHs with ALFs; studies that answer the question: given the different regulatory environments and institutional purposes, what are the differences in NHs and ALFs as places for dying? Is either setting preferable as a place for dying under certain condition (e.g., type of terminal condition, presence of certain symptoms, specifically needed symptom management therapies)? What are unique and common challenges to providing EOL care, including use of hospice services, in ALFs versus NHs? What are organizational variables that might improve education and foster retention of the best possible licensed nursing and ancillary care staff in these settings?

Numerous policy questions are identified from this review of the literature. What is the relationship between the OBRA '87 mandates for

NH resident rehabilitation, and facilities' abilities to provide EOL care? Are modifications needed in the Minimum Data Set and Resident Assessment Protocols for EOL care, as suggested by Engles and colleagues (1998)? Given the limited and variable regulatory mandates for registered nurse supervision in ALFs, how is nursing care being delivered in these settings? What are experiences and outcomes related to delegation of nursing tasks such as medication administration and skin care by RNs to nonlicensed staff in ALFs? What are policy lessons to be learned by comparing highly regulated NHs with relatively unregulated ALFs that will promote these settings as places for dying?

This discussion has proposed an ambitious research agenda. Because elderly residents in these settings experience multiple functional limitations and require chronic illness management across prolonged time spans, nursing is the appropriate discipline to lead a multidisciplinary effort to develop programs of research on NHs and ALFs as places for dying for elders.

REFERENCES

Primary Resources

Baer, W. M., & Hanson, L. C. (2000). Families' perception of the added value of hospice in the nursing home. *Journal of the America Geriatrics Society, 48*, 879–882.

Bradley, E. H., Walker, L., Blechner, J. D., & Wetle, T. (1997). Assessing capacity to participate in discussions of advance directives in nursing homes: Findings from a study of the Patient Self Determination Act. *Journal of the American Geriatrics Society, 45*(1), 79–83.

Castle, N. G. (1998). Innovations in dying in the nursing home: The impact of market characteristics. *Omega, 36*(3), 227–241.

Clare, J., & DeBellis, A. (1997). Palliative care in South Australian nursing homes. *Australian Journal of Advanced Nursing, 14*(4), 20–29.

Engle, V. F., Fox-Hill, E., & Graney, M. J. (1998). The experience of living-dying in a nursing home: Self-reports of black and white older adults. *Journal of the American Geriatrics Society, 46*, 1091–1096.

Ersek, M., Kraybill, B. M., & Hansberry, J. (1999). Investigating the educational needs of licensed nursing staff and certified nursing assistants in nursing homes regarding end-of-life care. *American Journal of Hospice & Palliative Care, 16*, 573–582.

Forbes, S., Bern-Klug, M., & Gessert, C. (2000). End-of-life decision making for nursing home residents with dementia. *Journal of Nursing Scholarship, 32*(3), 251–258.

Froggatt, K. (2000). Evaluating a palliative care education project in nursing homes. *International Journal of Palliative Nursing, 6,* 140–146.

Gibbs, G. (1995). Nurses in private nursing homes: A study of their knowledge and attitudes to pain management in palliative care. *Palliative Medicine, 9,* 245–253.

Hanson, L. C. & Henderson, M. (2000). Care of the dying in long-term care settings. *Clinics in Geriatric Medicine, 16*(2), 225–237.

Hanson, L. C., Danis, M., & Garrett, J. (1997). What is wrong with EOL care? Opinions of bereaved family members. *Journal of the American Geriatrics Society, 45,* 1339–1344.

Jones, B., Nackerud, L., & Boyle, D. (1997). Differential utilization of hospice services in nursing homes. *Hospice Journal, 12*(3), 41–57.

Katz, J., Komaromy, C., & Sidell, M. (1999). Understanding palliative care in residential and nursing homes. *International Journal of Palliative Nursing, 5*(2), 58–64.

Kayser-Jones, J. (2000). A case study of the death of an older woman in a nursing home: Are nursing care practices in compliance with ethical guidelines? *Journal of Gerontology Nursing,* 48–54.

Kayser-Jones, J. (1995). Decision making in the treatment of acute illness in nursing homes: Framing the decision problem, treatment plan, and outcome. *Medical Anthropology Quarterly, 9*(2), 236–56.

Komaromy, C., Sidell, M., & Katz, J. T. (2000). The quality of terminal care in residential and nursing homes. *International Journal of Palliative Nursing, 6*(4), 192–200.

Kovach, C. R., Wilson, S. A., & Noonan, P. E. (1996). The effects of hospice interventions on behaviors, discomfort, and physical complications of end-stage dementia nursing home residents. *American Journal of Alzheimer's Disease, 11*(4), 7–15.

Levin, J. R., Wenger, N. S., Ouslander, J. G., Zellman, G., Schnelle, J. F., Hirsch, S. H., & Reuben, D. B. (1999). Life-sustaining treatment decisions for nursing home residents: Who discusses, who decides and what is decided? *Journal of the American Geriatrics Society, 47*(1), 82–87.

Lurie, N., Pheley, A. M., Miles, S. H., & Bannick-Mohrland, S. (1992). Attitudes toward discussing life-sustaining treatments in extended care facility patients. *American Geriatrics Society, 40,* 1205–1208.

Mitty, E. L. (2000, November). End-of-life planning and care in assisted living facilities. In M. Mezey (Chair), *Improving end-of-life care: Nursing homes, assisted living, and transitions from nursing homes to hospitals.* Symposium conducted at the 53rd Annual Scientific Meeting of the Gerontological Society of America, Washington, DC.

Palker, N. B., & Nettles-Carlson, B. (1995). The prevalence of advance directives: Lessons from a nursing home. *Nurse Practitioner, 20*(2), 7–21.

Patterson, C., Molloy, W., Jubelius, R., Guyatt, G. H., & Bedard, M. (1997). Provisional educational needs of health care providers in palliative care in three nursing homes in Ontario. *Journal of Palliative Care, 13*(3), 13–17.

Petrisek, A. C., & Mor, V. (1999). Hospice in nursing homes: A facility-level analysis of the distribution of hospice beneficiaries. *Gerontologist, 39,* 279–290.

Wilson, S. A., & Daley, B. J. (1998). Attachment/detachment: Forces influencing care of the dying in long-term care. *Journal of Palliative Medicine, 1*(1), 21–34.

Wilson, S. A., & Daley, B. J. (1999). Family perspectives on dying in long-term care settings. *Journal of Gerontological Nursing,* 19–25.

Secondary Resources

Allen, K. G. (1999). *Assisted living: Quality-of-care and consumer protection issues in four states.* (GAO/T-HEHS-99-111). Washington, DC: U.S. General Accounting Office.

Brock, D., & Foley, D. (1998). Demography & epidemiology of dying in the U.S. with emphasis on deaths of older persons. *Hospice Journal, 13*(1/2), 49–60.

Dickoff, J., James, P., & Wiedenbach, E. (1968). Theory in a practice discipline, Part 1: Practice oriented theory. *Nursing Research, 17*(5), 415–435.

Engle, V. F. (1998). Care of the living, care of the dying: Re-conceptualizing nursing home care. *Journal of the American Geriatrics Society, 46*(46), 1172–1174.

Field, M. M., & Cassel, C. K. (Eds.). (1997). *Approaching death: Improving care at the end of life.* Washington, DC: National Academy Press.

Hawes, C., Rose, M., & Phillips, C. (1999). *A national study of assisted living for the frail elderly: Results of a national survey of facilities.* Washington, DC: U.S. Department of Health and Human Services.

Kane, R. A. (1995). Expanding the home care concept: Blurring distinctions among home care, institutional care, and other long-term-care services. *Milbank Quarterly, 73*(2), 161–187.

Keay, T. J. (1999). Palliative care in the nursing home. *Generations, 23*(1), 96–98.

Kolcaba, K. Y. (1995). The art of comfort care. *Image: The Journal of Nursing Scholarship, 27*(4), 287–289.

Last Acts. (1997, December). *Precepts of palliative care.* [On-line]. Electronic Newsletter of Last Acts Campaign. Available http://www.lastacts.org.

Manard, B. B., & Cameron, R. (1997). *A national study of assisted living for the frail elderly: Report on in-depth interviews with developers.* Washington, DC: U.S. Department of Health and Human Services.

Mezey, M., Miller, L. L., & Linton-Nelson, L. (1999). Caring for caregivers of frail elders at the end of life. *Generations, 23*(1), 44–52.

Mollica, R. (1998). *State assisted living policy.* Washington, DC: U.S. Department of Health and Human Services, National Academy for State Health Policy.

Moss, M. S. (2001). End of life in nursing homes. In M. P. Lawton (Vol. Ed.), *Annual review of gerontology and geriatrics* (Vol. 20, pp. 224–258). New York: Springer Publishing Co.

National Center for Assisted Living. (2001). *Guiding principles for assisted living.* [On-line]. Available http://www.ncal.org/about/concepts.htm

Phillips, C. D., Hawes, C., Spry, K., & Rose, M. (2000). *Residents leaving assisted living: Descriptive and analytical results from a national survey.* Washington, DC: U.S. Department of Health and Human Services.

Rubenstein, R. L. (2001). The ethnography of the end of life: The nursing home and other residential settings. In M. P. Lawton (Vol. Ed.), *Annual review of gerontology and geriatrics* (Vol. 20, pp. 259–272). New York: Springer Publishing Co.

Sheehy, E. (2000, November). Assisted living: To regulate or not to regulate? That is the question. In J. Franks (Chair), *Assisted living: To regulate or not to regulate— that is the question*. Symposium conducted at the 53rd Annual Scientific Meeting of the Gerontological Society of America, Washington, DC.

Strahan, G. W. (1997). An overview of nursing homes and their current residents: Data from the 1995 National Nursing Home Survey. *Advance data from vital and health statistics, 280*. Hyattsville, MD: National Center for Health Statistics.

Teno, J. M., McNiff, K., & Lynn, J. (2001). Measuring quality of medical care for dying persons and their families: Preliminary suggestions for accountability. In M. P. Lawton (Ed.). *Annual review of gerontology and geriatrics* (pp. 20, 97–119). New York: Springer Publishing Co.

Wilson, K. B. (1995). Assisted living as a model of care delivery. In L. M. Gamroth, J. Semradek, & E. M. Tornquist (Eds.), *Enhancing autonomy in long-term care: Concepts and strategies* (pp. 139–154). New York: Springer Publishing Co.

PART III

Public Health, Social, and Scientific Trends

Chapter 9

Home Health Services Research

ELIZABETH A. MADIGAN, SUSAN TULLAI-MCGUINNESS, AND
DONNA FELBER NEFF

ABSTRACT

This chapter reviews 69 published research reports of home health care from a health services perspective by nurse researchers and researchers from other disciplines. Reports were identified through searches of the National Library of Medicine (MEDLINE), and the Cumulative Index to Nursing and Allied Health Literature and Social Sciences Citation Index using the following search terms: *home health care*, *health services research*, and *elders*. Within the major areas identified, the following additional terms were specified: *resource use* and *outcomes*. Reports were included if published between 1995 and 2001, used samples age 65 and older, performed in the U.S., and published in English. Studies of all types were included. The key findings follow: (a) Most studies were atheoretical. If a theoretical model was used, it was most often the Andersen Behavioral Model. (b) Few conclusions can be drawn about resource use—increasing age and higher severity of health related problems are associated with higher numbers of home visits. The variety of measures of resource use and the study approaches (large national data sets versus single or several agency samples) limits the ability to draw conclusions on resource use. (c) There is a growing body of evidence on rehospitalization of home health care patients which indicates rehospitalization is prevalent but largely not predictable. (d) Patient outcomes research is inconclusive at this point, primarily because there are few studies that examine patient outcomes using a consistent set of measures. The main recommendations are: to study rehospitalization using a more profile-based approach to determine visit patterns that may be effective, to further specify the kinds of outcomes that may be achieved as a result of home health care and which patients might be expected to achieve positive outcomes, and to examine the integration of home health care with the broader community-based services.

Keywords: health services research, home care services, access to health care, hospital readmission, health resources

Although home health care services are predicted to be the largest growing segment of health care over the next several decades, the home health care industry has changed dramatically in the last few years, primarily as a result of changes in reimbursement and regulation in the Medicare program and also in managed care. The impact of these changes has been substantial—more than 25% of all home health care agencies nationwide have closed since 1997 (National Association for Home Care, 2001). In addition to agency closures, there has been a 14% reduction in the number of patients seen by home care agencies and a 30% reduction in the number of home visits for those patients who do receive home health care services (National Association for Home Care, 2001).

From a health services research perspective, the regulatory change that has had the most impact has been the change from a fee-for-service payment system for Medicare home care to a prospective payment system with case mix adjustment (Department of Health and Human Services, Health Care Financing Administration, 2000). The case mix adjustment is based on the collection of standardized data on home health care at admission, at discharge/end of care, and at periodic interim points. While Medicare home health care represents only 40% of all expenditures for home health care, it is twice the expenditure of the next highest category, out-of-pocket payment. Thus, as Medicare home health care goes, so goes the remainder of the home health care segment of the health system.

For some time there has been a shift from acute inpatient care to community-based acute and/or chronic care. This shift has provided additional opportunities for nursing in that much of community-based care is nursing care. This is certainly true for home health care where more than 84% of home health care patients received nursing care and most (72%) of these patients were over 65 years of age (Haupt, 1998; Munson, 1999). Among the opportunities for nursing is research within home health care.

Within health care research, including nursing research, there is increasing focus on the "continuum" of care versus "silos" of care—hospital *or* home health care *or* long term care. The continuum of care approach is particularly important for elders who consume larger amounts of health care services and dollars compared with other age groups. Increasing numbers of nurse researchers are incorporating a health services research perspective. Health services research, with its focus on health system variables, can provide context for nursing research, even for very clinically oriented research, and also can provide additional explanation for nursing research findings.

One of the challenges inherent in evaluating systems of health care is the terminology. In particular, there is confusion regarding the terms *home care* and *home health care*. Home care has been used as the broader term encompassing any service provided in the home, including home-maintenance services, home-delivered meals, and some smaller scope of health care services. Home care, as the term is generally defined, is primarily a social service system often designed to prevent or delay placement in a nursing home. Home health care, then, is more specific and refers to the delivery of health care services in the home—primarily nursing (RN and LPN), rehabilitative therapy (physical and occupational therapy, speech and language pathology), and social work. The focus of home health care is focused on illness and the remediation of illness. There are some patients who use services from both systems at the same time while other patients move between systems. Part of the difficulty with the definitions is that the scope and services available from the home care system are often geographic, either state or locality based. Home health care, particularly under Medicare, has fewer geographic variations. The fragmentation of the systems presents challenges for the users and providers of the systems as well as the researchers who study the systems.

In summary, home health care remains a nursing intensive system, providing care to a predominantly elder population, and has undergone dramatic change in the last few years. These three aspects (nursing intensive, elder focus, dramatic change) provide an impetus for the evaluation of home health care for elders from a health services perspective.

Thus, the questions to be addressed in this chapter include:

1. What theoretical frameworks have been used to study home health care from a health services research perspective?
2. How has home health care resource use been defined?
3. What individual, organizational, and policy factors are associated with the use of home health care services?
4. What are the outcomes of home health care?
5. What research is needed to develop the knowledge base about home health care from a health services research prospective?

METHOD

A systematic search strategy was used to identify relevant research literature on home health care from a health services perspective. The strategy involved the searching of three databases—MEDLINE from the National Library of Medicine, the Cumulative Index to Nursing and Allied Health Literature (CINAHL), and the Social Sciences Citation Index, and was not limited to nursing research. The primary search terms used included: *home health care, health services research,* and *elders.* Within the major areas identified—*resource use* and *outcomes*—more specific searches were done to identify studies within the area that may not have been found using the primary search terms. We focused our search to include primarily home health care services—that is, skilled services. Due to the nature of the patient populations, some studies that were focused primarily on supportive, in-home care (paraprofessional) also had skilled services included as well.

A total of 69 articles were chosen that met the additional inclusion criteria of published in peer-reviewed, English language journals; U.S. studies; and published between 1995 and 2001. The criterion limiting the articles to U.S. studies reflects the nation-specific effects of the health system. Other countries have health systems that differ dramatically from the U.S. and health services research done in these countries reflects the orientation and philosophy of the particular health care system. In addition, economic forces drive health services decisions in many cases, and the economic systems for the financing and delivery of health care also vary widely by country.

The time frame of 6 years was designed to capture the rapid evolution of health care delivery and financing services in home health care. While there was a flurry of research in the 1980s on the topic of community-based and long-term home health care, the overall health system was such that those findings are likely not generalizable to the current health system.

RESULTS

What Theoretical Frameworks Have Been Used to Study Home Health Care From a Health Services Research Perspective?

The behavioral model of utilization, or health services utilization model, is the framework that is most frequently used to describe and explain the use of home health care services. Initially the model was developed by Andersen (1968) to assist in understanding the family's use of health care services, but was later adapted to study health care utilization by an individual (Andersen & Newman, 1973). Utilization of health care services is conceptualized as the result of the interaction of predisposing, enabling, and need for care factors. In its most recent versions (Andersen, 1995), the model has been expanded to include environmental characteristics, health behavior, and outcomes while retaining the population characteristics (predisposing, enabling, and need). In the research reviewed here, the Andersen model has been used by several researchers (Dansky, Brannon, Shea, Vasey, & Dirani, 1998; Fortinsy & Madigan, 1997; Proctor, Morrow-Howell, & Kaplan, 1996).

The transitional model, as first described by Brooten (Brooten et al., 1986) has been used to guide studies evaluating the use of advanced practice nurses (APNs) for patients with particular conditions (Naylor et al., 1999a; Naylor & McCauley, 1999b) (See also Naylor in chapter 5 of this volume).

The transitional model was designed using APNs, and thus is valuable for studies and practice involving APN care. The transitional model is a nursing model and has not yet been used by other disciplines. The Andersen model is more abstract and has been used to study a variety of health services in addition to home health care. The Andersen model provides a venue to evaluate environmental or larger health care system factors, patient and family factors, use of health services, and health outcomes. The broad applications of the model in health services research reflect the level of abstractness and the inclusion of important health services research concepts—use of health services and outcomes in particular. The decision between the two models, then, is driven by the kind of health service to be examined, the type of provider, the desired level of abstractness, and the utility for direct application to practice.

In the majority of the studies reviewed here, there was no explicit theoretical model. As will be further explained in the description and evaluation of the studies, the lack of an explicit theoretical model is one explanation for the disparate selection of concepts, variables, and measures. The interrelationships between the independent variables, and between the independent variables and dependent variables, are not clearly defined within the bodies of literature reviewed. The development of additional models for examination of home health care services might provide more conceptual and empirical clarity to the body of science.

How Has Home Health Care Resource Use Been Defined?

In general, the body of research factors associated with the use of home health care is small and diverse. While the research literature on resource use is more developed than that on outcomes, there are few conclusions that can be drawn. If one of the purposes of health services research is to inform policy and the formation of policy, then the scattershot approach to scientific evaluation of home health care from a health services perspective has limited utility for policy purposes. For example, there is not yet a critical mass of studies that would allow for conclusions to be drawn about the effectiveness of particular interventions or even to say with any degree of confidence whether better patient outcomes are achieved with a higher number of home health care visits. One of the challenges within this body of scientific literature is to define the use of home health care services, referred to here as *resource use*. Thus, this section is divided into definitions of resource use for home health care services and the individual, organizational, and policy factors that are associated with the use of home health care services. Finally, studies were included only if they included skilled home health care services versus only paraprofessional services.

DEFINING RESOURCE USE

The literature shows great variability in measurement of resource use, differing in amount and type. Resource use by home care patients has been measured by the number of nursing, therapy, social work, and aide visits over an episode of care (Adams, Corbett, & Michel, 2000; Anderson, Pena, & Helms, 1998; Fortinsky & Madigan, 1997; Swan, Black, Benjamin, & Fox, 1995; Torrez, Estes, & Linkens, 1997); the number of Medicare HMO & Medicare fee-for-service RN, home care aide, medical social work, and therapy visits, as well as length of stay (Adams & Kramer, 1996; Madigan, Schott, & Matthews, 2001); number of Medicare home care visits for 1 year (Dansky et al., 1998); Medicare home health users and home health visits per user for each of 3 years (Cohen & Tumlinson, 1997); Medicare HMO home health care visits over 18 months (Murphy & Hepworth, 1996); expenditures over 30 months (Experton, Zili, Branch, Ozminkowski, & Mellon-Lacey, 1997); use of at least one visiting nurse service or home health service in 10 years (Ozawa & Tseng, 1999); use of in-home services (Slivinske, Fitch, & Wingerson, 1998); number of RN and home care aide visits over 6 months (Hays & Willborn, 1996); a visiting nurse visit during 1 year (Clark & Dellasega, 1998); number and type of home health care services in a Medicaid waiver program (Diwan, Berger, & Manns, 1997); and first use of home care services (Cagney & Agree, 1999). In addition, there has been some observation of intensity of visits which is generally the number of visits divided by the length of stay in days (Anderson et al., 1998; Fortinsky & Madigan, 1997; Madigan & Fortinsky, 1999) and hours of care over the episode (Madigan & Fortinsky, 1999).

Although the decisions around definitions of resource use are a function of the study purpose, the disparity between definitions makes it difficult to compare across samples, even within the commonly studied Medicare home health care population. Not only do the definitions vary in what counts as a visit, but also in what defines an episode of care. Because the resources are consumed or provided over an episode, varying definitions make it difficult to ascertain whether study findings are due to the phenomena under study or the definitional differences. In addition, there is little scientific evidence to guide practice on the best profiles of home health care contacts, whether those contacts are home visits or some kind of telehealth (phone or computer-based) initiative. The current regulation for prospective payment under Medicare home health care may simplify the definitions of resource use in that the episodes of care for Medicare patients are specified.

RESOURCE USE—TRAJECTORIES

Home health care services cannot be studied in isolation—patients come into home health care from a variety of sources and depart home health care for a variety of reasons. The entries and exits have been referred to as the trajectory of care (Fortinsky & Madigan, 1997). Patients most commonly enter home health care from the acute care institution or a subacute or rehabilitation facility. Entry into home health care often occurs following a hospital stay. From 59% to 82% of patients are admitted to home health care from a hospital stay (Anderson, Hanson, & DeVilder, 1996; Fortinsky & Madigan, 1997). Fewer admissions come from long-term care facilities with one study finding that only 11% of those in long-term care facilities in one state are discharged home (Chapin, Wilkinson, Rachlin, Levy, & Lindbloom, 1998). For those patients with hip fractures discharged from rehabilitation units, more than 60% received home health care (Intrator & Berg, 1998). Fewer patients are directly admitted into home health care from the community, although there are not regulations that preclude this point of entry.

The research evidence on hospital discharge planning specific to home health care has focused on the evaluation of three areas—the referral patterns for home health care services, the actual delivery of home health care following referral, and the effectiveness of models of discharge planning. Naylor and colleagues found that, of high-risk patients who were discharged from a hospital, only 44% were actually referred to home health care (Naylor et al., 1999a). Similarly, Castro and colleagues found that 45% of 194 patients visiting an ED were eligible for home care services but were not referred (Castro, Anderson, Hanson, & Helms, 1998). When examining specific diagnostic patient groups, Narsavage and Naylor (2000) found that patients who were referred for home health care services during a hospital stay were more likely to have both heart failure and COPD (as opposed to just one of the diagnoses), require the use of a home health aide, and be unmarried. Kane and colleagues (1998; 2000) found that the proportion of patients discharged from an acute care setting and referred for home health care varied by the diagnosis; 38% of patients with chronic obstructive pulmonary disease were referred while only 14% of those with a hip fracture were referred. Most patients with hip fractures (> 50%) were referred to a nursing home or a rehabilitation center post hospital stay. In a separate study of primarily elders, of those referred for home health care, most (65%) were referred for skilled nursing care and fewer (28%) for home health aide (Pohl, Collins, & Given, 1995).

There are ethnicity differences in discharge planning between African-Americans and Whites in that African Americans are more likely to pursue home health care services post-discharge than nursing home care (Morrow-Howell, Chadiha, Proctor, Hourd-Bryant, & Dore, 1996). This has been found despite the finding by the same research team that African-Americans were found to be more functionally and cognitively impaired at the time of hospital discharge (Proctor et al., 1997).

While referral patterns are important for patients who may be eligible for services, there is also a second step following referral—do patients receive home health care services once they are referred? One group found that 91% of patients referred for home health care received services following referral (Simon, Showers, Blumenfield, Holden, & Wu, 1995).

In evaluating the effectiveness of a multidisciplinary approach using a standardized assessment instrument for discharge planning, Rosswurm and Lanham (1998) found that the intervention did not change the rehospitalization or emergency department visit rate, but the intervention group received more home care services than the control group.

Haupt (1998), in describing a national sample of home health care patients, found that exits from home health care occur because patients are better and able to assume their own care (29%), no longer need services

(21%), require a higher or different level of care such as nursing home, hospice, or hospital (28%), or death (4%). There are a variety of other reasons for discharge that occur more rarely.

What Individual, Organizational, and Policy Factors Are Associated with the Use of Home Health Care Services?

There is a body of literature that focuses on the factors associated with use of home health care services, for both predicting which patients will enter into home health care as well as the volume of services that the patient will receive once home care has started. These factors can be divided into individual factors, organizational factors, and policy factors.

INDIVIDUAL FACTORS

Several studies have examined the relationship between individual patient/ family factors and home health care resource use including: gender, age, race, marital status, education, income, geographic location, caregivers, household living arrangements, payor source, hospitalizations, and functional status.

Many studies found no gender differences in the use or volume of services (Kenney & Rajan, 2000; Lee & Mills, 2000; Murphy & Hepworth, 1996; Ozawa & Tseng, 1999; Swan et al., 1995; Torrez et al., 1997). Male gender was found to be associated with both a shorter and longer length of stay in home health care (Anderson et al., 1998; Swan et al., 1995, respectively), more home health visits (Dansky et al., 1998), and fewer nursing and more aide visits (Anderson et al., 1998).

Increasing age is a useful predictor for visiting nurse services (Ozawa & Tseng, 1999; Swan et al., 1995), home health services (Hays & Willborn, 1996; Ozawa & Tseng, 1999), Medicare home care visits (Dansky et al., 1998; Kenney & Rajan, 2000; Murphy & Hepworth, 1996), and home health expenditures (Experton et al., 1997). At the same time, the older old were less likely to receive physical therapy (Swan et al., 1995). Either no effect or a limited effect of age has been found by others (Cohen & Tumlinson, 1997; Lee & Mills, 2000; Torrez et al., 1997).

The effect of race on use of services is inconclusive. Race was not found to be a predictor of home health use (Dansky et al., 1998; Guild, Ledwin, Sanford, & Winter, 1994; Lee & Mills, 2000), number of Medicare home health visits (Kenney & Rajan, 2000), or in use of RN services compared with RN and HHA services (Hays & Willborn, 1996). Ozawa and Tseng (1999) found that non-Whites were less likely to use visiting nurse services, but found no difference in use of home health services. Cagney and Agree (1999) found that Whites have an 8% greater risk than Blacks by the time they reach 80 of using home health care services. But, when controlling for health status, family structure, and social class, they did not find a significant difference in use between Whites and Blacks.

Similarly, the effects of marital status are inconclusive. The likelihood of using visiting nurse services and home health services was higher for widows and the separated or divorced (Ozawa & Tseng, 1999). These findings are consistent with Kenney and Rajan (2000) who found that married enrollees used fewer Medicare home health visits. However, there was no difference in use by those who were never married (Ozawa & Tseng, 1999) or not married (Dansky et al., 1998). Hays and Willborn (1996) found no significant difference in marital status between those who use RN services and those who use RN and HHA services.

Few studies examined relationships between home health care resource use and education level or income level. Education was not found to be a predictor of the number of Medicare home health visits (Kenney & Rajan, 2000). The effect of income is mixed—income was not related to use of home health care services in one study (Ozawa & Tseng, 1999). Other studies have found that lower income is associated with higher use by age 80 (Cagney & Agree, 1999).

The effect of geographic location suggests that a rural residence is associated with more resource use. Cohen and Tumlinson (1997) found a significant and negative relationship between those living in urban areas and Medicare home health use in only one (1991) of three years (1991–1993) studied. Consistent with these findings, Dansky and colleagues (1998), in a study of 6,956 Medicare beneficiaries from five geographic categories, found residents living in metropolitan areas were as likely to receive at least one home health visit as those in rural areas, but those in rural areas had a larger number of mean visits per person. In a smaller study of 106 elders (Clark & Dellasega, 1998), no differences were found in home care use between urban and rural dwellers. Researchers have also examined geographic location in a larger context and found that enrollees in the northeast had higher use of Medicare home health visits than those in the west and Midwest (Kenney & Rajan, 2000), suggesting an area variation effect.

The number of caregivers, regardless of relationship, has not been found to be related to the amount or number of services (Swan et al.,

1995). Having a daughter predicts earlier use of home health, while for Blacks, having grandchildren decreased the risk for use of home health care (Cagney & Agree, 1999). Gender of the caregiver was not a predictor of use of home health care services.

Part of the confusion related to the number of helpers is the operational distinction between those who are caregivers and household size. Household size was found to be a significant predictor of Medicare home health service use (Dansky et al., 1998) yet Hays and Willborn (1996) found no significant difference in living arrangements between those who use RN services and those who use RN and HHA services.

Discussions on the impact of payor source are complicated in that the number of payers may or may not have an effect on resource use depending on the type of service under discussion. For example, having more than Medicare for traditional Medicare home health care confers no benefits in terms of qualifying patients for additional services. The effect of having Medicaid on resource use varies. When comparing patients with Medicare and those with Medicaid, no differences were found in the use of home health care (Ozawa & Tseng, 1999), the amount of service use (Swan et al., 1995), or in the amount of expenditures of home health services (Experton et al., 1997). Dual beneficiaries (those with both Medicare and Medicaid) have been found to have a higher probability of visiting nurse services (Ozawa & Tseng, 1999), were longer-term users of services (Freedman, 1999), and had more visits (Dansky et al., 1998; Kenney & Rajan, 2000). The effect of HMO coverage is less clear. In one study, those with Medicare HMO coverage received 71% fewer home health care visits than those with traditional Medicare (Experton et al., 1997), yet other studies found no differences (Adams et al., 1996; Torrez et al., 1997).

Physical health status is often conceptualized by measurement of functional dependency or health status, and severity of illness. Reflecting the incongruent measurements of resource use, findings concerning the relationship between functional dependency and resource use are inconclusive. Functional dependency is most often measured by activities of daily living (ADLs) and instrumental activities of daily living (IADLs), although the actual measures used vary between studies.

In some studies, functional dependency as measured by ADLs was found to be a significant predictor of the number of services used (Torrez et al., 1997), the type of service (Slivinske et al., 1998), and the number of visits (Dansky et al., 1998; Kenney & Rajan, 2000; Torrez et al., 1997).

Dansky and colleagues (1998) found that impairments in both ADLs and IADLs were highest in the most rural residents. Other researchers have found that only IADL impairment is associated with the number of visits (Kenney & Rajan, 2000).

When examining functional dependency and resource use by specific discipline, functional dependency has been found to reduce the likelihood of skilled nursing, with no evidence of effects on number of visits (Swan et al., 1995). The probability of respondents with two ADL problems using visiting nurse services was 2.8 times the probability of those with no ADL problems but no significance was found between ADL problems and use of home health services versus nursing service (Ozawa & Tseng, 1999).

Grabbe and colleagues (1995) provide a different level of detail suggesting that the odds-ratio for functional status cannot be independently interpreted. Functional impairment as the primary risk factor for receiving either a nurse or a homemaker aide during the last year of life was moderated by the living situation and the number of informal caregivers.

The number of health impairments has been found to be positively related to the use of in-home services, visiting nurse services (Ozawa & Tseng, 1999), and the number of home health visits (Kenney & Rajan, 2000). There is a positive relationship between severity of illness and numbers of visits—visits were found to be more likely among patients with at least moderately acute medical problems, but successively higher levels of medical acuity are not shown to affect likelihood or volume of visits. This finding, however, was attributed to one of the agencies within the study targeting patients for rehabilitation (Swan et al., 1995). In another work, health status was not found to be a predictor of number of different services or visits received (Torrez et al., 1997). However, fair or poor self-reported health status was found to be a predictor of home health use (Dansky et al., 1998; Slivinske et al., 1998) and number of visits (Kenney & Rajan, 2000).

The type of provider has been found to vary by patient medical diagnosis wherein patients with heart failure were more likely to receive RN visits while patients with total hip replacements were more likely to receive physical therapy visits. No difference was found in intensity or length of care between the types of providers (O'Sullivan & Volicer, 1997).

ORGANIZATIONAL FACTORS

Agency characteristics alone explain only 9% of the variance in the type of services provided with those receiving services from a for-profit agency having significantly higher numbers for different services, but not for numbers of visits (Torrez et al., 1997). Cohen and Tumlinson (1997) found no significant difference in the proportion of proprietary (for-profit) agencies and use of home health care services. However, when agencies are owned by hospitals, it has been found that patients are 21% more likely to be referred to home health care, with an even higher likelihood (57%) if the hospital is urban (Dansky, Milliron, & Gamm, 1996).

POLICY FACTORS

In studying data from all states with Medicaid programs, Cohen and Tumlinson (1997) found that the number of Medicare home health users is higher in states with greater fiscal pressure concerning their Medicaid budgets and fewer state personal care programs. States without personal care aide programs had an average of 15 more Medicare home health users per enrollee. However, when excluding New York, a state that consumes 51% of all Medicaid home health and personal care expenditures, it was found that Medicaid spending on home health and personal care had a negative but not significant impact on the use of Medicare home health services (Kenney & Rajan, 2000).

Market factors include such variables as the number of long-term care beds and labor availability. The ratio of home health aides to population was found to be a positive predictor in the number of visits over 1 year (Dansky et al., 1998). Cohen and Tumlinson (1997) found that as the number of skilled nursing facilities decreased, the number of home health users increased and for 2 of the 3 years studied, as the number of home care agencies increased, the number of users increased. In contrast, Kenny and Rajan (2000) found the number of nursing home beds and home care agencies were not indicators of Medicare home care visits.

In summary, some patient factors (increasing age and severity of health related problems) and some agency or market factors (nursing home bed numbers) have been found to be associated with higher likelihood of using home health services or using more services. The ability to draw conclusions is hampered by the diversity in the ways use and volume have been measured. In some cases, the services are primarily health care services (nursing, therapy, social work, home care aide) while in others the services are primarily supportive services (homemaking, chore, transportation, and meals). Some studies combine both types. In addition, the time frames over which the use of resources has been measured limit the ability to compare across studies. Finally, some of the studies within this section are based on large national or regional data sets while others involve primary data collection from one or a small number of agencies. Although organizational and market factor comparisons would be valuable from a health services research perspective, it may not be a variable of interest within a study that is more clinically focused. In general, much of the research in this area has been descriptive and explanatory. There is a dearth of research evidence on intervention studies that are designed to determine optimal service profiles for both the type of provider and the timing of the care.

What Are the Outcomes of Home Health Care?

From a health services perspective, outcomes of home health care include service utilization outcomes, patient outcomes, and satisfaction with care. Each will be discussed in detail.

SERVICE UTILIZATION OUTCOMES

Service utilization outcomes are challenging to evaluate because home health care is provided for a variety of populations by several levels of health care providers (paraprofessional and health care professionals). Thus, expectations that home health care can serve as a substitute for more expensive institutional care (hospital, nursing home) is not realistic across populations of home health care patients. Indeed, there is increasing focus on the issue of targeting home health care services to those who are most likely to benefit (Benjamin, 1999; Greene, Ondrich, & Ladtika, 1998; Kane et al., 1998). Policy and programmatic activities currently have a venue for targeting under the Medicaid waiver programs for home and community based care (HCBC). In evaluating the HCBC programs, there is evidence that targeting home care services to those at higher risk of nursing home placement (older, living alone, higher levels of functional impairment) and increasing the skill mix to a higher level of nursing care would provide an overall cost reduction (Greene et al., 1998). In a capitated HCBC program in Arizona, elders receiving services from a HCBC program were more likely to be placed in a nursing home if they were older, male, and had Alzheimer's disease (Bauer, 1996). Almost one-third of the patients were placed in a nursing home, even after receiving HCBC services.

These recent studies, with their focus on targeting HCBC, grow out of the Channeling and OnLok experiments of the 1980s that were designed to evaluate whether supportive in-home services, primarily paraprofessional, could replace the more expensive nursing home care. The Greene and colleagues (1998) study findings suggest that movement from a primarily paraprofessional model to a more skilled and nursing-intensive program bears further study. At the same time, changes in the health care system, for example a reduction in hospital length of stay, may also substantially contribute to study findings.

A second utilization outcome is rehospitalization, where there is evidence that from 12% to more than 40% of home health care patients require a subsequent hospital stay (Anderson et al., 1996; Dennis, Blue, Stahl, Benge, & Shaw, 1996; Hoskins, Walton-Moss, Clark, Schroeder, & Thiel, 1999; Madigan, Schott, & Matthews, 2001; Moulton, McGrane, Beck, Holland, & Christopher, 1998; Naylor et al., 1999b; Proctor, Morrow-Howell, Li, & Dore, 2000; Redeker & Brassard, 1996). Martens and Mellor (1997), in examining a patient population with heart failure at hospital discharge, found that patients receiving home health care were significantly less likely to be rehospitalized over a 90-day period than those patients who did not receive home health care. However, a significant reduction in hospitalization was not found for shorter periods of time.

Evidence on rehospitalization indicates that 30% to 48% of home health care patients are rehospitalized because they develop a new problem (Anderson et al., 1996; Anderson, Helms, Hanson, & DeVilder, 1999; Madigan et al., 2001), an existing problem worsens (38–64%) or, for patients following cardiac surgery, they have surgical complications and higher functional impairment. The most critical period for rehospitalization is within the first 4 weeks of home health care—for all types of patients, the average length of home health care stay is 27 days before a rehospitalization occurs (Anderson et al., 1996). For elders, the time period is shorter—a mean of 13 to 18 days (Anderson et al., 1996; Madigan et al., 2001). Within the diagnostic category of cardiac disease, half of the rehospitalizations of elders with heart failure occurred within 24 days (Hoskins et al., 1999). In examining medical cardiac and surgical cardiac patients, Naylor and colleagues (1999b) found that 28% and 42% of rehospitalizations, respectively, occurred within 42 days following discharge.

The research findings are inconclusive on factors predictive of rehospitalization from home health care. A retrospective study (Hoskins et al., 1999) found that patients with heart failure who were rehospitalized took more medications, and were more likely to have home health aide care, longer home health care lengths of stay, and prior rehospitalization. In a prospective study, Madigan and colleagues (2001) found that neither demographic, illness-related, nor functional status factors were predictive of a subsequent rehospitalization for patients with heart failure. Dennis and colleagues (1996), in a smaller sample study (Hoskins et al., 1999), found that the number of nursing visits was inversely correlated with rehospitalization.

Research on rehospitalization from the home health care perspective has been limited by methodologic issues on how long patients are followed after an index hospitalization and critical questions about the length of time following an index hospital stay that truly reflect issues related to that index hospital stay. In addition, the reasons for rehospitalization can be patient specific (decline in health status, development of a new problem), reflective of a family/caregiver issue wherein the family feels unable to care for the patient, or a function of health system determinants, such as premature hospital discharge. The latter is based primarily on provider judgment and may differ widely between physicians and home health care nurses as well as between hospital personnel and home health care personnel, regardless of discipline. The research within this area is not sufficiently developed to determine reasons for rehospitalization, including determination of premature hospital discharge.

Anderson and colleagues' (1996) development of the Hospital Readmission Inventory provided consistency across several studies of rehospitalization (Anderson et al., 1996; Madigan et al., 2001), allowing some conclusions to be drawn regarding patient rehospitalization. Further use of the same instrument in various studies would contribute to the comparability of findings and a clearer view on the issue of rehospitalization.

PATIENT OUTCOMES

Patient outcomes have been evaluated as part of randomized clinical trials (Naylor et al., 1999a; Naylor et al., 1999b) as well as with home care as it was provided by home health care agencies (Fortinsky & Madigan, 1997; Holtzman, Chen, & Kane, 1998; Lee & Mills, 2000; Penrod, Kane, Finch, & Kane, 1998). Naylor, using the transitional model of care with advanced practice nurses in an RCT providing comprehensive discharge planning and follow-up care to patients with heart failure, found no difference in functional status or depression outcomes. Similarly, Tinetti and colleagues (1999) found no advantage to providing a multicomponent home rehabilitation program to elders with hip fractures—there were no differences in gait and balance measures and lower extremity strength between the intervention and control groups. Of note, there were significant cost savings in using the APN model of care, significant reductions in subsequent hospital stays, as well as reductions in lengths of stay for subsequent rehospitalizations (Naylor et al., 1999a).

When studying home care as it is provided by home health care agencies, a more natural experiment, the relationships between patient outcomes and the numbers of visits have not been found to be linear. Patients receiving more visits did not improve in functional ability (Adams et al., 2000; Fortinsky & Madigan, 1997; Penrod et al., 1998). In fact, more RN visits were strongly related to a decline in patient ambulation, bathing, and self-medication (Adams et al., 2000). The findings from this body of research suggest that perhaps these patients were chronically and functionally impaired and would not be expected to improve in function. Indeed, for patients who were frail or with a progressive chronic illness, a functional outcome of functional stability (no decline in function) might be considered a "good" outcome. The current instruments used to measure change in outcomes may not be sufficiently sensitive to detect change or the measures used may not be reflective of the impact home health care has on patient status. Further development and refinement of the instrumentation could more clearly demonstrate the value of home health care services and allow for a better targeting of care.

Dansky and colleagues (1996), comparing those who received home health care and those who did not with regard to reported health problems and unmet needs after hospital discharge, found significantly more health problems and unmet needs for those who did not receive nursing, but only for those who were 80 years and older. Similarly, Chadiha and colleagues (1995) found that although African Americans received fewer hours of formal (i.e., paid) care, there were no differences in the numbers of unmet needs between African Americans and Whites when controlling for marital status, chronic conditions, socioeconomic status, age, and gender. Hadley and colleagues (2000) found that users of home health care services did improve more than nonusers of home health care services when adequate control for prior (prehospital) function is added. Home health care patients with better prognoses used fewer resources and had better discharge outcomes (Lee & Mills, 2000).

Examination of the effect of payer on outcomes, particularly comparing traditional Medicare with managed care, found that the substantial improvement in health and functional status for traditional Medicare patients observed in the early 1990s did not persist (Adams, Kramer, & Wilson, 1995; Holtzman et al., 1998; Madigan, 2001). In a study of home health care patients from one agency, Adams and colleagues (1995) found no differences between the groups in ADL management, mobility, or condition-specific abilities. Holtzman and colleagues (1998) studied patients with stroke, COPD, CHF, hip replacement, or hip fracture and found there were no differences in functional ability or hospital readmission. Madigan (2001), in a study of patients with wound and skin problems, found there were no differences in functional or wound healing outcomes between the two groups.

Outcome studies within health services research on home health care are in an early state. As the theoretical, methodological, and analytic aspects of outcome studies improve, it is expected that there will be more in-depth examination of combinations of factors that contribute to patient outcomes. One of the challenges inherent in studying home health care outcomes is that the patient populations are very diverse and, in some cases, improvement in health-related or functional status is not expected because of the normal trajectory of illness. There is not sufficient information on the outcomes that could be expected, the best measures for these outcomes, or what factors contribute to improvement in patient outcomes.

What Research Is Needed to Develop the Knowledge Base About Home Health Care From a Health Services Research Prospective?

There are several trends that are apparent in the research efforts to date. First, there is an interest in rehospitalization from the home health care perspective. However, simply studying rehospitalization from home health care is likely not sufficient to determine the causes and to test interventions to reduce rehospitalization. Studies on rehospitalization allude to premature hospital discharge but rarely evaluate readiness for discharge and what happens if patients are discharged prematurely, with or without home health care. While rehospitalization is monetarily expensive to the health system, it also often takes a significant toll on patients and families, which is a societal cost. The finding that rehospitalizations are due to the development of a new problem (Anderson et al., 1996; Madigan et al., 2001) suggests that further examination of what constitutes a new problem is merited. The research evidence in this body of work is clear that there are critical time points during which to deploy home health care resources—the first 3 to 4 weeks for many kinds of patients. However, there is little research to guide practice on the timing and frequency of these home visits to determine if some visit patterns are more effective than others. Under the current reimbursement system, where agencies are no longer presented with the incentive to maximize the delivery of services, there may be patterns of contacts, not just home visits but also phone calls or telehealth initiatives (see Jones and Brennan in chapter 10 of this volume) that are effective in reducing rehospitalization and improving patient outcomes.

The second trend is the relationships between resource use and patient outcomes. The lack of a positive correlation between the two suggests several areas for further research. One possibility is that outcomes for home health care patients depends on whether the patient has the possibility to improve. In some cases, improvement may not be possible or expected, and maintenance of an existing condition could be a "positive" outcome. For example, patients with advanced heart failure may not achieve functional independence. However, stability of the condition may be considered a successful outcome attained with the assistance of home health care nursing. In other cases, following joint arthroplasty for example, functional improvement may be expected and used as a barometer of the quality and effectiveness of home health care services. Research to date in this area of inquiry has been relatively simple from a theoretical perspective with probably insufficient attention to other kinds of factors that can influence the relationship between resource use and patient outcomes. For example, there is evidence that there are market factors that influence the use of home health care services, primarily evidence on substitution of skilled nursing home care for home health care. Yet little has been done to examine, for example, the influence of the supply of nursing home beds on the relationship between patient outcomes and resource use.

The third trend is the articulation of the long-term home and community-based care system (primarily a social service system) with the home health care system (more focused on illness and remediation of illness). As technological advances and demographic changes continue, it is likely that some combination of long-term and short-term services could be most effective in optimizing patient outcomes. In part, the return to an integration of services recalls agency operations from the past, in that home health care agencies historically provided services to both kinds of patients and often moved patients from the post-acute to the long-term care system within the same agency structure. At the same time, the return to a more integrated system reflects some of the goals of the Medicare managed care initiative to provide all health care services under one system. Finally, a return to a more integrated system suggests that the fragmentation, driven by regulatory and economic pressures, may have been a misguided strategy. Innovative programs that target services to patients most likely to benefit from care and that provide the right level of service at the right time could be developed and tested empirically prior to widespread adoption.

CONCLUSIONS

As was previously suggested in the discussion of the theoretical framework and demonstrated in the section on predictors of resource use, the development and refinement of conceptual models would provide guidance on what variables and measures to examine in the area of resource use. Certainly the scale of the studies, from small relatively circumscribed samples to large national samples provides important rigor. Without one or several overarching frameworks, the interrelationships among independent variables and then with the dependent variables are haphazard and cannot be easily compared from one study to another. Certainly the Andersen Behavioral Model is one such framework to consider; it is not without its criticisms, however. The development and refinement of additional models specific to home health care, such as the Transitional Model, holds promise for explanation and to guide research and practice efforts.

From a methodological perspective, the measurement of the concepts and variables has been disparate, preventing researchers from drawing conclusions across studies. For example, the study of resource use has been relatively extensive and it may be time to begin to measure resource use in a systematic manner. In this instance, the regulatory changes with the prospective payment system may facilitate this movement in that there are now regulations around the definition of a home health care episode—what constitutes an admission and what concludes the episode? Further innovation on how to measure home health care resources, in addition to the visit metric, is in order. Again, health system changes provide an impetus to consider other types of resources that may be scientifically important, such as phone calls and telehealth contacts. Similarly, with the measurement of outcomes, the standardized Outcomes Assessment Information Set (OASIS) provides a more systematic way to measure changes in health and functional status over the episode of care. The caveat is that the resource use and OASIS measures have been developed for purposes other than research and may need further psychometric evaluation (Madigan & Fortinsky, 2000).

Finally, attention to patient groups who may be underserved by home health care services merits examination. There is some evidence to suggest that there may be disparities in resource use based on ethnicity, although the evidence is inconclusive. Other groups that may be at risk for being underserved include the rural patient, related to agency closure statistics (General Accounting Office, 1999). With the fragmentation of health care services between the home health care and home care systems, there may be patients who might benefit from home health care services but do not qualify, based on income or functional ability, for long-term home health care. Certainly patients who cannot pay out of pocket for home health care, the second highest category of expenditure, are at risk for being underserved.

Home health care services, in some iteration and delivery model, will continue to evolve. Nursing science can make a substantial contribution to the development of the theoretical and empirical underpinnings of the scientific progress in this area, as well as integrate the findings of the scientific inquiry into care delivery.

REFERENCES

Adams, C. E., Corbett, C. F., & Michel, Y. (2000). Service utilization and outcomes in rural homehealth agencies. *Outcomes Management for Nursing Practice, 4*(2), 63–68.

Adams, C. E., & Kramer, S. (1996). Home health resource utilization: Health maintenance organization versus fee-for-service subscribers. *Journal of Nursing Administration, 26*(2), 20–27.

Adams, C. E., Kramer, S., & Wilson, M. (1995). Home health quality outcomes: Fee-for-service versus health maintenance organization enrollees. *Journal of Nursing Administration, 25*(11), 27–34.

Andersen, R. M. (1968). *A behavioral model of families' use of health services.* Chicago, IL: Center for Health Administration Studies, University of Chicago.

Andersen, R. M. (1995). Revisiting the behavioral model and access to medical care: Does it matter? *Journal of Health and Social Behavior, 36,* 1–10.

Andersen, R. M., & Newman, J. F. (1973). Societal and individual determinants of medical care utilization in the United States. *Milbank Memorial Fund Quarterly Journal,* 95–124.

Anderson, M. A., Hanson, K. S., & DeVilder, N. W. (1996). Hospital readmission during home care: A pilot study. *Journal of Community Health Nursing, 13*(1), 1–12.

Anderson, M. A., Helms, L. B., Hanson, K. S., & DeVilder, N. W. (1999). Unplanned hospital readmissions: A home care perspective. *Nursing Research, 48,* 299–307.

Anderson, M. A., Pena, R. A., & Helms, L. B. (1998). Home care utilization by congestive heart failure patients: A pilot study. *Public Health Nursing, 15,* 146–162.

Bauer, E. J. (1996). Transitions from home to nursing home in a capitated long-term care program: The role of individual support systems. *Health Services Research, 31,* 309–326.

Benjamin, A. E. (1999). A normative analysis of home care goals. *Journal of Aging and Health, 11,* 445–468.

Brooten, D., Kumar, S., Brown, L. P., Butts, P., Finkler, S. A., Bakewell-Sachs, S., Gibbons, A., & Delivoria-Papadopoulos, M. (1986). A randomized clinical trial of early hospital discharge and home follow-up of very-low-birth-weight infants. *New England Journal of Medicine, 315,* 934–939.

Cagney, K. A., & Agree, E. M. (1999). Racial differences in skilled nursing care and home health use: The mediating effects of family structure and social class. *Journal of Gerontology, 54B,* S223–S236.

Castro, J. M., Anderson, M. A., Hanson, K. S., & Helms, L. B. (1998). Home care referral after emergency department discharge. *Journal of Emergency Nursing, 24,* 127–132.

Chadiha, L. A., Proctor, E. K., Morrow-Howell, N., Darkwa, O. K., & Dore, P. (1995). Post-hospital home care for African-American and white elderly. *Gerontologist, 35,* 233–239.

Chapin, R., Wilkinson, D. S., Rachlin, R., Levy, M., & Lindbloom, R. (1998). Going home: Community reentry of light care nursing facility residents age 65 and over. *Journal of Health Care Finance, 25*(2), 35–48.

Clark, D., & Dellasega, C. (1998). Unmet health care needs: Comparison of rural and urban senior center attendees. *Journal of Gerontological Nursing, 24*(12), 24–33.

Cohen, M. A., & Tumlinson, A. (1997). Understanding the state variation in Medicare home health care. *Medical Care, 36,* 618–633.

Dansky, K. H., Brannon, D., Shea, D. G., Vasey, J., & Dirani, R. (1998). Profiles of hospital, physician, and home health service use by older persons in rural areas. *Gerontologist, 38,* 320–330.

Dansky, K. H., Milliron, M., & Gamm, L. (1996). Understanding hospital referrals to home health agencies. *Hospital & Health Services Administration, 41,* 331–342.

Dennis, L. I., Blue, C. L., Stahl, S. M., Benge, M. E., & Shaw, C. J. (1996). The relationship between hospital readmissions of Medicare beneficiaries with chronic illnesses and home care nursing interventions. *Home Healthcare Nurse, 14,* 303–309.

Department of Health and Human Services, Health Care Financing Administration (2000). Outcome and assessment information set: Implementation manual [Online]. Available: http://www.hcfa.gov/medicaid/oasis/oasisdat.htm

Diwan, S., Berger, C., & Manns, E. K. (1997). Composition of the home care service package: Predictors of type, volume, and mix of services provided to poor and frail older people. *The Gerontological Society of America, 37,* 169–181.

Experton, B., Zili, L., Branch, L. G., Ozminkowski, R. J., & Mellon-Lacey, D. M. (1997). The impact of payor/provider type on health care use and expenditures among the frail elderly. *American Journal of Public Health, 87,* 210–216.

Fortinsky, R. H., & Madigan, E. A. (1997). Home care resource consumption and patient outcomes: What are the relationships? *Home Health Care Services Quarterly, 16*(3), 55–73.

Freedman, V. A. (1999). Long-term admissions to home health agencies: A life table analysis. *Gerontologist, 39*(1), 16–24.

General Accounting Office. (1999). *Medicare home health agencies: Closures continue, with little evidence beneficiary access is impaired* (Rep. No. GAO/HEHS-99-120). Washington, DC: Author.

Grabbe, L., Demi, A. S., Whittington, F., Jones, J. M., Branch, L. G., & Lambert, R. (1995). Functional status and the use of formal home care in the year before death. *Journal of Aging and Health, 7,* 339–364.

Greene, V. L., Ondrich, J., & Ladtika, S. (1998). Can home care services achieve cost savings in long-term care for older people? *Journals of Gerontology, Series B: Psychological Sciences and Social Sciences, 53B,* S228–S238.

Guild, S. D., Ledwin, R. W., Sanford, D. M., & Winter, T. (1994). Development of an innovative nursing care delivery system. *Journal of Nursing Administration, 24*(3), 23–29.

Hadley, J., Rabin, D., Epstein, A., Stein, S., & Rimes, C. (2000). Posthospitalization home health care use and changes in functional status in a Medicare population. *Medical Care, 38,* 494–507.

Haupt, B. J. (1998). *An overview of home health and hospice care patients: 1966 national home and hospice survey* (Rep. No. 297). Washington, DC: U.S. Department of Health and Human Services, CDC, National Center for Health Services.

Hays, B. J., & Willborn, E. H. (1996). Characteristics of clients who receive home health aide service. *Public Health Nursing, 13*(1), 58–64.

Holtzman, J., Chen, Q., & Kane, R. (1998). The effect of HMO status on the outcomes of home-care after hospitalization in a Medicare population. *Journal of American Geriatrics Society, 46,* 629–634.

Hoskins, L. M., Walton-Moss, B., Clark, H. M., Schroeder, M. A., & Thiel, L. (1999). Predictors of hospital readmission among the elderly with congestive heart failure. *Home Healthcare Nurse, 17,* 373–381.

Intrator, O., & Berg, K. (1998). Benefits of home health care after inpatient rehabilitation for hip fracture: Health service use by Medicare beneficiaries, 1987–1992. *Archives of Physical Medicine and Rehabilitation, 79,* 1195–1199.

Kane, R. L., Chen, Q., Finch, M., Blewett, L., Burns, R., & Moskowitz, M. (1998). Functional outcomes of posthospital care for stroke and hip fracture patients under Medicare. *Journal of the American Geriatrics Society, 46,* 1525–1533.

Kane, R. L., Chen, Q., Finch, M., Blewett, L., Burns, R., & Moskowitz, M. (2000). The optimal outcomes of post-hospital care under Medicare. *Health Services Research, 35,* 615–661.

Kenney, G., & Rajan, S. (2000). Understanding dual enrollees' use of Medicare home health services: The effects of differences in Medicaid home care programs. *Medical Care, 38*(1), 90–98.

Lee, T., & Mills, M. E. (2000). Analysis of patient profile in predicting home care resource utilization and outcomes. *Journal of Nursing Administration, 30*(2), 67–75.

Madigan, E. A. (2001). Comparison of home health care outcomes and service use for patients with wound/skin diagnoses. *Outcomes Management for Nursing Practice, 5,* 63–69.

Madigan, E. A., & Fortinsky, R. H. (1999). Alternative measures of resource consumption in home care episodes. *Public Health Nursing, 16,* 198–204.

Madigan, E. A., & Fortinsky, R. H. (2000). Additional psychometric evaluation of the Outcomes and Assessment Information Set (OASIS). *Home Health Care Services Quarterly, 18,* 49–62.

Madigan, E. A., Schott, D., & Matthews, C. R. (2001). Rehospitalization among home healthcare patients: Results of a prospective study. *Home Healthcare Nurse, 19,* 298–305.

Martens, K. H., & Mellor, S. D. (1997). A study of the relationship between home care services and hospital readmission of patients with congestive heart failure. *Home Healthcare Nurse, 15,* 123–129.

Morrow-Howell, N., Chadiah, L., Proctor, E. K., Hourd-Bryant, M., & Dore, P. (1996). Racial differences in discharge panning. *Health and Social Work, 21,* 131.

Moulton, P. J., McGrane, A. M., Beck, T. L., Holland, N. L., & Christopher, M. A. (1998). Research corner. Utilization of home health care services by elderly patients with heart failure. *Home Health Care Management and Practice, 10,* 66–73.

Munson, M. L. (1999). Characteristics of elderly home health care users: Data from the 1996 National Home and Hospice Care Survey. (Rep. No. 309). Washington, DC: U.S. Department of Health and Human Services, CDC, National Center for Health Services.

Murphy, J. F., & Hepworth, J. T. (1996). Age and gender differences in health services utilization. *Research in Nursing & Health, 19,* 323–329.

Narsavage, G. L., & Naylor, M. D. (2000). Factors associated with referral of elderly individuals with cardiac and pulmonary disorders for home care services following hospital discharge. *Journal of Gerontological Nursing, 26*(5), 14–20.

National Association for Home Care. (2001). *Crisis in home care: Dismantling of the Medicare home health benefit.* Washington, DC: Author.

Naylor, M. D., Brooten, D., Campbell, R., Jacobsen, B. S., Mezey, M. D., Pauly, M. V., & Schwartz, J. S. (1999a). Comprehensive discharge planning and home follow-up of hospitalized elders: A randomized clinical trial. *Journal of the American Medical Association, 281,* 613–620.

Naylor, M. D., & McCauley, K. M. (1999b). The effects of a discharge planning and home follow-up intervention on elders hospitalized with common medical and surgical cardiac conditions. *Journal of Cardiovascular Nursing, 14*(1), 44–54.

O'Sullivan, M. J., & Volicer, B. (1997). Factors associated with achievement of goals for home health care. *Home Health Care Services Quarterly, 16*(3), 21–34.

Ozawa, M. N., & Tseng, H. (1999). Utilization of formal services during the 10 years after retirement. *Journal of Gerontological Social Work, 31*(1/2), 3–20.

Penrod, J. D., Kane, R. L., Finch, M. D., & Kane, R. A. (1998). Effects of post-hospital Medicare home health and informal care on patient functional status. *Health Services Research, 33*(3 Pt 1), 513–529.

Pohl, J. M., Collins, C., & Given, C. W. (1995). Beyond patient dependency: Family characteristics and access of elderly patients to home care services following hospital discharge. *Home Health Care Services Quarterly, 15*(4), 33–47.

Proctor, E. K., Morrow-Howell, N., Chadiha, L., Braverman, A. C., Darkwa, O., & Dore, P. (1997). Physical and cognitive functioning among chronically ill African-American and white elderly in home care following hospital discharge. *Medical Care, 35,* 782–791.

Proctor, E. K., Morrow-Howell, N., & Kaplan, S. J. (1996). Implementation of discharge plans for chronically ill elders discharged home. *Health and Social Work, 21*(1), 30–40.

Proctor, E. K., Morrow-Howell, N., Li, H., & Dore, P. (2000). Adequacy of home care and hospital readmission for elderly congestive heart failure patients. *Health and Social Work, 25,* 87–96.

Redeker, N. S., & Brassard, A. B. (1996). Health patterns of cardiac surgery clients using home health care services. *Public Health Nursing, 13,* 394–403.

Rosswurm, M. A., & Lanham, D. M. (1998). Discharge planning for elderly patients. *Journal of Gerontological Nursing, 24*(5), 14–21.

Simon, E. P., Showers, N., Blumenfield, S., Holden, G., & Wu, X. (1995). Delivery of home care services after discharge: What really happens. *Health and Social Work, 20*(1), 5–14.

Slivinske, L. R., Fitch, V. L., & Wingerson, N. W. (1998). The effect of functional disability on service utilization. *Health and Social Work, 23,* 175–185.

Swan, J. H., Black, L., Benjamin, A. E., & Fox, P. (1995). Use of covered services in Medicare home health care. *Home Health Care Services Quarterly, 15*(4), 1–18.

Tinetti, M. E., Baker, D. I., Gottschalk, M., Williams, C. S., Pollack, D., Garrett, P., Gill, T. M., Marottoli, R. A., & Acampora, D. (1999). Home-based multicomponent rehabilitation program for older persons after hip fracture: A randomized trial. *Archives of Physical Medicine and Rehabilitation, 80,* 916–922.

Torrez, D. J., Estes, C., & Linkens, K. (1997). The impact of a decade of policy on home health care utilization. *Home Health Care Services Quarterly, 16*(4), 35–56.

Chapter 10

Telehealth Interventions to Improve Clinical Nursing of Elders

JOSETTE F. JONES AND PATRICIA FLATLEY BRENNAN

ABSTRACT

This chapter reviews reports of research conducted worldwide from 1966 to January 2001 on telehealth interventions in clinical nursing for elders. Reports were identified through a systematic search of MEDLINE, CINAHL, PsychInfo, ERIC, and ACM using the search terms *Telemedicine* or *Health Information Networks*, *Nursing*, and *Research*, and were restricted to those published in English. Reports of research using interactive computer technology to assess or intervene with nursing problems commonly observed in persons age 65 and older were sought. Only published reports presenting the findings of an exploratory or experimental study and exploring the association between one intervention variable and technology were included. The search resulted in 18 research reports describing eight research projects. Due to the preponderance of demonstrations and feasibility reports, the dearth of experimental investigations, and the heterogeneous nature of the few studies identified, statistical summarization was not attempted. Telehealth interventions have the potential to improve the clinical nursing care of elders because they provide alternative, equivalent approaches to assess key indicators of the physical and psychological state of elders; are acceptable to nurses, elders, and family caregivers; and may prove less costly than face-to-face interventions. Telehealth approaches provide not only acceptable substitutes for discrete nursing actions but also can serve as a context within which a large range of professional gerontological nursing services can be delivered in a manner that is timely and convenient for elders.

Keywords: telehealth, nursing informatics, gerontological nursing, home care, nursing practice, computer-mediated communication

The marked increase in the absolute and relative number of older people leads to changes in society's perceptions and expectations about health and health care delivery and taxes institutionally based approaches to meeting nursing care needs (Carlson, 1998). Judicious, but widespread, use of computer technology is one plausible solution to some of the current challenges in health care. A philosophy of patient-centered care, including greater attention to the needs, desires, and resources of the patient and greater reliance on self-management, complements the movement of care from institutions to communities, and demands that technology-based interventions not only facilitate the actions of professionals, but also support the needs of patients (Brennan, Moore, & Smyth, 1991; Gerteis, Edgman-Levitan, Walker, Stoke, & Delbanco, 1993). Although the impact of these changes pervades the entire health care system, special attention is needed to determine the extent to which telehealth interventions improve clinical nursing for elders.

Gerontological nursing practice encompasses the delivery of services by nurses, focused on helping the older client maintain an adaptive behavior, promoting optimal health and well-being, maximizing independent functioning, and enhancing quality of life (International Council of Nurses, 1999). Features of professional gerontological nursing practice can be described as a patient-centered, active, and shared process that enables the elder to adapt to those changing life circumstances with an emphasis on the individual's potential to achieve his or her desired health choices (American Nurses Association, 1995). Key components include assessment of psychological and physiological status, rapid intervention, and ongoing counseling and support. Gerontological nurses are challenged to provide their older patients and their families with professional nursing care that is suited to the situation of the older client. However, in an era of constrained human resources and increasing demands for residence-centered, rather than institution-centered care, traditional models of gerontological nursing practice must be augmented with technologies that transcend space and time, allowing gerontological nurses to provide support and services to the patient at a time and place convenient to the patient.

The defining aspect of telehealth is the use of electronic signals to transfer various types of information from one site to another (American Nurses Association, 1999). Information ranges from clinical records to health promotion instructions to still images of wounds and motion images demonstrating exercise routines. This broad definition includes several means of transmission, including telephone and fax transmissions, interactive video and audio, store-and-forward technology, patient monitoring equipment, electronic patient records, electronic libraries and databases, the Internet and intranets, the World Wide Web, electronic mail systems, decision and care planning support systems, and electronic documentation systems. Telehealth is used interchangeably with telemedicine, and every so often the term "telenursing" surfaces. The term "telehealth" is embraced as the more encompassing concept.

Most nurses have already employed telehealth interventions without realizing it. Examples include telephoning or faxing a patient status report, telephone triage, and home health visits via telecommunication for monitoring and designing Websites to educate patients. While much attention has been paid to technology and innovative equipment for enhancing access to and availability of health care services for patients, regardless of where they live, very little work has addressed the efficiency and effectiveness of their applications. An exception is the use of the telephone for consultations. Randomized clinical trials have established the efficacy of telephone consultation to improve patients' outcomes across a broad spectrum of patient populations, including elders with complex drug regimens, caregivers of Alzheimer's patients, and patients with chronic diseases such as arthritis and cardiac diseases (Balas et al., 1997). Studies of interactive teleconsultations have been performed throughout the world and most suggest that health care delivery via these technologies is acceptable to patients in a wide variety of circumstances (Balas et al., 1997; Crouch & Dale, 1998a; Crouch & Dale, 1998b). By addressing the feasibility of electronic media as a pathway to provide valued health services, rather than examining the impact of these approaches, most studies have raised more questions than they have answered (Mair & Whitten, 2000).

This integrated review examines the impact of telehealth on the clinical nursing of elders and answers two questions:

1. To what extent do telehealth applications support essential components of nursing care of elders?
2. To what extent do telehealth applications support the professional dimensions of gerontological nursing practice?

METHOD

Problem Formulation

Telehealth is broadly defined as the use of interactive computer or communications technology for the provision of health care over a short or long distance (American Nurses Association, 1999). Nursing intervention is defined as action based on a scientific rationale that is executed to benefit the client in a predicted way related to the nursing diagnosis and the stated goals (CINAHL, 2000) and includes both assessment and treatment of patient's condition.

Criteria for inclusion of reports were: a focus on nursing intervention using interactive technology targeting problems commonly observed in persons age 65 and older and the findings of an exploratory or experimental study. Research on telehealth applications addressing health care more broadly were excluded, as were published reviews.

Data Collection

The following bibliographic databases were searched: MEDLINE (1966–Feb 2001), the Cumulative Index of Nursing and Allied Health Literature (CINAHL, 1982–Feb 2001), PsychInfo (1975–Feb 2001), ERIC (1966–Feb 2001), and ACM (1985–Feb 2001). Next, the work of known investigators, identified as holding significant NIH funding for inquiry in the area of nursing informatics, was examined for the presence of experimental studies. These searches were complemented by evaluations of previous review articles, citation tracking, and serendipitous discoveries.

A first search was performed in Medline, using the search term *telehealth*. The MEDLINE search routine matched the term telehealth to the medical subject heading *telemedicine*. Next, the subject headings *nursing* and *research* were explored. A Boolean combination of these three concepts was performed, limiting to results to age 65 and over. The same procedure was repeated in CINAHL, PsychInfo, ERIC, and ACM.

Additional reports were sought by examining bibliographic database entries of the works of known investigators. The terms, such as *Computer Communication Networks*, used to index these works were used in consequent searches. Additionally, cross-database searches were re-executed, this time using the combination of *Computer Communication Networks, Nursing*, and *Research*. This resulted in a few more reports.

Evaluation and Data Points

Culling the literature described above resulted in 117 articles. After reading the abstracts and skimming through the articles based on the inclusion and exclusion criteria, 39 articles were identified for more in-depth review. Articles were critically read by three researchers and grouped according to their focus: 18 were related to research, four were prior research reviews, eight clarified the conceptualization of telehealth, six reported on implementation issues, and four did not meet all inclusion criteria. The resulting 18 research articles describe eight research projects. Table 10.1 lists projects and their key characteristics.

Following is a brief overview of the eight projects; four projects were reported in multiple papers and are presented here as integrated sets. Two projects characterized the nature of home care services that could be delivered via telehealth applications (Allen et al., 1999; Wootton et al., 1998a), and telephone (Huber & Blanchfield, 1999). Three projects evaluated the efficacy of telehealth applications for conducting health assessments of elders, including patients with congestive heart failure (CHF) (Jenkins & McSweeney, 2001), patients with leg ulcers (Johnson-Mekota et al., 2001), and mental status assessment (Ball & Puffett, 1998). Two experimental evaluations of telehealth applications for direct care delivery occurred, one addressing the caregivers of persons with Alzheimer's disease (Bass, Brennan, & McCarthy, 1998; Brennan et al., 1991; Brennan, Moore, & Smyth, 1992; Brennan et al., 1995; Brennan, Overholt, Casper, & Calvitti, 1995; Casper, Calvitti, Brennan, & Overholt, 1995) and the other examining interventions addressing self-esteem and depression in elderly clients (Heyn Billipp, 2001). Finally, one project examined patients' perceptions of uses and benefits of telehealth (Whitten et al., 1997).

A relational database in Access™ (Figure 10.1) was developed to assist in the coding and evaluation of the data. We employed models from nursing informatics to characterize the interventions and organize the information related to projects, published reports, and samples. The ACCESS tables allowed for a descriptive analysis of the article, a definition of nursing interventions based on the type definition of nursing (Bakken, Cashen, & O'Brien, 1999) and Nursing Intervention Classification (NIC) terminology (Bulechek & McCloskey, 1999); and a description of the means of delivery of the intervention, including human factor characteristics. The ACCESS tables also captured the statistical hypotheses, the variables, and their measurements. The conceptualization of research problems and hypotheses by Haber (1998) guided the design of the tables. Two nursing team members read the articles, summarized key aspects in

TABLE 10.1 Summary of Research Projects

Project	Research goals	Nursing intervention	Participants/units of analysis	Research design
Analysis of the suitability of home health visits for telemedicine	Suitability of home health visits for telehealth in the US and in the UK	Self-care assistance, medical management, health system guidance, etc.	Clinical records of home health visits ($N = 906$ [US]; $N = 839$ [UK])	Retrospective review
Telephone nursing interventions in ambulatory care	Capturing of nursing diagnosis and interventions related to nursing care during telephone consultations	Telephone consultation	Adult clients of a medical ambulatory clinic ($N = 152$)	Retrospective review
The effects of computer networks on self-esteem and depression	Assessment of psychosocial effects of interactive computer use on self-esteem and depression	Self-esteem enhancement/ mood management	Home care pages 65 years and older ($N = 40$)	Randomized prospective trial
Physical assessment of CHF via in-home interactive communication	Equivalence of face-to-face and interactive video nursing assessment of CHF	Nursing assessment	CHF home care patients, 65 years and older ($N = 28$)	Cross-over design

TABLE 10.1 (*continued*)

Project	Research goals	Nursing intervention	Participants/units of analysis	Research design
Chronic wound management using interactive video technology	Examination of accuracy of wound management using interactive video technology, its related costs and providers and patient satisfaction	Wound management	Residents of a long-term care facility ($N = 13$)	Pair wise comparison
Effects of computer networks on caregivers of persons with Alzheimer's disease	Effectiveness of computer network on caregivers of Alzheimer's patients perceptions of social support and the impact on their decision making skills	Social Support	Caregivers of Alzheimer patients ($N = 102$)	Randomized field experience
Assessment of cognitive functioning in elderly using different communication modes	Equivalence of assessment of cognitive functioning in elderly using face-to-face, fax, and videoconferencing	Nursing Assessment	Residents from an old-age psychiatry service (1) CAMCOG test ($N = 8$) (2) MMSE ($N = 99$)	Structured interview
Survey of patients' perceptions of uses and benefits of telehealth	Surveying patients perceptions of uses and benefits of telehealth	(No specific intervention mentioned)	Survey of patients receiving home telenursing ($N = 22$)	Semi-structured interview

299

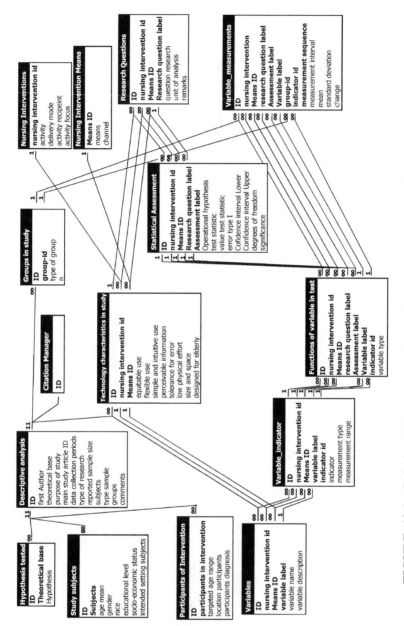
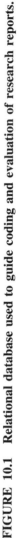

FIGURE 10.1 Relational database used to guide coding and evaluation of research reports.

300

the ACCESS database, and discussed the structure and findings. Iterative discussions resolved report interpretations and coding decisions.

Analysis and Interpretation

The purpose of the studies, the exploratory nature of most reports, and the small number of participants included in each sample precluded statistical summarization. However, the rich set of approaches and intervention studies permits qualitative summarization of the state of telehealth interventions to support clinical nursing of elders. Studies varied by recruitment method, subject characteristics, study design, time frame, setting, measurement of effects, and intervention focus. A broad, qualitative overview of the data, including a critical review of the findings, is reported. Statistical results reported in this chapter are the values reported by the authors. Table 10.2 summarizes a critical review of each article.

RESULTS

To What Extent Do Telehealth Applications Support Essential Components of Nursing Care of Elders?

It can be inferred from the reports reviewed that telehealth applications support the essential components of nursing care for elders. Although most research is in its infancy, the following statements can be made.

TELEHEALTH VISITS CAN SUBSTITUTE FOR FACE-TO-FACE NURSING CARE HOME VISITS

Two sets of studies examined the nature of clinical services that could be delivered via telehealth. A retrospective review of nursing clinical records was used to determine what percentage of home health nursing could be done by telehealth (Allen et al., 1999; Wootton et al., 1998a; Wootton et al., 1998b; Allen et al., 1999). Forty-six percent of the home visits could reasonably be replaced by telehealth visits (Allen et al., 1999). Significant factors determining the substitutability of home visits with telehealth visits included primary diagnosis, the number of interventions, and age.

Primary diagnoses appropriate for telehealth visits are chronic airway obstruction, heart failure, essential hypertension, neuromuscular diseases,

TABLE 10.2 Critical Review of the Reports

Author	Purpose	Project	Research approach	Key findings	Limitations
Allen, A., Doolittle, G. C, Boysen, C. D., Komoroski, K., Wolf, M., Collins, B., & Patterson, J. D. (1999)	Suitability of home health visits for telehealth	Analysis of the suitability of home health visits for telemedicine	Retrospective review of nursing charts by four observers (*N* = 906) 54-item coding scale	46% of on-site nursing visits could reasonably be replaced by telehealth visits Possible use of telehealth visits is determined by primary diagnosis, number of interventions and patient age	Retrospective review of chart does not reflect the individual patient's suitability Chart may report only hands-on interventions Not all determinants of suitability for telehealth were assessed
Ball & Puffet (1998)	Equivalence of assessment cognitive functioning using different modes of communication	Assessment of cognitive functioning in elderly using different communication modes	Structured interview (*N* = 11) CAMCOG test	CAMCOG can be performed reliable via videoconferencing with some modification for visual stimuli	Small sample size Technical difficulties with equipment Use of aide at remote site

302

TABLE 10.2 (*continued*)

Author	Purpose	Project	Research approach	Key findings	Limitations
Ball, Tyrell, & Long (1999)	Equivalence of assessment cognitive functioning using different modes of communication	Assessment of cognitive functioning in elderly using different communication modes	Structured interview (*N* = 99) Minimal Mental State Examination (MMSE) Three raters	Equivalence of assessment cognitive functioning using different modes of communication	Differences in presentation of visual stimuli by diverse examiners may be a confounding variable
Bass, D. M., Brennan, P. F., & McCarthy, C. (1998)	Effectiveness of computer network on caregiver strain	Effects of computer networks caregivers of persons with Alzheimer's disease	Randomized field experience (*N* = 96)	Reduction in four types of care-related strain: physical, emotional, relationship strain, and activity restriction	Many variables not considered in analysis such as content of information, user mix, etc.
Brennan (1996)	Effectiveness of computer network as nursing intervention	Effects of computer networks caregivers of persons with Alzheimer's disease	Randomized field experience (*N* = 102)	Computer networks provide a pathway for communication between nurses and patients	

(continued)

303

TABLE 10.2 *(continued)*

Author	Purpose	Project	Research approach	Key findings	Limitations
Brennan, Moore, & Smyth (1991)	Feasibility of computer network for delivering nursing services	Effects of computer networks caregivers of persons with Alzheimer's disease	Randomized field experience (N = 22)	Feasibility of computer networks as a mechanism for delivering nursing services	Preliminary examination
Brennan, Moore, & Smyth (1992)	Assess use of computer networks by caregivers	Effects of computer networks caregivers of persons with Alzheimer's disease	Randomized field experience (N = 47)	Effective use of computer networks to meet social support needs of home caregivers	Pilot study
Brennan, Moore, & Smyth (1995)	Effectiveness of computer network on social support and decision making	Effects of computer networks caregivers of persons with Alzheimer's disease	Randomized field experience (N = 102)	Computer networks enhanced decision-making confidence, decision-making skills unaffected, no changes in social isolation	Psychometrics of instruments used to measure social isolation

TABLE 10.2 *(continued)*

Author	Purpose	Project	Research approach	Key findings	Limitations
Brennan, P. F., Overholt, J. L., Casper, G., & Calvitti, A. (1995)	Demonstrate pattern of use of computer network	Effects of computer networks caregivers of persons with Alzheimer's disease	Observation (N = 1)	Case-study of pattern of use	Single observation of atypical example
Casper, G. R., Calvitti, A., Brennan, P. F., & Overholt, J. L. (1995)	Effectiveness of computer network on decision making skills	Effects of computer networks caregivers of persons with Alzheimer's disease	Randomized field experience (N = 102)	Access to computer networks increased decision-making confidence, but not decision-making skills	

(continued)

TABLE 10.2 *(continued)*

Author	Purpose	Project	Research approach	Key findings	Limitations
Gardner, S. E., Frantz, R. A., Pringle Specht, J. K., Jonhson-Mekota, J. L., Buresh, K. A., Wakefield, B., & Flanagan J. (2001)	Equivalence of face-to-face wound management and interactive video wound management	Chronic wound management using interactive video technology	Paired observation (N = 13)	Agreement for three of the nine wound characteristics was 100%; five characteristics had an agreement between 77% and 92%, while one characteristic (epithelial tissue) had only a 54% agreement	Confounding variable: nurse at remote site directed the videotaping. The taped session reflected a biased assessment procedure
Heyn Billip (2001)	Assess psychosocial effects of computer use on self-esteem and depression	The effects of computer networks on self-esteem and depression	Randomized prospective trial (N = 40) One control group, three experimental groups	Interactive computer use was associated with change self-esteem but has no effect on depression	Small sample size Homogeneity of study population

TABLE 10.2 (*continued*)

Author	Purpose	Project	Research approach	Key findings	Limitations
Huber & Blanchfield (1999)	Identifying the dimensions of the nurse's role during phone consultation	Telephone nursing interventions in ambulatory care	Retrospective review ($N = 152$) Tea	Nurses have an appropriate role in telephone interactions and standardized nursing languages can be used. Diagnoses mostly captured are altered health maintenance, knowledge deficit and health seeking behavior. Nursing interventions captured are: self-care assistance, medical management, guidance, and emotional support	Differences in nurses' knowledge and use of standardized nursing languages Not all nursing interventions are captured (e.g., family support)

(*continued*)

307

TABLE 10.2 *(continued)*

Author	Purpose	Project	Research approach	Key findings	Limitations
Jenkins & McSweeney (2001)	Equivalence of face-to-face and interactive video nursing assessment	Physical assessment of CHF via in-home interactive communication	Cross-over design ($N = 28$)	Few significant differences between face-to face assessment and two-way audio video assessment of CHF. Inspiratory wheeze, ankle edema, and pedal edema are more frequently detected during face-to-face assessment; nail color abnormality was more frequently picked up during telehealth assessment	Small sample size Homogeneity of population

TABLE 10.2 *(continued)*

Author	Purpose	Project	Research approach	Key findings	Limitations
Johnson-Mekota, J. L., Maas, M., Buresh, K. A., Gardner, S. E., Frantz, R. A., Specht, J. K., Wakefield, B., & Flanagan, J. (2001)	Assessment of patient and provider satisfaction with telehealth care	Chronic wound management using interactive video technology	Exit interview (Patients: $N = 11$) (Nurses: $N = 10$)	Nurses and most patients were 'very satisfied' with the both services	Artificial setting which leads to hypothetical judgment
Pringle Specht, Wakefield, & Flanagan (2001)	Cost analysis of telehealth wound management	Chronic wound management using interactive video technology	Descriptive study ($N = 15$)	The average cost of a telehealth wound consultation is less compared to face-to-face consultation	Very basic cost analysis

(continued)

TABLE 10.2 (*continued*)

Author	Purpose	Project	Research approach	Key findings	Limitations
Whitten, Mair, & Collins (1997)	Suitability of home health visits for telehealth	Survey of patients' perceptions of uses and benefits of telehealth	Semi-structured phone interview (*N* = 22 [phase 1]) (*N* = 9 [phase 2])	Technology is not an issue for elderly, nor did it have negative effects on communications. Elders have no particular worries or excitement about telenursing	Small sample size Selection of subjects was based on location and not on nursing services received
Wootton, R., Loane, M., Mair, F., Allen, A., Doolittle, G., Begley, M., McLernan, A., Moutray, M., & Harrisson, S. (1998a)	Suitability of home health visits for telehealth	Analysis of the suitability of home health visits for telemedicine	Retrospective review (*N* = 1745)	Telehealth may have a role in the delivery of home health care since about 45% of the site visits can be replaced with telehealth visits in the United States compared to 15% in the United Kingdom.	Retrospective review of chart does not reflect the individual patient's suitability Chart may report only hands-on interventions Not all determinants of suitability for telehealth were assessed

urinary tract disorders, and joint disorders. Visits with fewer interventions were rated more suitable for telehealth visits than visits with more interventions ($F_{(2,903)} = 444$, $p < .001$). Types of intervention rated as inappropriate for telehealth were: visits involving intravenous, intramuscular, intradermal, and subcutaneous administration of fluid and medication. From the 152 visits involving wound management, only 3 were considered appropriate for telehealth consultation. Older patients were judged to be better candidates for telehealth than younger patients ($F_{(2,899)} = 11.2$, $p < .001$), with no differences for gender, duration of visits, seasonal variations, distance traveled, or geographical location.

Although the efficacy of telephone consultation has been shown to improve patients' outcomes including elders (Balas et al., 1997), little is known about the type and extent of nursing interventions that occur during teleconsultations. A pilot study (Huber & Blanchfield, 1999) was conducted in two cities to explore whether nursing diagnoses and interventions could be captured during telephone interactions. Diagnoses identified were listed as health maintenance altered (43%), primarily related to upper respiratory tract, flu-like symptoms, and dizziness; pain (18%) related to abdominal and lower back pain; knowledge deficit (16%) related to drug regimen; and knowledge deficit (8%) to treatments; health-seeking behavior (7%); and individual NANDA diagnosis (8%). Most frequently checked nursing interventions were self-care assistance ($n = 109$), medical management ($n = 56$), health system guidance ($n = 54$), emotional support ($n = 38$), and pain management ($n = 28$). The duration of the phone interaction ranged from less than five minutes (64%) to 20 minutes (4%), with no record of time for about 25%.

Results of these two studies indicate that nurses perceive that telehealth visits can substitute for face-to-face care for some problems. Results suggest that telehealth home health visits not only facilitate nursing care but specifically support the care of elders. Caution is required in interpreting these results because some are based on retrospective reviews of clinical records. Information can only be as accurate as the data. It is necessary to question the extent to which nursing notes really reflect the encounter (Wootton et al., 1998a) and not only report hands-on interventions. Hence, the results may underestimate the appropriateness of telehealth home health visits. More investigation is warranted to define the real potential of telehealth in nursing care for the elders.

TELEHEALTH ASSESSMENTS YIELD FINDINGS CONSISTENT TO FACE-TO-FACE ASSESSMENTS

Two sets of studies examined the equivalence of physical assessments conducted in traditional face-to-face modes and via telehealth modes. The efficacy of telehealth was tested for equivalence of face-to-face nursing assessment of home care patients with CHF (Jenkins & McSweeney, 2001). Results indicated few significant differences between the face-to-face assessment and the telehealth assessment for cardiac problems. Inspiratory wheeze ($p = .01$), ankle edema ($p = .024$) and pedal edema ($p = .099$) were more frequently detected during face-to-face examination, while nail-color abnormality ($p = .048$) was picked up more often during telehealth examination.

The accuracy of wound assessment using interactive video communication systems (Gardner et al., 2001) compared with in-person consultation revealed that agreement for three of the nine wound characteristics was 100%, five characteristics had an agreement rate between 77% and 92%, whereas one characteristic (epithelial tissue) had only 54% agreement.

These two studies suggest the feasibility and substitutability of face-to-face physical assessment by two-way, in-home audio-video assessment. Both research projects employed a crossover design to control for patient parameters. The CHF assessment study employed 12 nurses—6 in each treatment group—although the latter study only used 1 nurse for both treatments, rendering it difficult to apply statistical summarization. The extent of agreement between nurses' assessments (Kappa coefficients) in the CHF assessment is claimed to be significant, but an exact value is not reported (Jenkins & McSweeney, 2001). The wound assessment study did not calculate the extent of agreement under the two conditions (Johnson-Mekota et al., 2001). Although taped sessions were used and assessments were made after a substantial period of time to avoid confounding variables such as memory and recall (Johnson-Mekota et al., 2001), other confounding variables are introduced by the use of a second nurse expert that directed the videotaping. The taped session consequently reflected a biased assessment procedure arising from the fact that the second nurse expert may have inadvertently directed the focal point of the assessment, thus aiding the nurse conducting the assessment via video. The use of homogenous and relatively small sample size in both projects hampers the generalization of the findings beyond patients with this specific problem, but the results should be used to generate new questions and encourage more investigation.

The feasibility and reliability of telehealth mechanisms for assessing cognitive function was assessed in two studies. In one study, researchers compared the results of face-to-face and video assessments of elders' cognitive functioning using a structured interview (CAMDEX-CAMCOG)

(Ball & Puffett, 1998). In a follow-up study, Ball and colleagues evaluated the scoring of the Mini-Mental State Exam (MMSE) using the phone, face-to-face, fax, and videoconferencing methods (Ball, Tyrrell, & Long, 1999).

In both studies researchers found that written parts of cognitive functioning of elderly can be assessed reliably using fax and videoconferencing. The results, though, are less clear when visual stimuli or intricate graphs are transmitted over low-resolution video. Sentences could be interpreted reliably, but the interpretation of graphs was less reliable (Ball et al., 1999). Patients had difficulty interpreting visual stimuli using video, and the presence of a second investigator to represent the stimuli at the remote site was required (Ball & Puffett, 1998). The need for further investigation, higher resolution video technology, and different forms of cognitive testing is apparent if clinicians want to use this technology for assessment and management of elderly people with cognitive problems who do not have easy access to health care providers.

ELDERS WILL ACCEPT TELEHEALTH TECHNOLOGY

Several studies examined patient and nurse satisfaction with telehealth technology. A convenience sample of 22 subjects involved in telehealth home visits (cable television-based interactive video) were interviewed about their perceptions of telehealth visits during the time of the visits and 3 months after (Whitten et al., 1997). Contrary to expectations, adapting to the use of telehealth equipment was not a problem for the subjects (Whitten et al., 1997). Similar findings are reported by Brennan and colleagues (1991). Patients did not express worry or experience difficulties adapting to the use of electronic media for communicating. Whitten and colleagues (1997) also reported that perceptions about what telehealth was able to do for patients changed over time: 25% (compared with 45% during the initial interview) felt that this service could act as a security tool in case of problems, 50% (versus 41%) felt it really did not contribute to their health needs in any way, and 13% (versus 14%) reported that it acted as a tool to address their medical conditions.

The apparent decline in the value gained from the telehealth intervention over that reported by Whitten and colleagues (1997) stands in contrast to the earlier, more positive evaluations found by Brennan's group (1995) and in the various projects assessing the equivalence of telehealth and face-to-face assessments of CHF (Johnson-Menkota et al., 2001). Three explanations can be offered for this discrepancy: (a) the timing of the satisfaction assessment (Whitten's group interviewed patients long after care services had terminated, while Brennan and colleagues (1995) and Jenkins and McSweeney (2001) measured satisfaction at the end of the intervention), (b) instrumentation differences, and (c) the integration between the telehealth application and the standard process of care.

TELEHEALTH CONSULTATIONS MAY COST LESS THAN FACE-TO-FACE ASSESSMENTS

A corollary study to the wound management study (Pringle Specht, Wakefield, & Flanagan, 2001) examined cost minimization from the perspective of the consulting agency, the referring agency, and the patient. The cost of the telehealth chronic wound clinic was estimated at an average of $136.16 (acute care perspective) versus $246.28 for the face-to-face consultation. If the cost also includes the line and equipment, a telehealth consultation totals $213.36. Telehealth consultation avoids travel time for the consultant ($36.66) and transportation of the patient from the long-term care facility to the clinic ($191.28). Patients spend, on average, 20 minutes in telehealth consultation compared with the average of 8.5 hours they needed to travel back and forth. Although in this study cost savings were realized and patients benefited, more cost-benefit studies are needed to determine when and under what circumstances the cost of telehealth consultations, including equipment, maintenance, and depreciation, offsets the cost of face-to-face consultation.

Within the limits of the small sample sizes and narrow, focused evaluations, it is possible to conclude that telehealth provides equivalent, alternative, and potentially beneficial approaches to accomplishing some of the important components of nursing care of elders. For specific, discrete nursing interventions, such as assessment of wounds and certain other clinical problems, telehealth mechanisms provide results equivalent to face-to-face encounters and may do so at lower cost. Additional benefits include a lower burden of care experienced by the patient. Elders find telehealth interventions acceptable although no long-term, positive advantage of the approach was perceived by some participants.

To What Extent Do Telehealth Applications Support the Professional Dimensions of Gerontological Nursing Practice?

Demonstrating that discrete components of nursing interventions can occur in a safe and reliable fashion in a telehealth environment provides necessary, but not sufficient, support for the use of telehealth to improve the nursing care of elders. To do so requires a more comprehensive view of the professional dimensions of gerontological nursing practice and examination of the ability of telehealth interventions to provide a rich environment for the delivery of nursing care to elders. The results of the exploration of telephone communication between patients and nurses (Huber & Blanchfield, 1999) give some indication of the importance and role of nurses in telephone interactions with elders related to self-care assistance, health system guidance, emotional support, and medication management. A key component of the professional practice of gerontological nursing encompasses supporting family caregivers in the process of care for elders.

Although previous studies have supported that telehealth provides an acceptable substitute for discrete nursing procedures and actions, the next studies demonstrate that telehealth also provides a context within which a full range of gerontological nursing services can be delivered. Both projects investigated the delivery of supportive nursing interventions— interventions tailored to the needs and characteristics of the client. The first project, ComputerLink, was aimed at family caregivers of Alzheimer's patients (Brennan et al., 1995); the second was designed to reduce depression and increase self-esteem in older patients (Heyn Billipp, 2001).

Caregiver participants with access to ComputerLink showed improved confidence in decision-making, $F(1,93) = 9.73, p < .01$; however, decision-making skills did not improve, $F(1,95) = 1.69, p = .20$, nor was perceived isolation reduced, $F(1,95) = .43, p = .51$, compared with the participants in the control group (Brennan et al., 1995; Casper et al., 1995). While no differential decline in caregiver health status occurred ($z = .33; p < .01$), secondary analysis of the original data revealed that some caregivers experienced mitigation of certain types of caregiver strain, such as physical, emotional, and relationship strain, and activity restriction (Bass et al., 1998). A multiple regression analysis enhanced by factor analytic characterizations of ComputerLink use demonstrated that access to ComputerLink significantly reduced relationship strain for spouses ($b = -1.58$). The conditional mean change in relationship strain after 1 year was $-.78$ for the experimental group, whereas the control group showed no change (Bass et al., 1998). In contrast, nonspouse caregivers showed a small increase (.30), whereas the control group showed a decrease ($-.85$) in relationship strain. Noteworthy, also, is that ComputerLink access led to significantly greater reduction in emotional strain (difference in mean change = −.52 compared with .97 for less support) and activity restriction (difference in mean change = −1.16 compared with .81 for less support) for caregivers with more informal support. Analysis of the frequency of use and use patterns within the experimental group indicates a significant interaction of the use of the communication service with physical strain ($b = -.04$; $p \leq .01$), relationship strain ($b = -.02$; $p \leq .05$), and activity restriction ($b = -.05$; $p \leq .05$).

The ComputerLink research demonstrated that computer networks provide pathways to deliver tailored care and serve as discrete nursing interventions (Brennan, 1996) such as assistance in care management, teaching, and consultation. Because this study was one of the first systematic evaluations of the impact on decision making, social isolation, and certain types of caregiver strains, it should be considered exploratory (Bass et al., 1998). The impact of the manner in which information was provided to the user (e.g,. standardized, tailored, or individualized) was not considered in the study, nor was the impact of the interactions between the participants and the nurse moderator on the outcome variables. Except for Brennan (1996), the effect of the computer network on communicative behaviors and interactions between the nurse and other health care providers remains unexplored. Other potential benefits of computer networks for social, functional, and health purposes, such as improved knowledge of caregiving, positive caregiving consequences, increased self-esteem, and the use of health care services, were not considered (Bass et al., 1998).

Heyn Billipp (2001) examined whether a telehealth application could help improve self-esteem and reduce depression in home-dwelling elders using a 3-month randomized prospective trial design. The researcher found a statistically significant association between computer use and positive self-esteem ($p = .02$), but not for depression ($p = .71$). The author noted that interactive computer use alone did not change scores relating to depression or self-esteem.

Although the studies related to ComputerLink suggest that computer networks exist both as a way to provide discrete nursing interventions and to deliver nursing care (Brennan, 1996), Heyn Billipp's work can be described as a preliminary efficacy study of computer use as a nursing intervention for self-esteem enhancement and mood management in elders. The small sample size and the homogeneity of the sample, however, limit the generalizability of the findings (Heyn Billipp, 2001). Effects of modifiers, such as nurse presence, nurse–subject interaction, and the type of information exchanged, were not accounted for in this study.

As one moves from the procedure—specific equivalence of telehealth approaches with specific nursing activities—to a more broad-based view, evidence supports the employment of telehealth approaches as a context within which professional nursing practice can be delivered. The two projects presented depicted telehealth as a delivery model, which allows nurses to design interventions that are adaptive to the user's needs and characteristics as they emerge during the intervention, rather than an assessment tool focused on a single activity. This approach to nursing interventions is congruent with the philosophy of a patient-centered approach to gerontological nursing.

DISCUSSION

Determining the value of telehealth interventions to improve the clinical care of elders requires that research demonstrate that (a) telehealth approaches serve as acceptable, equivalent alternatives to key components of gerontological nursing care; and (b) telehealth approaches provide a robust environment to support the professional dimensions of gerontological nursing practice. Preliminary evidence exists to support both of these requirements. Nurses can identify many face-to-face assessment activities that can be mediated by technology, and they have good evidence of the equivalence of selected technology-mediated assessments with those occurring in traditional face-to-face encounters. Experimental evidence also indicates that nurses can construct and employ a telehealth environment to address the professional dimensions of nursing practice, including assessment and intervention with psychological problems, caregiver support, and clinical coaching. Preliminary evidence also shows that positive health outcomes arise from the use of telehealth interventions for the care of elders.

It is important to examine gerontological nursing practice for specific components that are not amenable to delivery via telehealth approaches. Certainly any gerontological nursing intervention that requires the physical presence and psychomotor skills of the nurse is not suitable for delivery via telehealth intervention.

Unstudied are many candidate situations where telehealth may be of value. For example, the absence of studies examining the use of telehealth approaches in emergency situations leaves unanswered whether these situations are completely unsuitable for telehealth strategies. It is plausible that appropriate deployment of telehealth interventions in the context of comprehensive gerontological nursing care may provide timely interventions that ultimately reduce the number of situations that escalate to emergency status.

Research examining telehealth in support of the clinical nursing of elders is in its infancy, with most projects, save Brennan's ComputerLink work, occurring during the past 5 years. This relative youth is a consequence both of the state of telehealth applications and the expectations of nurses regarding the nature of appropriate interventions. The literature that has been reviewed revealed greater attention to the application of telehealth as a tool for assessment by nurses who care for elders. Such attention is appropriate, given the growing evidence of positive effects of early interventions in disease management. An important fact is that the findings from the studies demonstrate the effectiveness of telehealth assessment strategies for complex and meaningful patient problems. Thus, the use of telehealth approaches for clinical assessment, while not ready for wide-scale clinical deployment, shows great promise in assisting nurses in this most important component of the nursing process. Telehealth assessment strategies must build on face-to-face assessment approaches with appropriate modifications for the nature of asynchronous, technology-mediated care. Nurses trained to assess the nonverbal cues of patients must identify, interpret, and incorporate the electronic correlates of those nonverbal indicators. Future research is needed to identify the circumstances in which telehealth assessment provides reliable data and those that should serve as indicators of the need for further face-to-face evaluation.

Preliminary investigations into the use of telehealth for delivery of professional nursing interventions demonstrate the feasibility of the approach and the potential for not only social benefits but also health improvement among elders. However, across all of the studies, a persistent theme emerges: the telehealth innovations that work the best are those that complement existing nursing approaches. This important finding calls for an end to isolated telehealth application evaluations and initiation of a series of studies wherein the telehealth innovation is examined as a component of, not apart from, the nursing intervention.

Certainly much technical work remains. Human-factor considerations of device design, interface layout, and navigation strategies have not been systematically addressed in any of the studies to date. Creation of telehealth applications that capitalize on the strengths of technology features to compensate for physical, cognitive, or social limitations of elders, requires intensive collaboration between clinical nursing investigators, engineers, computer scientists, and the elders themselves. Principles unique to the various modes of telehealth must be characterized and their contribution to the project outcomes made explicit. Pragmatic information that defines and benefits the future delivery of telehealth nursing care for elders is needed, such as the effect of this method of delivery on the nurse-patient relationship. Not only is it useful to explore the impact of telehealth on the professional dimensions of gerontological nursing, but also how professional dimensions of gerontological nursing affect the use of tele-health. More investigation is warranted to define the real potential of telehealth in nursing care of elders.

Methodological considerations also require attention. Most studies were exploratory using a small homogeneous sample that allowed detecting the impact of the telehealth application without too many confounding variables. This approach seems appropriate since randomized clinical trials, the gold standard of many clinical intervention evaluations, may prove infeasible or even undesirable as methods to determine the impact of telehealth applications in the clinical nursing of elders. As can be inferred from this review, research instruments measuring the unique components of telehealth applications are needed.

Finally, our nursing informatics approach to an integrated review of (1) the use of standardized terminology and type representation models of nursing practice, (2) the selection of the search terms in accordance with the subject headings of the bibliographic databases, and (3) the construction of a relational database, is innovative. Our initial impression was satisfactory, but the approach needs some further exploration and refinement.

ACKNOWLEDGMENTS

Support for preparation for this review came from the National Institute of Nursing Research (T32 3223), J. Jones, Predoctoral Trainee, and Patricia Flatley Brennan, Program Director.

REFERENCES

Allen, A., Doolittle, G. C., Boysen, C. D., Komoroski, K., Wolf, M., Collins, B., & Patterson, J. D. (1999). An analysis of the suitability of home health visits for telemedicine. *Journal of Telemedicine & Telecare, 5*(2), 90–96.

American Nurses Association. (1995). *Standards and Scope of Gerontological Nursing Practice*. Washington, DC: Author.

American Nurses Association. (1999). *Core principles on telehealth. Report of the Interdisciplinary Telehealth Standards Working Group. March 25, 1998*. Washington, DC: Author.

Bakken, S., Cashen, M. S., Mendonca, E. A., O'Brien, A., & Zieniewicz J. (2000). Representing nursing activities within a concept-oriented terminology system. *Journal of the American Medical Informatics Association, 7*(1), 81–90.

Bakken, S., Cashen, M. S., & O'Brien, A. (1999). Evaluation of a type definition for representing nursing activities within a concept-based terminologic system. *AMIA Annual Symposium Proceedings* (pp. 17–21). Washington, DC: AMIA.

Balas, E. A., Jaffrey, R., Kuperman, G. J., Boren, S. A., Brown, G. D., Pinciroli, F., & Mitchell, J. A. (1997). Electronic communication with patients: Evaluation of distance medicine technology. *Journal of the American Medical Association, 278*, 152–159.

Ball, C., & Puffett, A. (1998). The assessment of cognitive function in elderly using videoconferencing. *Journal of Telemedicine & Telecare, 4* (Supplement 1), 36–38.

Ball, C., Tyrrell, J., & Long, C. (1999). Scoring written material from the mini-mental state examination: a comparison of face-to-face, fax and video-linked scoring. *Journal of Telemedicine & Telecare, 5*(4), 253–256.

Bass, D. M., Brennan, P. F., & McCarthy, C. (1998). The buffering effect of computer support network on caregiver strain. *Journal of Aging and Health, 10*(1), 20–43.

Brennan, P. F. (1996). The future of clinical communication in an electronic environment. *Holistic Nursing Practice, 11*(1), 97–104.

Brennan, P. F., Moore, S. M., & Smyth, K. A. (1991). Computerlink: Electronic support for the home caregiver. *Advances in Nursing Science, 13*(4), 14–27.

Brennan, P. F., Moore, S. M., & Smyth, K. A. (1992). Alzheimer's disease caregivers' uses of a computer network. *Western Journal of Nursing Research, 14*(5), 662–673.

Brennan, P. F., Moore, S. M., & Smyth, K. A. (1995). The effects of a special computer network on caregivers of persons with Alzheimer's disease. *Nursing Research, 44*(3), 166–172.

Brennan, P. F., Overholt, J. L., Casper, G. R., & Calviti, A. (1995). Elders using a community network: Profile of a champion. *MEDINFO'95 Proceedings, 1545*. Vancouver: IMIA.

Bulechek, G. M., & McCloskey, J. C. (1999). *Nursing Intervention Classification (NIC): Effective nursing treatments* (3rd ed.). Philadelphia: W. B. Saunders.

Carlson, E. (1998). Emerging roles for the gerontological nurse practitioner. *Journal of the American Academy of Nurse Practitioners, 10*(9), 403–405.

Casper, G. R., Calviti, A., Brennan, P. F., & Overholt, J. L. (1995). ComputerLink: The impact of a computer network on Alzheimer's caregivers' decision-making confidence and skill. *MEDINFO'95 Proceedings, 1546*. Vancouver: IMIA.

Chaffee, M. (1999). A telehealth odyssey. *American Journal of Nursing, 99*(7), 27–32.

Cooper, H. (1989). *Integrating research: A guide for literature review* (2nd ed.). (Applied Social Research Methods Series No. 2). Newbury Park, CA: Sage.

Cooper, H., & Hedges, L. V. (1994). *Handbook of research synthesis*. New York: Russell Sage Foundation.

Crouch, R., & Dale, J. (1998a). Telephone triage—identifying the demand (Part 1). *Nursing Standard, 12*(34), 33–38.

Crouch, R., & Dale, J. (1998b). Telephone triage—how good are the decisions? (Part 2). *Nursing Standard, 12*(35), 33–39.

Fulmer, T., & Abraham, I. L. (1998). Rethinking geriatric nursing. *Nursing Clinics of North America, 33*(3), 387–394.

Gardner, S. E., Frantz, R. A., Pringle Specht, J. K., Jonhson-Mekota, J. L., Buresh, K. A., Wakefield, B., & Flanagan J. (2001). How accurate are chronic wound assessments using interactive video technology? *Journal of Gerontological Nursing, 27*(1), 15–20.

Gerteis, M., Edgman-Levitan, S., Walker, J. D., Stoke D. M., & Delbanco, T. L. (1993). What patients really want. *Health Management Quarterly, 15*(3), 2–6.

Gray, J. E., Safran, C., Davis, R. B., Pompilio-Weitzner, G., Stewart, J. E., Zaccagnini, L., & Pursley, D. (2000). Baby CareLink: Using the Internet and telemedicine to improve care for high-risk infants. *Pediatrics, 106*(6), 1318–1324.

Haber, J. (1998). Research problems and hypotheses. In G. LoBiondo-Wood & J. Haber (Eds.), *Nursing research: methods, critical appraisal, and utilization* (4th ed., pp. 59–91). St. Louis, MO: Mosby Yearbooks.

Heyn Billipp, S. (2001). The psychosocial impact of interactive computer use within a vulnerable elderly population: A report on a randomized prospective trial in a home health care setting. *Public Health Nursing, 18*(2), 138–145.

Huber, D. L., & Blanchfield, K. (1999). Telephone nursing interventions in ambulatory care. *Journal of Nursing Administration, 29*(3), 38–44.

International Council of Nurses. (1999). International Council of Nurses on healthy ageing. *Nursing Standards, 13*(41), 31.

Jenkins, R. L., & McSweeney, M. (2001). Assessing elderly patients with congestive heart failure via in-home interactive telecommunication. *Journal of Gerontological Nursing, 27*(1), 21–27.

Johnson-Mekota, J. L., Maas, M., Buresh, K. A., Gardner, S. E., Frantz, R. A., Pringle Specht, J. K., Wakefield, B., & Flanagan, J. (2001). A nursing application of telecommunication: Measurements of satisfaction for patients and providers. *Journal of Gerontological Nursing, 27*(1), 28–33.

Mair, F., & Whitten, P. (2000). Systematic review of studies of patient satisfaction with telemedicine. *British Medical Journal, 320*(7248), 1517–1520.

Perednia, D. A., & Allen, A. (1995). Telemedicine technology and clinical applications. *Journal of the American Medical Association, 273*(6), 483–488.

Pringle Specht, J. K., Wakefield, B., & Flanagan, J. (2001). Evaluating the cost of one telehealth application connecting an acute and long-term care setting. *Journal of Gerontological Nursing, 27*(1), 34–39.

Wakefield, B., Flanagan, J., & Pringle Specht, J. K. (2001). Telehealth: An opportunity for gerontological practice. *Journal of Gerontological Nursing, 27*(1), 10–14.

Whitten, P., Mair, F., & Collins, B. (1997). Home telenursing in Kansas: Patients' perceptions of uses and benefits. *Journal of Telemedicine & Telecare, 3*(Suppl 1), 67–69.

Wootton, R., Loane, M., Mair, F., Allen, A., Doolittle, G., Begley, M., McLernan, A., Moutray, M., & Harrisson, S. (1998a). A joint U.S.-U.K. study of home telenursing. *Journal of Telemedicine & Telecare, 4*(Suppl. 1), 83–85.
Wootton, R., Loane, M., Mair, F., Moutray, M., Harrisson, S., Sivananthan, S., Allen, A., Doolittle, G., & McLernan, A. (1998b). The potential for telemedicine in home nursing. *Journal of Telemedicine & Telecare, 4*(4), 214–218.

Chapter 11

Genetics and Gerontological Nursing: A Need to Stimulate Research

LORRAINE FRAZIER AND SHARON K. OSTWALD

ABSTRACT

The purpose of this chapter is to discuss how genetics will affect gerontological nursing. The chapter will answer two questions: (1) Which aspects of genetics will be most relevant to future gerontological nursing practice? and (2) What will be the impact of genetics on the future of gerontological nursing education and research? MEDLINE was searched for relevant articles from 1995 to 2001 using the key words *aging, genetics, geriatrics, nursing education, research,* and *gerontology.* CRISP was searched using the thesaurus terms *education/ planning, genetics, health education, model design/development, psychological model, pubic health curriculum, behavioral/social science research,* and *research nursing/genetics.* A total of 101 nursing and nonnursing articles were reviewed. Research reports were selected if they focused on issues related to gerontological nursing. Articles were reviewed that had application to genetic nursing, complex diseases, and genetics.

The evolution of the science of genetics will revolutionize gerontological nursing and affect future nursing education and research as the concepts of genetic science and the technology they generate are translated into everyday clinical practice. Genetic discoveries in common complex diseases will affect care provided by gerontological nurses in the 21st century. Gerontological nurses must move quickly to recognize this genetic paradigm shift and to incorporate genetics issues into their nursing practice.

Keywords: aging, genetics, geriatrics, gerontology, nursing education, nursing research, disease management, pharmacogenetics

323

The most dramatic scientific breakthrough of the 20th century was arguably the mapping of the human genome. We know that diseases can occur from individual gene mutations, gene-to-gene interactions, and the interactions of single or multiple genes with the environment (Collins, 1999; Motulsky, 2001). These discoveries are already affecting the prevention, diagnosis, and treatment of disease and are predicted to have a significant impact on the delivery of health care in the 21st century. The rapidity of the scientific discoveries is demonstrated by the mapping of chromosome 21. In 1980, a dozen human genes were sequenced, while in May 2000, researchers reported mapping 225 genes on chromosome 21 (Hattori et al., 2000).

Nurses in all settings will care for clients with genetic concerns, whether these are related to testing, screening, counseling, or treatment options (Scanlon & Fibison, 1995). Therefore, over 2 million nurses in the United States must become informed about these revolutionary changes or face becoming obsolete. According to Lea, Anderson, and Monsen (1998), "the goal is for nurses to be informed about genetics so that they can better understand people as whole persons whose growth and development, human response patterns, and biopsychosocial processes are affected by, and have an effect on, human DNA" (p. 77). It is not enough for nurses to be educated generally about genetics. Instead, all specialties need to view their work "through a new genetic/developmental/environ-mental lens" (Eisenberg, 1998). Traditionally, gerontological nurses have provided holistic care to elders and their families. To continue to do this, gerontological nurses need to gain expertise and be integrated into the genetics community so that they can become partners with those who are leading the genetic paradigm shift in health care (Anderson, Monsen, Prows, Tinley, & Jenkins, 2000; Collins, 1999).

The purpose of this chapter is to discuss how genetics will affect gerontological nursing. The chapter addresses two questions.

1. Which aspects of genetics will be most relevant to future geronto-logical nursing practice?
2. What will be the impact of genetics on the future of gerontological nursing education and research?

METHODS

In preparation for developing the chapter, MEDLINE was searched for relevant articles 1995 to 2001 using the key words *genetics, nursing education, research, aging, geriatric,* and *gerontology.* CRISP was searched using the thesaurus terms *education/planning, genetics, health education, model design/development, psychological model, public health curriculum, behavioral/social science research,* and *research nursing/genetics.* One hundred and one articles were reviewed. Nursing articles and articles from other disciplines were included in the search.

RESULTS

Which Aspects of Genetics Will Be Most Relevant to Future Gerontological Nursing Practice?

The aspect of genetics that will be most relevant to gerontological nursing in the future will be the influence that it has on nursing practice. As the new era of genetics dawns, the roles in which gerontological nurses have traditionally excelled will take on even greater importance: health assessment, health education and counseling, health promotion, disease prevention, management of complex treatment regimes, including medication monitoring, and patient advocacy. Nurse clinicians, researchers, and policymakers who are appropriately trained in genetics will be needed to bridge the gap between genetic science, cultural values, and human diversity (Anderson et al., 2000). Lashley (2000) outlined a number of assumptions related to genetics that inform nursing practice and that have clear implications for gerontological nurses.

HEALTH ASSESSMENT

A thorough assessment of the patient is basic to the development of an effective treatment plan. The advent of genetic medicine makes some parts of the gerontological health assessment even more important. Nurses will need to construct a family tree that covers at least three generations to gather information about diseases that may have genetic components, especially those with a late adult onset. In the era of genetic medicine, the family history, including identification of cultural and ethnic background, assessment of maternal reproductive health history, and identification of physical or developmental conditions within the family takes on increasing importance (Lea et al., 1998). Environmental and occupational exposures over the lifespan are also important, but are sometimes minimized for the older retired person. These historical findings may suggest directions for the physical examination and for laboratory tests. Lashley (2000) suggests that nurses begin to think of a mutant gene as an etiologic agent. Findings on the physical and laboratory examinations, such as high blood pressure or hypercholesteremia, also suggest that a genetic link may be present in the patient. New genetic testing will allow the confirmation of these suspicions. In the 21st century treatment of one individual will be linked with the treatment of a family. As Feetham (1999) stated, "Through the consideration of genetic testing less tangible family stories of illness and premature death may be transformed to facts, concerns about etiology, and evidence of risk" (p. 319).

HEALTH EDUCATION AND COUNSELING

Gerontological nurses are recognized as trusted sources of information; the exploding availability of information on the Internet will challenge nurses to keep abreast of new developments and their implications for clients. In the future, increasing numbers of consumers will access genetic information through sources such as the Internet. Nurses' roles will change from givers of information to interpreters of information. Nurses who can help older persons and their families sift through the available information, consider options, and make wise choices will be in great demand.

HEALTH PROMOTION AND DISEASE PREVENTION

Although physicians have focused on the treatment and cure of disease, gerontological nurses have focused on promoting health and on preventing disease and excessive disability within the geriatric population. The relatively new field of molecular epidemiological research seeks to estimate genetic risks in small groups of people who can then be targeted with specific health-promotion and disease-prevention interventions before the disease occurs (Shimokata et al., 2000).

More people are expected to live longer and in better health. Thus, the focus on self-care will take on greater importance. Gerontological nurses will need to have thorough knowledge of the lifestyle modifications that can help the older population make the most of the greater longevity they are expected to achieve by the middle of the 21st century (Flower et al., 2000). Gerontological nurses with skill in leading interdisciplinary teams will be in demand to put together lifestyle modification teams to help elders to achieve a higher quality of life. As always, new pharmaceuticals and dietary products may make traditional advice obsolete and nurses will need to keep abreast of the changes in drugs and food products. Increasing importance will be placed on environmental factors and the reduction of disparities due to poverty. Gerontological nurses will need to work with communities to ensure that elders live in environments where social and environmental supports necessary to support health are maintained.

COMPLEX CARE MANAGEMENT

With the advent of new gene and pharmaceutical therapies, fewer patients will need hospitalization. Elders who are hospitalized can expect to be there for shorter periods of time and to experience fewer side effects. Complications such as infection may decrease due to the use of genetic testing. It may be possible to determine which patients are genetically susceptible to infection and to develop effective, individualized preventive plans.

Gerontological nurse practitioners, working closely with physicians and geneticists in outpatient settings, will have a major role in monitoring complex medical regimes. These nurses will need to be skillful communicators, have knowledge of molecular biology, and be technologically competent. They can expect to use sophisticated technology to monitor patients following medical regimes that do not currently exist. Genotyping will allow personalized therapy, and both screening tests and treatments will be matched to the individual's genetic background (Sander, 1999). Futuristic thinkers predict that increasing numbers of patients will be monitored electronically with information transmitted to a remote computer. Monitoring devices are expected to become smaller and less obtrusive. Flower and colleagues (2000) suggest the use of "smart clothing," bras and belts that monitor vital signs, and "smart dust," small sensors that travel in the blood stream and monitor blood chemistry and hemodynamic flow and pressure. These sensors will transmit to remote locations thousands of molecular indicators from bodily fluids, such as RNA expression, protein expression, protein modification, and concentration of metabolites (Sander, 1999). This kind of molecular profiling will allow nurses using advanced electronic technology and protocols to initiate immediate therapy.

MEDICATION MONITORING

Pharmacogenetics will have implications for the gerontological nurse's role in medication management. Pharmacogenetics is not a new phenomenon in genetic research. In 1957, Vogel described pharmacogenetics as "the study of the role of genetics in drug response" (Vogel, 1959). The science of pharmacogenetics is based on the premise that the individual's phenotypic expression, or individual variation, of proteins may alter a drug's effect (Meyer, 1992). Without knowledge of individual variations in drug response, current therapy uses a "one size fits all" approach to drug treatment that results in increased adverse side effects and decreased drug response in patients. This is particularly problematic for elders, who consume more medications, on average, than any other age group, and who often have altered absorption and secretion rates due to multiple diseases, medication interactions, and the aging process.

Pharmacogenetics will help eliminate trial and error approaches to drug treatment by revolutionizing the way we medicate patients through individualized drug treatment. Pharmacogenetics will answer the questions of why drugs react differently in different patients, and will eventually be able to predict those differences. Clinicians will be able to prescribe drugs that are individualized for the patient. For example, patients with high blood pressure will receive a hypertensive drug that is suitable for their genetic makeup rather than a traditional step-therapy approach that is now recommended.

According to Lindpainter (1999), the development of targets for the pharmacogenetics of complex diseases will have long-term, mid-term, and short-term impact on health care. In the long term, as we gain understanding of how pharmacogenetics works, we will understand the differences between individuals with the same disease (Turner, Schwartz, Chapman, Hall, & Boerwinkle, 1999). The gerontological nurse will need to understand the genetic tests that will be commonly used in the clinical area to monitor and adjust individual pharmacological therapy. To provide appropriate patient and family education, the gerontological nurse will need to understand the pharmacokinetics of those drugs.

A midterm impact of the molecular genetic approach to pharmacogenetics is that genetically selected drugs will be more efficient. The potential for increased efficacy, along with individualized patient education on person-specific drug therapy, may lead to increased patient compliance with drug regimes. It will be important that the gerontological nurse prepare the patient to accept and try the new individualized medication with the understanding that this different approach may be more beneficial than previous nonpersonalized drug therapy regimes. Nurses will need to support the patient and family with genetic consulting and genetic education as these new therapies are implemented in the clinical arena.

One short-term implication of pharmacogenetics that is of particular interest to the gerontological nurse is that pharmacogenetic therapies of the future may reduce adverse reactions to drugs by either the selection of the appropriate drug, or by the selection of the appropriate dose of the drug for the patient. In other words, new risk-stratification approaches will be developed for drug treatment based on pharmacogenetic testing. A result of the new genetic drugs, according to Lindpainter (1999), may be an increase in the cost of medication, although most of the literature proposes that new pharmacogenetic therapy, by being more efficient, will increase the health of the population. The proposed increase in the cost of medications to elders, who have fixed incomes, can also result in decreased compliance.

The health-care system is likely to benefit financially by the improved efficiency of pharmacotherapy. Increasingly effective drugs, prescribed to the appropriate population to prevent complications and control chronic disease processes, will result in less blanket prescribing by clinicians and in less money being spent on drugs that are ineffective. The health of the population will also be affected by pharmacogenetics. With increasingly targeted treatment, chronic disease should produce fewer complications leading to a decrease in morbidity and mortality rates. Lower morbidity will result in decreased clinic and hospital visits and therefore decreased costs. Later trends in pharmacogenetics may include gene therapy where normal or modified genes will be inserted into the cells of patients to prevent or treat diseases (Jacobs & Deatrick, 1999). Physical means of administering gene therapy may include microinjection and electroporation. Gerontological nurses will need to keep abreast of the new technology as it becomes commonplace in clinical practice.

ADVOCACY

Genetics strikes at the core of what it means to be human. Thus, an individual's value and belief system cannot be ignored in the health-care decision-making process, if we are to respect an individual's personhood. Anderson (1998) suggests that nurses play a special role in genetics when they narrate a patient's story to their interdisciplinary team of colleagues who may never have stopped to hear the patient's voice. She says, "this means giving genuine respect to that person's essence of humaness" (p. 69).

Ethical dilemmas are not new to gerontological nurses. Nurses have always felt an obligation to advocate the rights of individuals and families within the health-care system. As a result of the genetic revolution, humans face new threats based on their genotype: legal and financial discrimination from insurance companies and employers, disruption of their family and social relationships, loss of autonomy, threats to personal identity, limited availability and access to services, and limited therapeutic interventions (Donaldson, 1997; Monsen, 2000; Scanlon & Fibison, 1995). Discussions of genetic medicine are inevitably accompanied by discussions of new legal and ethical dilemmas. The Ethical, Legal, and Social Implications (ELSI) program is a government sponsored forum for addressing these issues concurrently with the new discoveries of the Human Genome Project (HGP) (National Human Genome Research Institute, 2000). Two additional sources are helpful to nurses, "The Code for Nurses with Interpretive Statements," the code of professional ethics for American nurses, and the "Statement on Scope and Standards of Genetics Clinical Nursing Practice" developed by the American Nurses Association and the International Society of Nurses in Genetics (1998).

The Presidential Symposium at the 1999 Gerontological Society of America Scientific Meeting was titled, "Genomic Geriatrics and Gerontology Science: Practice, Policy, and Ethics" (McGarry & Kleyman, 2000). There was disagreement among the experts on the panel regarding the extent to which genetic counseling will be used with elders due to costs and patient acceptance. Clients and their families have concerns about genetic testing and not everyone wants to know whether they will develop a specific disease in the future, especially if there is no cure for the disease (for example, Alzheimer's) (Saver, 1999). Others are concerned about the family dynamics if some members are shown to have a mutant gene and others are not. Will the one with the disease be isolated or will the survivors feel guilty?

As genetic testing extends beyond testing for single genes to testing for multiple genes which may predispose individuals to chronic diseases later in life, who will decide who should, and who should not, be tested, who will pay for testing, and who will have access to the results? We are in a transitional period in the genetics revolution because the technology to do genetic testing, especially for late-onset adult diseases, is proceeding at a much more rapid rate than the ability to cure the diseases that are discovered or to provide the legal protections against discrimination (McKinnon et al., 1997). Friedland expressed his concern that increased knowledge of genotypes would lead to segmentation of the market and that when the "once unknowable becomes known," discrimination will result (McGarry & Kleyman, 2000). In our society of electronic records, consumers are concerned about the confidentiality of their records. Will insurance companies and employers be able to access our genetic codes in the future? It is important that gerontological nurses ensure the patient's right to accept or refuse genetic testing, and that nurses seek to protect the individual's right to privacy.

Although the HGP will affect most aspects of gerontological nursing practice, the effect will need to go beyond practice. The changes in practice will lead to necessary changes in the education of gerontological nurses, as well as changes in nursing research.

What Will Be the Impact of Genetics on the Future of Gerontological Nursing Education and Research?

IMPACT ON GERONTOLOGICAL NURSING EDUCATION

Clinical application of genetic knowledge will change nursing practice, necessitating changes in the way we educate nurses. Korf (2000), Medical Director of Partners Center for Human Genetics and Associate Professor at Harvard Medical School said, "In truth, knowledge of the human genome will provide powerful insights into the pathophysiology of disease that will greatly enhance, but not replace, other approaches to our understanding of human biology and medicine" (p. 1). Some nurses were educated before the exciting breakthroughs in molecular genetics. Thus, nursing faces a dual challenge, educating the nurses of tomorrow who are in our educational institutions now, and providing continuing education that will enhance the practice of nurses in a wide range of settings.

Genetics has not been a major thread in nursing curricula, despite calls for its inclusion for the last 15 years (Anderson, 1996). It is imperative that nursing move quickly to prepare gerontological nurses for practice in this new genetic era. In 1997, Donaldson said, "Nurse educators and researchers need to create genetic health knowledge bridges now, before the nursing profession is stranded on the wrong side of a chasm of ignorance" (p. 279). If nurses are not prepared as full partners in clinical care, they will be shut out of the roles of education and counseling that have previously been central to the role of nursing in our health-care system. Gerontological nurses cannot depend on a limited number of specially trained genetic counselors, but must become conversant with genetic implications for their client group. Bernhardt, Geller, Doksum, and Metz (2000) found that with training and supervision, nurses were as effective as genetic counselors in providing education about genetic testing for breast cancer susceptibility. In addition, nurses and clients were more likely than genetic counselors and clients to perceive that a partnership had been established between them.

A 1996 national survey of genetics content in basic nursing preparatory programs in the United States found that 231 (76%) of the BSN programs, 294 (60%) of the ADN programs, and 52 (78%) of the hospital programs reported that they included genetics content in their programs (Hetteberg, Prows, Deets, Monsen, & Kenner, 1999). The survey found that 61% of the genetic content was in maternal/child courses, with only 15% in adult medical/surgical courses. Thirty-two textbooks, published between 1992 and 1997 and used in nursing education programs, were examined for genetic content (Monsen, 2000). While the number of text pages devoted to genetics and related topics varied, 47% of the texts had four or fewer pages. Four gerontology nursing texts were examined as a part of this study, and the mean number of pages devoted to genetics was 0.7. There was no content in the gerontology nursing texts on genetic basis for disease, genetic counseling, genetic screening, genetic testing, pharmacogenetics, gene mapping, genetic diagnosis, gene therapy, the Human Genome Project, social policy in genetics, or nursing roles in genetics (Monsen, 2000). Continued failure to add genetic content to nursing curricula could brand nursing as a technical workforce or an irrelevant profession (Donaldson, 1997).

This lack of focus on genetics within the gerontological nursing community reflects the historical reality that most of the single gene/chromosomal diseases were discovered during the prenatal and neonatal periods of life and these individuals did not live to be old. Even the proposed Practice-Based Genetics Curriculum for Nurse Educators (Lea & Lawson, 2000) is almost exclusively focused on maternal and child healthcare problems. However, new genetic discoveries are demonstrating that many common diseases seen in elders, such as adult-onset diabetes, arthritis, and heart disease, are caused by several genes or by genes interacting with external factors. The continuing discoveries of genes related to adult-onset diseases, as well as the multifactor nature of these genetic diseases, guarantees that genetics will play an increasing role in the prevention, diagnosis, and treatment of elders.

Clearly this knowledge base is essential for gerontological nurses of the 21st century and needs to become a part of basic nursing education curricula and continuing education programs. Gerontological nursing courses (basic, graduate, or continuing education) should teach nurses who work with elders about the genetic components of diseases and how to educate, manage, and support individuals and families who are undergoing screening or treatment for genetic-related diseases. Fortunately, the Internet offers the potential for self-directed study, as well as providing the basis for the development of course materials. A number of Internet sites contain up to date genetic information that will be of use to gerontological nurses, whether practitioners or faculty, who wish to remain informed about this rapidly changing world. In 1996, the American Nurses Association, the American Medical Association, and the National Human Genome Research Institute formed the National Coalition for Health Professional Education in Genetics (NCHPEG) that is now composed of more than 100 professional and lay organizations. In the late 1990s, leaders of the International Society of Nurses in Genetics (ISONG) collaborated with NCHPEG and the American Association of Colleges of Nursing (AACN) (Anderson et al., 2000). The result was the incorporation of core competencies related to genetic services in the AACN's revised *Essentials of Baccalaureate Education for Professional Nursing Practice* (American Association of Colleges of Nursing, 1998). Resources are available to help educators integrate genetics into their courses. (Refer to the sources listed under References.)

IMPACT ON GERONTOLOGICAL NURSING RESEARCH

Since the mid-1990s, the National Institute of Nursing Research (NINR) has been committed to increasing nursing research related to genetics. In 1997, NINR published a list of specific topics that were related to genetics, ranging from basic biological and behavioral studies to clinical and population studies (Sigmon, Grady, & Amende, 1997). In the summer of 2000, NINR offered their first 8-week summer institute to educate nursing faculty and advanced practice nurses about genetics.

Nurse researchers are needed to function as part of interdisciplinary teams with colleagues in the basic and quantitative sciences so that clinically relevant nursing questions can become a part of those that are answered by quantitative and predictive simulations. Nurse researchers can also evaluate short-term and long-term effects of genetic knowledge and technology on elders, their families, and communities. Nurses can make particular contributions to understanding the psychosocial and spiritual impact of genetic medicine on society (Lea et al., 1998). The National Institute of Nursing Research (2000) has stated one of its priority goals for the 21st century as the identification and support of research opportunities that will achieve scientific distinction and produce significant contributions to health in areas regarding implications of genetic advances. Desired areas of research include: reducing factors that increase the risk of disease, addressing issues related to genetic screening, and gene therapy techniques. Elders will be a major beneficiary of these genetic advances in the prevention, diagnosis, and treatment of chronic diseases. As gerontological nurses develop programs of research in genetics, nurses will develop a deeper understanding of the importance and meaning of incorporating genetics into the everyday care of elders.

CONCLUSIONS

Nurses are in the midst of a "genetic social revolution" in which human identity and health are being redefined on a daily basis (Donaldson, 1997). It may become possible, with the understanding of the genetic component of disease, to determine what environmental conditions predispose a certain genotype to develop diseases such as hypertension or Alzheimer's disease. DNA diagnostics in complex diseases will increase the quality and length of life. Science has moved from associating genes with rare diseases to the realization that there is a genetic component to all aspects of life, including common diseases (Johnson & Brensinger, 2000). Genes are now being cloned for major complex disease processes that include heart disease, hypertension, diabetes, osteoporosis, and prostate cancer. An understanding of the genetic basis of common complex diseases will lead to better diagnostic methods that will eventually result in a greater emphasis on early diagnosis and determination of predisposition (Smith, 2000). The use of this technology has the potential to increase the quality and length of life (Skolnick, 1999). Not only will diagnostics affect disease detection, but they will be used to understand disease progression, response to treatment, and how the penetrance of the disease alleles can be both increased and decreased by factors in the environment (Fears, Weatherall, & Poste, 1999).

Genetic discoveries in common complex diseases will affect care provided by gerontological nurses in this 21st century. Genetic tests will one day enable gerontological nurses to plan their interventions on a more individualized basis, thus providing better preventive treatment and decreasing morbidity and mortality in elderly patients. This "new" genetics will require genetic literacy for all health-care professionals (Collins, 1999; Feetham, 2000). Gerontological nurses must move quickly to recognize this genetic paradigm shift and to incorporate genetics into their nursing practice.

ACKNOWLEDGMENT

This work was supported in part by Grant NR 07574-01 from the National Institute for Nursing Research, National Institutes of Health.

REFERENCES

American Association of Colleges of Nursing. (1998). *Educational standard and special projects: Essentials of baccalaureate education for professional nursing practice.* Washington, DC: Author.

Anderson, G. (1998). Storytelling: A holistic foundation for genetic nursing. *Holistic Nursing Practice, 12*(3), 64–76.

Anderson, G., Monsen, R. B., Prows, C. A., Tinley, S., & Jenkins, J. (2000). Preparing the nursing profession for participation in a genetic paradigm in health care. *Nursing Outlook, 48*(1), 23–27.

Anderson, G. W. (1996). The evolution and status of genetics education in the United States 1983–1995. *IMAGE: Journal of Nursing Scholarship, 28,* 101–106.

Bernhardt, B., Geller, G., Doksum, T., & Metz, S. A. (2000). Evaluation of nurses and genetic counselors as providers of education about breast cancer susceptibility testing. *Oncology Nursing Forum, 27*(1), 33–39.

Collins, F. S. (1999). Shattuck lecture—medical and societal consequences of the Human Genome Project. *New England Journal of Medicine, 341*(1), 28–37.

Donaldson, S. K. (1997). The genetic social revolution and the professional status of nursing. *Nursing Outlook, 45,* 278–279.

Eisenberg, L. (1998). Chairman's summary of the conference: The implications of the new genetics for health professional education. New York: Josiah Macy Jr. Foundation.

Fears, R., Weatherall, D., & Poste, G. (1999). The impact of genetics on medical education and training. *British Medical Bulletin, 55,* 460–470.

Feetham, S. L. (1999). The future in nursing is genetics. *Journal of Child and Family Nursing, 2,* 318–321.

Feetham, S. L. (2000). The new genetics: Opportunities for nursing research and leadership. *Research in Nursing & Health, 23,* 257–259.

Flower, J., Dreifus, L. S., Bove, A. A., & Weintraub, W. S. (2000). Technological advances and the next 50 years of cardiology. *Journal of the American College of Cardiology, 35*(5 Suppl B), 81B–90B.

Guyton, A. C., Hall, J. E., Lohmeier, T. E., Jackson, T. E., & Kastner, P. R. (1981). Blood pressure regulation: Basic concepts. *Federation Proceedings, 40,* 2252–2256.

Hattori, M., Fujiyama, A., Taylor, T. D., Watanabe, H., Yada, T., Park, H. S., Toyoda, A., Ishii, K., Totoki, Y., Choi, D. K., Soeda, E., Ohki, M., Takagi, T., Sakaki, Y., Taudien, S., Blechschmidt, K., Polley, A., Menzel, U., Delabar, J., Kumpf, K., Lehmann, R., Patterson, D., Reichwald, K., Rump, A., Schillhabel, M., & Schudy, A. (2000). The DNA sequence of human chromosome 21: The chromosome 21 mapping and sequencing consortium. *Nature, 405,* 311–319.

Hetteberg, C. G., Prows, C. A., Deets, C., Monsen, R. B., & Kenner, C. A. (1999). National survey of genetics content in basic nursing preparatory programs in the United States. *Nursing Outlook, 47,* 168–180.

Jacobs, L. A., & Deatrick, J. A. (1999). The individual, the family, and genetic testing. *Journal of Professional Nursing, 15,* 313–324.

Johnson, K. A., & Brensinger, J. D. (2000). Genetic counseling and testing: Implications for clinical practice. *Nursing Clinics of North America, 35,* 615–626.

Korf, B. R. (2000). Medical education in the 'postgenomic era'. *Postgraduate Medicine, 108*(3), 15–18.

Ladislas, R. (2000). Cellular and molecular mechanisms of aging and age related diseases. *Pathology Oncology Research, 6*(1), 3–9.

Lashley, F. R. (2000). Genetics in nursing education. *Nursing Clinics of North America, 35,* 795–805.

Lea, D. H., Anderson, G., & Monsen, R. B. (1998). A multiciplicity of roles for genetic nursing: Building toward holistic practice. *Holistic Nursing Practice, 12*(3), 77–87.

Lea, D. H., & Lawson, M. T. (2000). A practice-based genetics curriculum for nurse educators: An innovative approach to integrating human genetics into nursing curricula. *Journal of Nursing Education, 39,* 418–421.

Lindpainter, K. (1999). Genetics in drug discovery and development: Challenge and promise of individualizing treatment in common complex disease. *British Medical Bulletin, 55,* 471–491.

McGarry, N., & Kleyman, P. (2000, January/February). Impact of human genome research debated. *Aging Today,* 1, 4.

McKinnon, W. C., Baty, B. J., Bennett, R. L., Magee, M., Neufeld-Kaiser, W. A., Peters, K. F., Sawyer, J. C., & Schneider, K. A. (1997). Predisposition genetic testing for late-onset disorders in adults. A position paper of the National Society of Genetic Counselors. *Journal of the American Medical Association, 278,* 1217–1220.

Meyer, U. (1992). Drugs in special patient groups: Clinical importance of genetics. In K. L. Melmon & H. F. Morrelli (Eds.), *Clinical pharmacology: Basic principle in therapeutics* (2nd ed., pp. 875–894). New York: McGraw-Hill.

Monsen, R. B. (2000). An international agenda for ethics in nursing and genetics. *Journal of Pediatric Nursing, 15,* 212–216.

Motulsky, A. G. (2001). 1999 ASHG Award for Excellence in Education: Some future directions in medical genetics. *American Journal of Human Genetics, 66,* 1190–1191.

National Human Genome Research Institute. (2000, October 20). ELSI: Ethical, legal, and social implications of human genetics research. Bethesda, MD: Author. Retrieved January 22, 2001 from the World Wide Web: http://www.nhgri.nih. gov/ELSI

Sander, C. (1999). Genomic medicine and the future of health care. *Science, 287,* 1977–1978.

Saver, C. (1999). Why genetics competency is a must: The Human Genome Project. *Imprint, 46*(3), 44–46.

Scanlon, C., & Fibison, W. (1995). *Managing genetic information: Implications for nursing practice.* Washington, DC: American Nurses Association.

Shimokata, H., Yamada, Y., Nakagawa, M., Okubo, R., Saido, T., Funakoshi, A., Miyasaka, K., Ohta, S., Tsujimoto, G., Tanaka, M., Ando, F., & Niino, N. (2000). Distribution of geriatric disease-related genotypes in the National Institute for Longevity Sciences, Longitudinal Study of Aging (NILS-LSA). *Journal of Epidemiology/Japan Epidemiological Association, 10*(1 Supp), S46–S55.

Sigmon, H. D., Grady, P. A., & Amende, L. M. (1997). The National Institute of Nursing Research explores opportunities in genetics research. *Nursing Outlook, 45,* 215–219.

Skolnick, M. H. (1999). The future of DNA diagnostics. *Disease Markers, 15,* 106–107.

Smith, R. (2000). Health care in the next millennium. *European Journal of Nuclear Medicine, 27*(1 Suppl), S17–S20.

The National Institute of Nursing Research. (2000, May). Strategic planning for the 21st century. Bethesda, MD: Author. Retrieved May 16, 2001 from the World Wide Web: http://www.nih.gov/ninr/a_mission.html

Turner, S., Schwartz, G., Chapman, A., Hall, W., & Boerwinkle, E. (1999). *Antihypertensive pharmacogenetics: Getting the right drug to the right patient.* Unpublished manuscript, Emory University, Atlanta, GA & University of Texas, Houston, TX.

Vogel, F. (1959). Moderne probleme der Humangenetik. *Ergebnisse der inneren Medizin und Kinderheilkunde, 12,* 52–125.

PART IV

Neglected Areas of Research in Gerontological Nursing

Chapter 12

Hearing Impairment

MARGARET I. WALLHAGEN

ABSTRACT

The purpose of this chapter is to review the literature on hearing impairment, specifically the impact of hearing impairment on the functioning of elders, interventions that minimize the impact of hearing loss on functioning, and identification of issues raised by the review for nursing research. Computerized (MEDLINE, PsychINFO, and CINAHL) and manual searches were used to obtain research reports from a range of disciplines. Research articles including elders ($\geq$ 60) and published between 1989 and 2001 were included. Twenty-five articles were selected for critical review, four written by nurses. The diversity of methodologies, the criteria used to define hearing impairment, the range of sample characteristics, and the assessment measures make comparisons across studies difficult. Most studies, however, support the negative impact of hearing impairment, especially on psychosocial functioning. Measures that are condition specific are generally more effective in capturing the impact of hearing loss than generic measures. Findings related to physical disability are less consistent. The results of intervention studies suggest that hearing devices can improve psychosocial and communication outcomes, but behavioral interventions have not shown long lasting benefit. For nurses to assist elders and their families manage the impact of hearing impairment, further research is needed in several areas that have been poorly explored. These include the dyadic experience of hearing impairment, the way in which culture influences the experience of hearing loss, the needs of hearing impaired individuals across settings, the long-term impact of ototoxic medications, and strategies to assist elders in coping with hearing impairment and utilizing available technologies.

Keywords: aging, disability, functioning, hearing impairment

Hearing impairment has been reported as the third most common chronic condition experienced by elders (Schick & Schick, 1994). However, prevalence data are based on studies using different sampling and assessment techniques, as well as different criteria for defining hearing loss. Approximately 30% of persons ≥ 65 (Ries, 1994), 33% of persons ≥ 70 (Campbell, Crews, Moriarty, Zack, & Blackman, 1999), and 50% of those ≥ 85 (USPHS, 1998) report hearing impairment. Using standardized audiometric testing, 45.9% of persons age 48–92 were found to be hearing impaired, a prevalence that increased significantly with age (OR = 1.88 for 5 years) and was greater for men than for women (OR = 4.42) (Cruickshanks, Wiley, et al., 1998). Data also indicate that individuals are reporting hearing impairment at increasingly younger ages (Benson & Marano, 1994; Ries, 1994; Wallhagen, Strawbridge, Cohen, & Kaplan, 1997).

Given its prevalence, hearing impairment should be of major concern to nursing. However, it has received relatively little attention from nurse researchers. The purpose of this chapter is to review the literature on hearing impairment, specifically addressing the following questions:

1. What is the impact of hearing impairment on the functioning of elders?
2. What interventions minimize the impact of hearing loss on functioning?
3. What are the central issues raised by the review for nursing research?

Included is a brief discussion of changes in hearing that occur with age, factors influencing age-related hearing loss, why hearing loss can affect functioning, and the design and methodological limitations of hearing impairment research.

METHOD

MEDLINE, PsychINFO, and CINAHL were searched using the subject headings or key words *hearing, hearing impairment, hearing disability, hearing loss,* and *deafness* as well as related subheadings. Limits narrowed the search to persons middle-aged or older. Reference lists were used to extend the search and obtain primary references. *Caregiving* was explored for data on the impact of hearing loss on family functioning. Specialty texts were used to provide material for the background review. The search focused on the years 1990–2001, but some studies included the span 1989–2001. Because of rapid changes in technology over the past decade, emphasis was placed on the past 5 years when reviewing articles on the benefits of hearing devices. Excluded from the critique were studies that did not focus on the impact of hearing loss on functioning; those focusing on youth-acquired or congenital deafness; occupational health in middle-aged individuals; spectral analysis, speech perception, or discrimination studies; cellular studies, such as those focusing on mitochondrial DNA; acoustic neuromas, Ménière's disease, cerumen impaction; all review articles; and research articles that did not provide adequate descriptive data regarding design or methodology or were based on a case study. The search identified eleven research reports by nurses published during the past 10 years and seven published during the past 5 years, three of which were from Great Britain. Seven of these studies were excluded from the review, three because they focused on cerumen impaction and four because their emphasis was on prevalence. A total of 25 published articles were selected for critical review.

BACKGROUND

Changes in Hearing with Age

Hearing loss can be classified as: (a) conductive, caused by conditions blocking sound waves from getting to the inner ear such as cerumen or otosclerosis; (b) sensorineural, caused by conditions that damage the inner ear, the auditory nerve, or both; (c) central, caused by damage at the level of the central nervous system; and (d) mixed, or a combination of conductive and sensorineural problems (Baloh, 1998; Sataloff & Sataloff, 1993). *Presbycusis*, the term used to refer to changes in hearing that occur with age, is considered a form of sensorineural hearing loss (Sataloff & Sataloff, 1993).

The sensory neural changes of presbycusis are grouped into four types (sensory, neural, metabolic, and cochlear conductive), each with distinct pathological findings. Patterns of hearing loss usually suggest that often more than one of these processes occur together (Fire, 1995; Roland & Marple, 1997). However, the most common deficit that characterizes presbycusis is loss of the ability to hear high-frequency sounds such as those produced by consonants (McCarthy & Sapp, 2000; Roland & Marple, 1997). Because consonants are important elements of word intelligibility, loss of high-frequency perception can make normal conversation difficult to understand, especially with background noise (Kenyon, Leidenheim, & Zwillenberg, 1998; Slawinski, Hartel, & Kline, 1993).

A simple diagnosis of presbycusis, however, does not provide adequate data about the extent of the disorder and how it is experienced (Kampfe & Smith, 1998). Hearing is a complex phenomenon involving interactions among the individual's central and peripheral auditory status, personal state, interpersonal relations, and environment (Kampfe & Smith, 1998). Thus, many issues raised by the experience of hearing loss are not adequately explained by testing only one component of this intricate process (Chmiel & Jerger, 1993, 1996). Further, while emphasis is usually placed on the sensorineural aspects of presbycusis, aging can impact structure and function throughout the auditory system; for example, decreased elasticity of the skin and cartilage of the external auditory canal can influence the fitting of a hearing aid and potentially lead to rejection (McCarthy & Sapp, 2000).

Controversy remains whether hearing loss is better explained by aging or by the accumulation of noxious environmental exposures (Roland & Marple, 1997). A longitudinal study of men ($n = 681$) and women ($n = 416$) with no evidence of noise induced deficits still found diminished hearing sensitivity with age (Pearson et al., 1995). Change in hearing level over a 10-year period was more than twice as fast in men than in women, but the rates of change in each gender began to converge after the age of 60 and were similar after age 80, suggesting that age has an independent effect on hearing impairment.

Factors Influencing Age-Related Hearing Loss

In addition to age, noise is considered one of the main causes of sensorineural hearing loss (Melnick, 1995). It causes a high frequency deficit similar to presbycusis, but with its own distinct audiometric pattern. Individual susceptibility to noise-induced hearing loss varies considerably (Henderson, Subramaniam, & Boettcher, 1993), and may be influenced by the presence of presbycusis (Shone, Altschuler, Miller, & Nuttall, 1991); previous or concurrent exposure to ototoxic substances (Morata, 1998), including medications (Brien, 1993; Carson, Prazma, Pulver, & Anderson, 1989); and protective auditory reflexes (Henderson et al., 1993). Physical activity may be protective, probably because of its positive effect on the cardiovascular system (Wallhagen et al., 1997).

Other factors implicated in hearing loss with age include a variety of medical conditions (Dalton, Cruickshanks, Klein, Klein, & Wiley, 1998; Duck, Prazma, Bennett, & Pillsbury, 1997; Gatland, Tucker, Chalstrey, Keene, & Baker, 1991; Hariri, Lakshmi, Larner, & Connolly, 1994; Lim & Stephens, 1991); elevated blood lipids (Pulec & Mendoza, 1997); cigarette smoking (Cruickshanks, Klein, et al., 1998); trauma (Fitzgerald, 1996); infections (Fuse, Inamura, Nakamura, Suzuki, & Auyagi, 1996; Kanazawa, Hagiwara, & Kitamura, 2000); nutritional status (Houston et al., 1999), and cerumen (Mahoney, 1993).

Although many of these relationships need further study, they may compound the effect of age on hearing loss and are often amenable to interventions. For example, cerumen is not an uncommon cause of hearing impairment and is readily corrected (Lewis-Cullinan & Janken, 1990). Ototoxic medications may be of special concern because of the multiple drugs that elders take concurrently over an extended period of time. The most clinically important known toxicities have been related to four classes of drugs: aminoglycosides, loop diuretics, antineoplastics, and nonsteroidal anti-inflammatory agents (Brien, 1993; Roland & Marple, 1997; Stypulkowski, 1990). Although ototoxicity is viewed as related to high serum levels and is frequently reversible, minimal data are available on the effects of long-term use of ototoxic agents at lower doses concurrently with other medications or with exposure to other agents impacting hearing, such as noise (Arslan, Orzan, & Santarelli, 1999; Mills et al., 1999).

Why Hearing Loss Influences Function

To appreciate the impact of hearing impairment, Ramsdell's (1970) delineation of three major functions of hearing is assistive: symbolic/social, warning/affective, and primitive/auditory background. The symbolic/social function is our ability to understand language and communicate with others. Studies have consistently shown that some of the major problems associated with the high-frequency hearing deficit commonly experienced by elders are speech misinterpretation and distortion of sounds. This deficit can significantly impact everyday functioning, social interactions, and relationships.

The warning/affective function emphasizes the essential nature of hearing in receiving information and environmental feedback, allowing us to escape danger, enjoy nature, and localize ourselves in space. Minimal data focus on the impact of hearing impairment on the loss of this function even though modern devices frequently utilize high-frequency sounds to inform; for example, microwaves, smoke detectors, phones, sirens. Hearing loss is sometimes listed in nursing texts as a risk factor for falls (Ebersole & Hess, 1998), but not all data support this association (Tinetti, Inouye, Gill, & Doucette, 1995).

The primitive/auditory background function includes the sounds that surround us but are not in the forefront of our attention. These sounds allow us to feel a part of our world. Ramsdell (1970) suggests that loss of this primitive/auditory background is a major reason for depression in those who are deaf. A quote from Tolson's (1999) work captures the potential importance of this function. A resident who had been provided a hearing aid and assisted in its use went on to note, "I had forgotten what it was like. Its [sic] like waking up. It is waking up and wanting to because there is something going on, chatting gives you something to think about. . . . You know what it's like. It's like living in a place where you can only look in, you know I mean you are not part of things, you are like a visitor on the outside watching everything going on" (p. 386).

Design and Methodological Limitations of Hearing Impairment Research

Design and methodological limitations of the research on hearing impairment make comparison across studies difficult. These include how hearing impairment is assessed and defined, whether general or hearing specific measures of functioning are used as outcome variables, whether studies are cross-sectional or longitudinal, and whether the sample represents the diversity of the current older population.

ASSESSMENT AND DEFINITION OF HEARING IMPAIRMENT

Several studies reviewed used self-report measures (Table 12.1), but items were not consistent across studies. Comparative studies provided support for the validity of self-report data. When self-report items were compared with clinical testing for hearing impairment, a scale derived from simple questions incorporating sociodemographic data along with reported hearing

TABLE 12.1 Measures of Hearing Impairment Used in Reviewed Studies

Type	Description	Examples	Pros	Cons
Audiometric (Gold Standard)	Pure Tone Average (PTA): Average thresholds in decibels at defined frequencies Impairment Levels: 0–25dB HL: Normal 25–40dB HL: Mild 40–60dB HL: Moderate 60–90dB HL: Severe > 90dB HL: Profound (Yellin, 1997)	Ventry-Weinstein Scale (VW) Impairment = 40dB HL at 1 or 2 kHz in both ears or 40dB HL at 1 and 2 kHz in one ear Speech Frequency PTA Impairment = Average threshold > 25dB HL at .5, 1, and 2 kHz in the better ear High Frequency PTA Impairment = Average threshold > 25dB HL at 1, 2, and 4 kHz in the better ear	Relatively objective and replicable	Affected by patient effort. Cannot quantify experience of hearing loss for subject. Assumes optimal testing environment.

(continued)

TABLE 12.1 *(continued)*

Type	Description	Examples	Pros	Cons
Physical exam	Whispered Voice (Free Voice): Words, numbers whispered from set distance behind subject with untested ear masked.	Impairment = Inability to repeat at least 50% of whispered words (Mulrow et al., 1991) 50% threshold approximates 30dB HL (Macphee, 1988)	Relatively easy to use and inexpensive compared with audiometric testing	Practitioner variability in loudness, voice frequency, words or numbers used, distance. Lack of consistency limits research utility.
Self-report	Questionnaire format. Subject evaluates own impairment.	Single item: e.g., trouble hearing or trouble hearing even with a hearing aid Multiple items: degree of trouble hearing in specific situations (telephone, noisy room, conversation)	Easy to use and inexpensive. Amenable to large surveys. Assesses subject's awareness and experience of hearing loss. Multiple items can approximate extent of loss.	Misses those who deny or are unaware of their hearing loss. Variation in specific items across studies.

difficulty (uncorrected) was an effective screen for hearing impairment (Reuben, Walsh, Moore, Damesyn, & Greendale, 1998). Further, clinical and self-report measures of hearing impairment were found to have relatively close agreement when used as predictors of subsequent disability (Rudberg, Furner, Dunn, & Cassel, 1993).

Even when more objective clinical measures are used, there is lack of agreement about what constitutes hearing impairment or loss (Rees, Duckert, & Carey, 1999) (Table 12.1). Although mild hearing impairment is defined as starting at > 25dBHL, Martin and Champlin (2000) argued that 15dBHL rather than 25dBHL should be the standard for the upper limits of normal hearing in adults because many people with losses between 15dB and 25dB complain of hearing problems. This is supported by the findings discussed below that even mild hearing impairment can have a negative impact on psychosocial functioning (Scherer & Frisina, 1998), and that standard assessments often fail to identify candidates for current forms of amplification (Sweetow, 1996).

Studies that incorporated audiometric assessments varied in the criteria defining hearing impairment. Tolson, in her study of institutionalized elders in Scotland, used ≥ 40dBHL as the cut-off, noting this was identified as a level at which hearing aid use might be most beneficial (Tolson & McIntosh, 1997; Tolson, Swan, & McIntosh, 1995). Bess, Lichtenstein, Logan, Burger, and Nelson (1989) defined the beginning of hearing loss as a ≥ 17dB average decibel loss at 500, 1000, and 2000 Hz in the better ear, and moderate, severe, and profound losses as those defined by a ≥ 40dB PTA. In contrast, Mulrow and colleagues (1990) defined hearing loss as a better ear threshold of ≥ 40dB at the single frequency of 2000 Hz. The differences in defined criteria for hearing impairment influence the sample included in the study and, potentially, the strength of any associations found. Further, as presbycusis often starts as a high-frequency deficit that may be expressed by a sharp drop-off, usually starting above 2000 Hz (Roland & Marple, 1997), early age-related losses could be missed if frequencies above 2000 Hz are not assessed.

Several studies attempting to identify the impact of hearing impairment in community-dwelling populations used the free-field or whispered-voice test (Carabellese et al., 1993; Keller, Morton, Thomas, & Potter, 1999), but it was not always carried out in the same manner. Carabellese and colleagues (1993) utilized a set of three random numbers, with hearing impairment defined as the inability to repeat all three numbers correctly or achieve greater than 50% success over three triplet sets of numbers. A group of 10 general practitioners carried out the assessments; interrater reliability (Cohen's kappa) was .66. Keller and colleagues (1999) used "an easily answered question." No interrater reliability was noted. Because the whispered test raises questions regarding standardization (Table 12.1), it should be used cautiously in research.

Measuring hearing impairment using audiometric assessments or self-reported impairment does not capture the total experience of being hearing impaired (Weinstein, Richards, & Montano, 1995). A number of hearing handicap measures have been developed to address the psychosocial, emotional, and situational sequellae of hearing impairment (Dillon, James, & Ginis, 1997; Mulrow & Lichtenstein, 1991; Saunders & Cienkowski, 1996; Ventry & Weinstein, 1982). While each taps into the experience of hearing impairment, they vary in their specific focus (situational, emotional, social). The Hearing Handicap Inventory for the Elderly (HHIE) (Ventry & Weinstein, 1982), one of the most commonly used tools, was specifically designed to address both emotional and social/situational issues in elders. Perceived hearing handicap may be important in determining acceptance or adaptation to hearing devices (Malinoff & Weinstein, 1989; Weinstein et al., 1995).

ASSESSMENT VARIABLES

Studies reviewed used a wide range of psychosocial and physiologic functioning variables to operationalize domains of quality of life, making comparisons difficult (Bess et al., 1989; Carabellese et al., 1993; Mulrow et al., 1990; Scherer & Frisina, 1998; Strawbridge, Wallhagen, Shema, & Kaplan, 2000; Tinetti et al., 1995; Wallhagen et al., 2001). A few studies focused on specific outcomes such as activities of daily living (ADLs), instrumental activities of daily living (IADLs), or related physical functioning measures (Dargent-Molina, Hays, & Breart, 1996; Keller et al., 1999; Reuben, Mui, Damesyn, Moore, & Greendale, 1999; Rudberg et al., 1993); loneliness and self-esteem (Chen, 1994; Dugan & Kivett, 1994); or how hearing impairment affected family or interpersonal relations (Hetu et al., 1993). Others focused on the relationship between the sensory impairment and cognitive functioning or cognitive decline (Anstey, Luszcz, & Sanchez, 2001; Baltes & Lindenberger, 1997; Gennis, Garry, Haaland, Yeo, & Goodwin, 1991; Lindenberger & Baltes, 1994; Luszcz & Bryan, 1999; Peters, Potter, & Scholer, 1988; Salthouse, Hambrick, & McGuthry, 1998; Salthouse, Hancock, Meinz, & Hambrick, 1996).

Many studies are cross-sectional which prevents causal interpretation (Bess et al., 1989; Carabellese et al., 1993; Dargent-Molina et al., 1996;

Keller et al., 1999; Kochkin & Rogin, 2000; Mulrow et al., 1990; Scherer & Frisina, 1998). With few exceptions, studies reviewed did not use a conceptual framework. Those that did were usually carried out by nurses, for example Tolson (1999), Tolson and McIntosh (1997), Chen (1994), and Zhan (2000) used Roy's Adaptation Model.

SAMPLE DIVERSITY

Studies rarely addressed the potential differential effect of hearing impairment on different ethnic groups, yet culture and health beliefs may influence participation in research studies as well as the response to hearing impairment and measures of psychosocial functioning. For example, Bess and colleagues (1989) found that Blacks were "somewhat less likely" (p. 124) than Whites to follow-up on the referral to the center, and the group that did not complete the questionnaire contained a greater proportion of Black female participants. However, no data are available on whether these differences were statistically significant and the small sample in this study would make subgroup analysis impossible.

Most studies focused on community-dwelling elders; few data were available on hearing loss in residents of long-term care settings. Tolson (1995) assessed a sample of 188 elders (94 men, 94 women) from fifteen long-stay wards in Scotland for pure tone sensitivity across the speech frequencies (0.5–4 kHz) using a portable audiometer; 70% were hearing impaired.

Variations in the measurement of hearing impairment, how dependent variables are defined and operationalized, and sample characteristics have to be considered in evaluating studies assessing the impact of hearing impairment as well as the benefits of treatment. Studies should describe their methodology thoroughly and, if possible, use more than one measurement of hearing impairment (i.e., self-report as well as audiometric testing) (Reuben et al., 1999).

RESULTS

What Is the Impact of Hearing Impairment on the Functioning of Elders?

PSYCHOSOCIAL AND PHYSICAL FUNCTIONING

Although differing significantly in their approach to the problem, studies support the negative impact of hearing impairment on psychosocial and physical functioning, although results varied in the strength of associations. In an early, frequently referenced, cross-sectional study of 153 (96 female, 57 male) elders ≥ 65 (Mean age = 72 years) from six primary care practices, Bess and colleagues (1989) found that level of hearing impairment was significantly associated with higher (worse) scores on all three Sickness Impact Profile (SIP) subscales. After controlling for demographic and health variables, each 10dB increase in hearing loss was associated with a 2.8-point increase in the physical subscale ($p < .001$), a 2.0-point increase in the psychosocial subscale ($p < .001$), and a 1.3-point increase in the overall scale score ($p < .02$).

Although the differences in the SIP scale scores in the Bess and colleagues study were small and raise issues regarding whether they were clinically significant, the results suggest a widespread negative impact with the strongest relationship occurring in the physical domain. However, subsequent data related to the impact of hearing impairment on function, as assessed by activities of daily living (ADL), instrumental activities of daily living (IADL), or related measures, are conflicting.

Focusing on persons referred to a geriatric assessment clinic, Keller and colleagues (1999) assessed 576 patients ranging in age from 56 to 102. Mean values for both ADL and IADL scores were significantly poorer for those with a hearing impairment than those without ($p = .001$). However, results of the ordinary least squares regression model with controls for gender, cognitive status, and comorbid disease (but not age), showed that while hearing impairment had an independent effect on IADL functioning ($p = .05$), only vision impairment had an effect on ADL performance. Sixty-four percent of the participants were cognitively impaired (MMSE ≤ 23), which may be related to the type of clinic setting and reason for referral, but raises issues regarding the assessment of hearing impairment, especially when a whispered test is used.

In a longitudinal study of measured (audiometry, VW criteria) and self-reported vision and hearing impairment, 5,444 men and women age 55 to 74 years old (Mean age 65.8 yrs; 83.6% White) were surveyed to assess the impact of sensory impairment on 10-year mortality and dependency in ADL, IADL, and Rosow-Breslau (RB) function (Reuben et al., 1999). After adjusting for length of follow-up, socio-demographic characteristics, and chronic conditions, both measured and self-reported hearing impairment were predictive of RB dependence (Relative Risk = 1.66 and 1.76, respectively) but not ADL or IADL dependence. Similarly, Rudberg and colleagues (1993) failed to find a relationship between hearing impairment and ADL disability across 4 years in a nationally representative sample of persons ≥ 70 years old. An analysis of data from a study conducted in 1975–1976 of 1,408 community-dwelling elders (≥ 65 yrs old), only those with impairments in vision, or both vision and hearing, experienced functional decline (LaForge, Spector, & Sternberg, 1992).

Contrary to the negative findings related to ADL impact, Tinetti and colleagues (1995) carried out a 1-year longitudinal study of 927 individuals ≥ 72 years old and found that hearing impairment was associated with subsequent urinary incontinence as well as ADL disability, but not with falls. Further, in a study that included both self-reported disability and objective measures of physical ability (chair stands, foot tapping, time to walk 6 m), Dargent-Molina and colleagues (1996) assessed the impact of both hearing and vision impairment on 1,210 community-dwelling women age 75 and older. Self-reported serious hearing difficulty, especially if supported by the observations of the nurse asking the questions, significantly increased the odds of dependency; wearing a hearing aid did not.

These studies suggest that basic ADLs may not be sensitive to the effects of hearing impairment, especially in community-dwelling elders or when the level of hearing impairment is not advanced. The RB assessment, which includes items on walking a quarter of a mile, climbing up and down at least 2 steps, and performing heavy chores, provides a better assessment of hearing impairment's influence on IADL functioning. At the same time, studies discussed below that included a broader array of outcome variables identified an impact of hearing impairment on both psychosocial and physical functioning, suggesting that additional research is warranted.

In a large community-based Italian study, Carabellese and colleagues (1993) assessed the impact of hearing and vision impairment on quality of life using the Self Evaluation of Life Function (SELF) scale (social domain); Beck Depression Inventory (affective domain); Mental Status Questionnaire (cognitive domain); and IADL (physical domain). Using logistic regression with controls for demographics, cognitive status, health, and other quality of life measures, subjects with hearing impairment were found to have a significantly higher risk of depression (OR = 1.76, CI 1.15–2.7) and IADL disability (OR = 2.1, CI 1.36–3.25) but not poorer social relationships.

Strawbridge and colleagues (2000), studied the 1-year impact of hearing impairment in a large (n = 2,461) community sample of persons aged ≥ 50 in 1994. Using logistic regression with controls for baseline functioning and chronic conditions as well as age, gender, and education, persons with moderate or more hearing impairment were found to be at significantly higher risk for: (a) poorer physical functioning on three measures (ADL [OR 1.85, CI 1.26–2.71], IADL [OR 1.37, CI 1.01–1.86], and physical performance [OR 1.98, CI 1.38–2.84]); (b) poorer mental health on five measures (depression [OR 2.05, CI 1.37–3.06], self-related mental health [OR 1.90, CI 1.30–2.78], little enjoyment of free time [OR 1.26, CI .96–1.66], difficulty paying attention [OR 1.99, CI 1.52–2.60], and not pleased with accomplishments [OR 1.34, CI 1.03–1.74]); and (c) poorer social functioning on three measures (not feeling close to others [OR 1.82, CI 1.33–2.50], feeling left out in a group [OR 1.96, CI 1.39–2.75], and feeling lonely or remote [OR 1.44, CI 1.10–1.88]). In this study, even a little hearing impairment was associated with greater risk for poorer ADL and IADL functioning, self-rated mental health, difficulty paying attention, feeling lonely or remote, and feeling left out in a group. A 5-year follow-up using additional analytic techniques provided further support for these findings (Wallhagen et al., 2001). In addition, Scherer and Frisina (1998) found that individuals with even mild hearing loss (12.8–41.3 dB HL) reported less satisfaction with their independence, and reduced emotional well-being.

These latter studies (Carabellese et al., 1993; Wallhagen et al., 2001) go beyond the impact of hearing impairment on physical functioning and support its impact on a range of psychosocial variables. The psychosocial impact of hearing impairment is further supported by additional studies focusing on a range of measures.

Mulroy and colleagues (1990) operationalized quality of life using two condition-specific measures, the HHIE and the Quantified Denver Scale of Communication (QDS), and four generic measures. Twenty-two percent ($n = 106$) of the 472 persons screened were hearing impaired. The hearing-impaired participants were compared with 98 individuals selected randomly from the remaining sample. Scores for the two condition-specific measures were significantly higher in subjects with a hearing impairment as compared with subjects who were not hearing impaired: HHIE mean score of 52.2 vs. 22.2 ($p = .0001$) and a QDS mean score of 61.8 vs. 40.0 ($p = .02$). Neither group differed in their mean scores on the generic measures.

Dugan and Kivett (1994) explored social and emotional isolation and its relationship to loneliness in 119 rural adults ≥ 65. Hearing was assessed with a single item ("How is your hearing?") with a 5-point response option ranging from totally deaf to excellent. Better hearing was significantly related to less loneliness (β = 0.21, $p \leq$ 0.05). Similarly, Chen (1994) carried out a small (n = 88, Male = 45, Female = 43) correlational study using a convenience sample of elders (65–90, Mean age = 74.9) recruited from retirement communities, speech and hearing centers, and ENT clinics. The criterion for entry into the study was a perceived hearing loss; how this was determined prior to distributing the questionnaires is not clear. Measures used included the HHIE, the UCLA Loneliness Scale, and the Rosenberg Global Self-Esteem Scale. Hearing handicap was associated with both loneliness (r = 0.23, p = .01) and lower self-esteem (r = .26, p = .008) in the total sample, but only in women in the subgroup analysis. The lack of controls and relatively small number in the subgroup analysis suggest results be viewed cautiously. However, the findings raise issues related to gender differences in the experience of hearing impairment and its impact.

FAMILY AND FRIENDS

Only one study published during the 1990s with adequate descriptive data could be located on the impact of hearing impairment on intimate relationships (Hetu et al., 1993). Interviews with the spouse of the person with hearing impairment highlighted the stress, effort/fatigue, frustration, anger, resentment, and guilt that can be experienced by the unimpaired partner.

SUMMARY OF HEARING LOSS IMPACT ON FUNCTIONING

Most studies support the negative impact of hearing impairment, especially on depression and psychosocial functioning. Measures that are more condition specific, such as the HHIE as opposed to generic measures, are generally more effective in capturing the impact of hearing loss. Findings related to physical disability are less consistent and are more difficult to explain. However, an area of growing interest is the relationship between sensory impairment, defined by visual and auditory acuity, and cognitive functioning (Baltes & Lindenberger, 1997; Salthouse et al., 1998; Salthouse et al., 1996). Luszcz and Bryan (1999) suggest that a decline in both cognitive and sensory functioning may occur secondary to a common underlying change in neurological integrity, the "common cause" hypothesis (Baltes & Lindenberger, 1997). If hearing impairment is representative of altered neurologic integrity, physical impairment may be another manifestation. Alternatively, if hearing impairment causes decreased social activity and increased isolation, alterations in physical functioning may be related to disuse. Additional longitudinal studies using standardized measures of hearing impairment and clearly defined outcome variables that are based on theoretical rationale are needed to further delineate relationships. At the same time, intervention studies add support to the negative impact of hearing impairment and the potential for appropriately designed interventions.

What Interventions Minimize the Impact of Hearing Loss?

SENSORY AIDS

Most intervention studies focused on the effects of hearing aid use. Because of the changing nature of technology, the generalizability of earlier findings may be questioned; yet both early and more recent data support the positive effect of sensory aids on functioning. Studies differ mainly in the range of outcomes affected by hearing aid use.

Mulroy and colleagues (1992) followed older veterans, most of whom were initially assessed for the impact of hearing impairment (Mulrow et al., 1990), to study the effects of hearing aid use at 6 weeks, and 4, 8 and 12 months. While the exact number of participants varied slightly across reports, of the initial 192 subjects, 162 appear to have completed all three assessments. As assessed by the HHIE, the QDS, and the Geriatric Depression Scale (GDS), significant improvements were seen in social and emotional functioning ($p = .0001$), communication ($p = .0001$), and depression ($p = .03$) at 6 months and maintained at 12. However, there were large standard deviations around the mean scores of the outcome variables, especially those related to hearing handicap and communication. Improvements in cognitive functioning were seen at 6 months but these returned to baseline at 12 months.

Taylor (1993) followed 58 elderly persons (65–81, Mean = 72) with at least mild sensorineural hearing loss on pure tone audiometric testing for 1 year after hearing-aid fitting. Hearing handicap was assessed using the HHIE. Improvement in audiometric test results after hearing aid use was initiated remained stable across the year. Hearing handicap dropped significantly at 3 weeks (total score from 33.8 to 8.77), rose again significantly at 3 months to 18.27, dropped to 12.65 at 6 months, and remained stable at 12 months (11.83). The pattern of early drop with a rise at 3 months suggests that 3 months may be an especially vulnerable time in adaptation to a hearing aid, although this may be less of a concern with newer technology.

In an analysis of data on the impact of hearing aid use, collected by the National Council on the Aging (NCOA) (1999), Kochkin and Rogin (2000) reported on the findings from a survey of 2,069 hearing impaired individuals and 1,710 family members. Participants were divided into five quintiles based on their level of hearing impairment (1 = least, 5 = most) as assessed by the Five Minute Hearing Test (FMHT), which correlates significantly with standard audiometric measures including speech reception and discrimination (Koike, Hurst, & Westmore, 1994). The mean age of the users and nonusers across quintiles ranged from 70–75, and the majority were male, married, and retired.

Measures assessed physical, emotional, mental, and social well-being, with both the hearing impaired individual and their family member responding to separate questionnaires. The greater the hearing impairment the greater the impact on almost all areas of self-assessed social, emotional, and physical health. Individuals who used hearing instruments, compared with those who did not, were more socially active; reported more interpersonal warmth and less interpersonal negativity; had fewer communication difficulties; experienced less frustration, anger, depression, self-criticism, and greater emotional stability; and reported better physical health.

The strengths of the NCOA study lie in its numbers and the range of variables assessed, as well as its inclusion of family members and friends. The data also suggest the progressive effects of increasing impairment and the fact that hearing aid use was associated with better functioning at all levels of hearing impairment even if scores were not as low as those with less hearing impairment. Limitations include the lack of baseline measures and controls. Further, while family members did report improved quality of life with hearing aid use, some data in the report suggest that family members experienced negative effects that were not improved by hearing aid use (such as finding it exhausting to cope with the hearing impaired person's needs). Nor did family and friends always agree with the hearing impaired person's assessment.

Sensory Aids with Environmental Manipulation

In studies carried out in long-term wards in Scotland, Tolson and McIntosh (1997) assessed the extent of hearing aid use, hearing impairment, policies related to the care of persons with hearing impairment, and the "listening environment," which included the dimension of hearing as well as aspects of the physical and social environment that promoted or limited opportunities or motivation to communicate. Of 700 residents from 29 wards, only 59 had hearing aids and only 9 of these were in working order. Of 221 residents from 15 wards reliably assessed by audiometry, 70% ($n = 131$) were considered potential hearing aid candidates, and of these 78% ($n = 103$) reported a positive attitude toward receiving one. However, the results of the environmental assessment suggested the ward was too noisy for hearing aid users and disabling for anyone trying to listen or carry on a conversation.

Based on these findings, Tolson and MacIntosh (1997) implemented a small feasibility study that provided hearing aids or personal communicators to eligible individuals, and familiarized the staff with the needs of hearing impaired persons and how to create a more conversation-friendly environment. The sample included 48 residents with a mean age of 81 (31 intervention; 17 nonintervention). Over 6 months the average quality of the listening environment improved by one category (4-point scale) and hearing aid ownership increased by 29%. However, no change in reported hearing handicap was found. Because of a large attrition in the sample (by 12 months 75% of the original sample had died), only 8 respondents were available for reassessment. Study participants emphasized the importance of a communication partner who was sensitive to their needs and provided companionship.

TRAINING IN COPING SKILLS

Andersson, Melin, Scott, and Lindberg (1995a) in Sweden focused on enhancing the skills necessary to deal with a hearing impairment. The study used a randomized, experimental, between-groups design that was carried out over 5 weeks and included applied relaxation, video self-modeling, problematic situations, and coping skills. Participants in the treatment group evidenced improved coping strategies as assessed by evaluations of video-recorded interactions and self-report. Given the small sample size ($n = 24$), results need to be viewed cautiously. Further, a 2-year follow-up evaluation evidenced a return toward baseline in coping skills (Andersson, Melin, Scott, & Lindberg, 1995b) suggesting that a one-time intervention may not be adequate. In addition, further data are needed on why specific coping strategies are used. In a sample of 61 hearing impaired adults (33 men, 28 women, mean age 75.5), Gomez and Madey (2001) explored whether the use of adaptive or maladaptive coping strategies was related to hearing loss, psychosocial variables, and perceived effectiveness of the coping strategy. The perceived effectiveness of the coping strategy was significantly related to the use of both adaptive (β = 0.42, $p < .01$) and maladaptive ($\beta = 0.34$, $p < .01$) strategies. Two psychosocial variables, social and emotional impact and personal adjustment to hearing loss, were also significantly related to the use of maladaptive strategies ($\beta = 0.34$, $p < .01$ and $\beta = -0.24$, $p < .05$, respectively). In the multiple regression model, clinically measured hearing loss was not significantly related to either adaptive or maladaptive strategies.

Based on Roy's Adaptation Model, Zhan (2000) hypothesized that hearing loss was a focal stimulus that initiates cognitive efforts to adapt, defined as the maintenance of self-consistency. Cognitive adaptation was assessed using Roy's Cognitive Adaptation Processing Scale (CAPS) and self-consistency was assessed using the Zhan and Shen Self-Consistency Scale (SCS). In a nonprobability study of 130 hearing impaired individuals (Mean age = 74; 55% female), she found that the CAPS was significantly related to the SCS ($r = .65$, $p < .01$), and that men had significantly higher SCS scores than women ($t = -2.06$, $p < .05$). Although the CAPS is noted to explain 48% of the variance in the SCS, and the results are used to discuss how nurses can facilitate effective adaptation in elders, the cross-sectional nature of the study precludes imputing causal order. At the same time, the results suggest that more data are needed regarding how elders view and process the meaning of hearing impairment and that further support the potential differences in how men and women experience hearing impairment (Chen, 1994).

Kricos and Holmes (1996) assessed the effects of analytic auditory training and active listening training for 78 elders with hearing impairment ranging in age from 52–85. All subjects were fitted with a hearing aid prior to the study and assigned on a rotating basis to one of three groups: no training ($n = 26$), analytic training ($n = 26$), and active listening training ($n = 26$). The effectiveness of the interventions was determined via measures of speech recognition, hearing handicap (HHIE), and psychosocial function (Communication Profile for the Hearing Impaired). Group differences at baseline were not discussed. No effects were found for analytic speech recognition drills. Active listening training improved auditory-visual recognition of speech in noise and select aspects of psychosocial functioning. The finding that active listening training improved recognition in noise, a major problem experienced by elders, is of potential importance. Given the small sample and apparent group differences, additional research in this area is warranted.

SUMMARY OF INTERVENTION STUDIES

The results of the intervention studies suggest that hearing devices can improve psychosocial and communication outcomes. However, behavioral interventions have not shown long-lasting benefit, and while the environment can have a significant impact, it is usually not taken into account. Further, in attempting to promote positive approaches to dealing with the effects of hearing loss, the meaning of the strategy and its perceived effectiveness for the individual need to be assessed.

DISCUSSION

Although the studies discussed above have methodological limitations and use a range of assessment instruments, most support the wide-ranging negative impact of hearing impairment, even when mild, on psychosocial and physiological functioning. The findings of studies specifically focused on impact are supported by those focused on the benefits of hearing instruments/aids. Most studies, however, did not attempt to isolate the specific etiology of the hearing impairment, such as attempting to distinguish pure sensory problems from problems created by alterations in both peripheral and central processes. Interventions may be differentially effective depending on the underlying deficit (Chmiel & Jerger, 1996), and solutions for central processing deficits are not as available. Further, although studies are available comparing the impact of hearing and vision impairments, few studies have addressed the impact of dual sensory losses, a not uncommon problem in older persons.

What Are the Central Issues for Nursing Research?

Nurses play a major role in assisting elders and their families in managing the impact of chronic illnesses. Yet, to accomplish this role with elders with a hearing impairment and their families, further research is needed in several areas that have been poorly explored. For example, nurses have been actively involved in assisting caregivers of persons with chronic conditions, and yet there are minimal data on the *dyadic experience of hearing impairment* and the ways that families negotiate changing relationships and changing communication patterns across time. Likewise, to facilitate acceptance of hearing devices, more data are needed on the way in which *culture* influences the experience of hearing loss and the acceptance of assistive devices or participation in programs aimed at developing coping strategies.

Research is also needed on the varying needs of hearing-impaired individuals *across settings*—community to residential to nursing home. The prevalence of hearing impairment is higher in nursing homes than community settings and can significantly influence residents' quality of life and ability to interact with others. Tolson's work strongly supports the potential impact that nursing interventions may have and the need for additional research (Tolson, 1997, 1999; Tolson & McIntosh, 1997; Tolson & Stephens, 1997; Tolson et al., 1995).

Fourth, while researchers have evaluated the impact of hearing aids on quality of life, minimal work has been done on the use of *other assistive devices* such as microphones, telephones or telephone attachments, telecommunicating devices (TDD), and special warning devices (Loovis, Schall, & Teter, 1997). Work by Jerger and colleagues (1996) suggests that elders may benefit from alternative amplification systems even if they choose conventional aids for daily use. This may be especially important since new technology has not yet been shown to overcome the adverse effects of noise on communication (Sweetow, 2000) and is expensive. Increasing attention is being given to the use of cochlear implants in elders (Buchman, Fucci, & Luxford, 1999; Cheng & Niparko, 1999). This area needs to be assessed for its potential long-term benefits for psychosocial and physiological outcomes. Nurses need to understand the options available to elders in order to facilitate decision making.

At the same time, *utilization of assistive devices* and hearing aids is far below identified need (Popelka et al., 1998). Sweetow (2000) notes that ownership of hearing aids has actually declined from 23.8% in 1984 to 20.4% in 1998. And the NCOA study (1999) found that a majority of individuals not using a hearing aid, even those with severe loss, felt that their hearing was not bad enough. Indeed, Wiley and colleagues (2000) found that, after adjusting for degree of hearing loss, reported hearing handicap decreased with age. Far more data are needed to understand how individuals experience hearing loss, why it is denied, and how to overcome the perceived stigma of using assistive devices. What must be considered is the difficulty adjusting to hearing aids. Hearing aid limitations include their current inability to return hearing to a prior level, potential to irritate the ear canal, distortion of feedback, potential to accentuate background noise, and need for ongoing care, which can be difficult for older persons with arthritis or decreased manual dexterity.

A closely related area is the *impact of other aural rehabilitation strategies.* Sweetow (2000) notes that an unfortunate consequence of more recent technology is the decrease in the amount of time spent in counseling and teaching hearing impaired individuals how to listen. Strategies that promote positive approaches to dealing with hearing impairment need to be further explored (Andersson et al., 1995a).

Fifth, as advanced practice nurses continue to increase their involvement in the management of chronic conditions, further data are needed on *the long-term use of medications.* Finally, data are needed on *how accomplished nurses are at meeting the needs of hearing impaired individuals.* In Tolson's work, nurses and care assistants often felt unprepared to take care of the hearing aids (Tolson & McIntosh, 1997). Thus, while nursing literature on the needs of hearing impaired individuals emphasizes the need for hearing aid use, the actual ability of care providers to implement this strategy may be limited.

Each of these areas needs further development to elicit the most effective strategies to assist hearing impaired elders. Nurse researchers as well as practitioners must be aware of the complex nature of hearing and the deficits that may occur with hearing loss across the life span. Further research is needed on the most effective way to measure hearing loss and hearing handicap, with attention paid to how the assessment measure actually addresses the area of concern and whether it will be sensitive to change across time. Given the extensive nature of hearing impairment in elders, its impact on psychosocial well-being, and the potential for significant improvements in quality of life through the use of advanced hearing technology and assistive devices, nurses have the potential to play important roles in this underexplored area.

REFERENCES

Andersson, G., Melin, L., Scott, B., & Lindberg, P. (1995a). An evaluation of a behavioural treatment approach to hearing impairment. *Behavioral Research and Therapy, 33*, 283–292.

Andersson, G., Melin, L., Scott, B., & Lindberg, P. (1995b). A two-year follow-up examination of a behavioral treatment approach to hearing tactics. *British Journal of Audiology, 29*, 347–354.

Anstey, K. J., Luszcz, M. A., & Sanchez, L. (2001). A reevaluation of the common factor theory of shared variance among age, sensory function, and cognitive function in older adults. *Journal of Gerontology: Psychological Sciences, 56B*, P3–P11.

Arslan, E., Orzan, E., & Santarelli, R. (1999). Global problem of drug-induced hearing loss. *Annals of the New York Academy of Sciences, 884*, 1–14.

Baloh, R. W. (1998). *Dizziness, hearing loss, and tinnitus.* Philadelphia: F. A. Davis.

Baltes, P. B., & Lindenberger, U. (1997). Emergence of a powerful connection between sensory and cognitive functions across the adult life span: A new window to the study of cognitive aging? *Psychology and Aging, 12*, 12–21.

Benson, V., & Marano, M. A. (1994). Current estimates from the National Health Interview Survey, 1993, *Vital and Health Statistics, Series 10, No. 190.* (Vol. DHHS Pub. No. 95-1518.). Washington, DC: U.S. Government Printing Office.

Bess, F. H., Lichtenstein, M. J., Logan, S. A., Burger, M. C., & Nelson, E. (1989). Hearing impairment as a determinant of function in the elderly. *Journal of the American Geriatrics Society, 37*, 123–128.

Brien, J. A. (1993). Ototoxicity associated with salicylates. *Drug Safety, 9*(2), 143–148.

Buchman, C. A., Fucci, M. J., & Luxford, W. M. (1999). Cochlear implants in the geriatric population: Benefits outweigh risks. *Ear, Nose, and Throat Journal, 78*, 489–494.

Campbell, V. A., Crews, J. E., Moriarty, D. G., Zack, M. M., & Blackman, D. K. (1999). Surveillance for sensory impairment, activity limitation, and health-related quality of life among older adults—United States, 1993–1997. *Morbidity and Mortality Weekly Report, CDC Surveillance Summaries, 48*, 131–156.

Carabellese, C., Appollonio, I., Rozzini, R., Bianchetti, A., Frisoni, G. B., Frattola, L., & Trabucchi, M. (1993). Sensory impairment and quality of life in a community elderly population. *Journal of the American Geriatrics Society, 41*, 401–407.

Carson, S. S., Prazma, J., Pulver, S. H., & Anderson, T. (1989). Combined effects of aspirin and noise in causing permanent hearing loss. *Archives of Otolaryngology— Head and Neck Surgery, 115*, 1070–1075.

Chen, H. L. (1994). Hearing in the elderly: Relation of hearing loss, loneliness, and self-esteem. *Journal of Gerontological Nursing, 20*(6), 22–28.

Cheng, A. K., & Niparko, J. K. (1999). Cost-utility of the cochlear implant in adults: A meta-analysis. *Archives of Otolaryngology—Head and Neck Surgery, 125*, 1214–1218.

Chmiel, R., & Jerger, J. (1993). Some factors affecting assessment of hearing handicap in the elderly. *Journal of the American Academy of Audiology, 4*, 249–257.

Chmiel, R., & Jerger, J. (1996). Hearing aid use, central auditory disorder, and hearing handicap in elderly persons. *Journal of the American Academy of Audiology, 7*, 190–202.

Cruickshanks, K. J., Klein, R., Klein, B. E., Wiley, T. L., Nondahl, D. M., & Tweed, T. S. (1998). Cigarette smoking and hearing loss: The epidemiology of hearing loss study. *Journal of the American Medical Association, 279*, 1715–1719.

Cruickshanks, K. J., Wiley, T. L., Tweed, T. S., Klein, B. E., Klein, R., Mares-Perlman, J. A., & Nondahl, D. M. (1998). Prevalence of hearing loss in older adults in Beaver Dam, Wisconsin: The Epidemiology of Hearing Loss Study. *American Journal of Epidemiology, 148*, 879–886.

Dalton, D. S., Cruickshanks, K. J., Klein, R., Klein, B. E., & Wiley, T. L. (1998). Association of NIDDM and hearing loss. *Diabetes Care, 21*, 1540–1544.

Dargent-Molina, P., Hays, M., & Breart, G. (1996). Sensory impairments and physical disability in aged women living at home. *International Journal of Epidemiology, 25*, 621–629.

Dillon, H., James, A., & Ginis, J. (1997). Client Oriented Scale of Improvement (COSI) and its relationship to several other measures of benefit and satisfaction provided by hearing aids. *Journal of the American Academy of Audiology, 8*(1), 27–43.

Duck, S. W., Prazma, J., Bennett, P. S., & Pillsbury, H. C. (1997). Interaction between hypertension and diabetes mellitus in the pathogenesis of sensorineural hearing loss. *Laryngoscope, 107*, 1596–1605.

Dugan, E., & Kivett, V. R. (1994). The importance of emotional and social isolation to loneliness among very old rural adults. *Gerontologist, 34*, 340–346.

Ebersole, P., & Hess, P. (1998). *Toward healthy aging* (5th ed.). St. Louis: Mosby.

Fire, K. M. (1995). Intervention with the elderly. In L. G. Wall (Ed.), *Hearing for the speech language pathologist and health care professional* (pp. 373–400). Boston: Butterworth Heinemann.

Fitzgerald, D. C. (1996). Head trauma: Hearing loss and dizziness. *Journal of Trauma: Injury, Infection, and Critical Care, 40*, 488–496.

Fuse, T., Inamura, H., Nakamura, T., Suzuki, T., & Auyagi, M. (1996). Bilateral hearing loss due to viral infection. *ORL: Journal of Oto-Rhino-Laryngology and Its Related Specialties, 58*, 175–177.

Gatland, D., Tucker, B., Chalstrey, S., Keene, M., & Baker, L. (1991). Hearing loss in chronic renal failure—hearing threshold changes following haemodialysis. *Journal of the Royal Society of Medicine, 84*, 587–589.

Gennis, V., Garry, P. J., Haaland, K. Y., Yeo, R. A., & Goodwin, J. S. (1991). Hearing and cognition in the elderly. New findings and a review of the literature. *Archives of Internal Medicine, 151*, 2259–2264.

Gomez, R. G., & Madey, S. F. (2001). Coping-with-hearing-loss model for older adults. *Journals of Gerontology: Series B: Psychological Sciences & Social Sciences, 56*, P223–P225.

Hariri, M. A., Lakshmi, M. V., Larner, S., & Connolly, M. J. (1994). Auditory problems in elderly patients with stroke. *Age and Ageing, 23*, 312–316.

Henderson, D., Subramaniam, M., & Boettcher, F. A. (1993). Individual susceptibility to noise-induced hearing loss: An old topic revisited. *Ear and Hearing, 14*, 152–168.

Hetu, R., Jones, L., & Getty, L. (1993). The impact of acquired hearing impairment on intimate relationships: Implications for rehabilitation. *Audiology, 32*, 363–381.

Houston, D. K., Johnson, M. A., Nozza, R. J., Gunter, E. W., Shea, K. J., Cutler, G. M., & Edmonds, J. T. (1999). Age-related hearing loss, vitamin B-12, and folate in elderly women. *American Journal of Clinical Nutrition, 69*, 564–571.

Jerger, J., Chmiel, R., Florin, E., Pirozzolo, F., & Wilson, N. (1996). Comparison of conventional amplification and an assistive listening device in elderly persons. *Ear and Hearing, 17*, 490–504.

Kampfe, C. M., & Smith, S. M. (1998). Intrapersonal aspects of hearing loss in persons who are older. *Journal of Rehabilitation, 64*(2), 24–28.

Kanazawa, T., Hagiwara, H., & Kitamura, K. (2000). Labyrinthine involvement and multiple perforations of the tympanic membrane in acute otitis media due to group A streptococcus. *Journal of Laryngology and Otology, 114*(1), 47–49.

Keller, B. K., Morton, J. L., Thomas, V. S., & Potter, J. F. (1999). The effect of visual and hearing impairments on functional status. *Journal of the American Geriatrics Society, 47*, 1319–1325.

Kenyon, E. L., Leidenheim, S. E., & Zwillenberg, S. (1998). Speech discrimination in the sensorineural hearing loss patients: How is it affected by background noise? *Military Medicine, 163*, 647–650.

Kochkin, S., & Rogin, C. M. (2000). Quantifying the obvious: The impact of hearing instruments on quality of life. *Hearing Review, 7*(1), 6–34.

Koike, K., Hurst, M., & Westmore, S. (1994). Correlation between the American Academy of Otolarnygology-Head and Neck Surgery five minute hearing test and standard audiologic data. *Otolaryngology-Head and Neck Surgery, 111*, 625–632.

Kricos, P. B., & Holmes, A. E. (1996). Efficacy of audiologic rehabilitation for older adults. *Journal of the American Academy of Audiology, 7*, 219–229.

LaForge, R. G., Spector, W. D., & Sternberg, J. (1992). The relationship of vision and hearing impairment to one-year mortality and functional decline. *Journal of Aging and Health*(Feb), 126–148.

Lewis-Cullinan, C., & Janken, J. K. (1990). Effect of cerumen removal on the hearing ability of geriatric patients. *Journal of Advanced Nursing, 15*, 594–600.

Lim, D. P., & Stephens, S. D. (1991). Clinical investigation of hearing loss in the elderly. *Clinical Otolaryngology, 16*, 288–293.

Lindenberger, U., & Baltes, P. B. (1994). Sensory functioning and intelligence in old age: A strong connection. *Psychology and Aging, 9*, 339–355.

Loovis, C. F., Schall, D. G., & Teter, D. L. (1997). The role of assistive devices in the rehabilitation of hearing impairment. *Otolaryngologic Clinics of North America, 30*(5), 803–847.

Luszcz, M. A., & Bryan, J. (1999). Toward understanding age-related memory loss in late adulthood. *Gerontology, 45*(1), 2–9.

Mahoney, D. F. (1993). Cerumen impaction: Prevalence and detection in nursing homes. *Journal of Gerontological Nursing, 19*(4), 23–30.

Malinoff, R. L., & Weinstein, B. E. (1989). Measurement of hearing aid benefit in the elderly. *Ear and Hearing, 10*, 354–356.

Martin, F. N., & Champlin, C. A. (2000). Reconsidering the limits of normal hearing. *Journal of the American Academy of Audiology, 11*(2), 64–66.

McCarthy, P. A., & Sapp, J. V. (2000). Rehabilitative needs of the aging population. In J. G. Alpiner & P. A. McCarthy (Eds.), *Rehabilitative audiology: Children and adults* (3rd ed.). Philadelphia: Lippincott Williams & Wilkins.

Melnick, W. (1995). Noise and hearing loss. In L. G. Wall (Ed.), *Hearing for the speech-language pathologist and health care professional* (pp. 401–413). Boston: Butterworth Heinemann.

Mills, J. H., Matthews, L. J., Lee, F. S., Dubno, J. R., Schulte, B. A., & Weber, P. C. (1999). Gender-specific effects of drugs on hearing levels of older persons. *Annals of the New York Academy of Sciences, 884*, 381–388.

Morata, T. C. (1998). Assessing occupational hearing loss: Beyond noise exposures. *Scandinavian Audiology, Supplementum, 48*, 111–116.

Mulrow, C. D., Aguilar, C., Endicott, J. E., Velez, R., Tuley, M. R., Charlip, W. S., & Hill, J. A. (1990). Association between hearing impairment and the quality of life of elderly individuals. *Journal of the American Geriatrics Society, 38*, 45–50.

Mulrow, C. D., & Lichtenstein, M. J. (1991). Screening for hearing impairment in the elderly: Rationale and strategy. *Journal of General Internal Medicine, 6,* 249–258.

Mulrow, C. D., Tuley, M. R., & Aguilar, C. (1992). Correlates of successful hearing aid use in older adults. *Ear and Hearing, 13,* 108–113.

Mulrow, C. D., Tuley, M. R., & Aguilar, C. (1992). Sustained benefits of hearing aids. *Journal of Speech and Hearing Research, 35,* 1402–1405.

The National Council on the Aging. (1999). *The consequences of untreated hearing loss in older persons—summary.* Washington, DC: Author.

Pearson, J. D., Morrell, C. H., Gordon-Salant, S., Brant, L. J., Metter, E. J., Klein, L. L., & Fozard, J. L. (1995). Gender differences in a longitudinal study of age-associated hearing loss. *Journal of the Acoustical Society of America, 97,* 1196–1205.

Peters, C. A., Potter, J. F., & Scholer, S. G. (1988). Hearing impairment as a predictor of cognitive decline in dementia. *Journal of the American Geriatrics Society, 36,* 981–986.

Popelka, M. M., Cruickshanks, K. J., Wiley, T. L., Tweed, T. S., Klein, B. E., & Klein, R. (1998). Low prevalence of hearing aid use among older adults with hearing loss: The Epidemiology of Hearing Loss Study. *Journal of the American Geriatrics Society, 46,* 1075–1078.

Pulec, J. L., & Mendoza, I. (1997). Progressive sensorineural hearing loss, subjective tinnitus and vertigo caused by elevated blood lipids. *Ear, Nose, and Throat Journal, 76,* 716–730.

Ramsdell, D. A. (1970). The psychology of the hard-of-hearing and the deafened adult. In H. Davis & S. R. Silverman (Eds.), *Hearing and deafness* (3rd ed., pp. 435–446). New York: Holt, Rinehart and Winston.

Rees, T. S., Duckert, L. G., & Carey, J. P. (1999). Auditory and vestibular dysfunction. In W. R. Hazzard, J. P. Blass, W. H. Ettinger, J. B. Halter, & J. G. Ouslander (Eds.), *Principles of geriatric medicine and gerontology* (3rd ed., pp. 617–631). New York: McGraw-Hill, Inc.

Reuben, D. B., Mui, S., Damesyn, M., Moore, A. A., & Greendale, G. A. (1999). The prognostic value of sensory impairment in older persons. *Journal of the American Geriatrics Society, 47,* 930–935.

Reuben, D. B., Walsh, K., Moore, A. A., Damesyn, M., & Greendale, G. A. (1998). Hearing loss in community-dwelling older persons: National prevalence data and identification using simple questions. *Journal of the American Geriatrics Society, 46,* 1008–1011.

Ries, P. W. (1994). Prevalence and characteristics of persons with hearing trouble: United States, 1990–91. *Vital and Health Statistics, Series 10: Data from the National Health Survey*(188), 1–75.

Roland, P. S., & Marple, B. F. (1997). Disorders of inner ear, eighth nerve, and CNS. In P. S. Roland, B. F. Marple, & W. L. Meyerhoff (Eds.), *Hearing loss* (pp. 195–256). New York: Thieme.

Rudberg, M. A., Furner, S. E., Dunn, J. E., & Cassel, C. K. (1993). The relationship of visual and hearing impairments to disability: An analysis using the longitudinal study of aging. *Journal of Gerontology, 48,* M261–M265.

Salthouse, T. A., Hambrick, D. Z., & McGuthry, K. E. (1998). Shared age-related influences on cognitive and non-cognitive variables. *Psychology and Aging, 13,* 486–500.

Salthouse, T. A., Hancock, H. E., Meinz, E. J., & Hambrick, D. Z. (1996). Interrelations of age, visual acuity, and cognitive functioning. *Journals of Gerontology, Series B, Psychological Sciences and Social Sciences, 51,* 317–330.

Sataloff, R. T., & Sataloff, J. (1993). *Occupational hearing loss* (2nd ed.). New York: Marcel Dekker.

Saunders, G. H., & Cienkowski, K. M. (1996). Refinement and psychometric evaluation of the Attitudes Toward Loss of Hearing Questionnaire. *Ear and Hearing, 17,* 505–517.

Scherer, M. J., & Frisina, D. R. (1998). Characteristics associated with marginal hearing loss and subjective well-being among a sample of older adults. *Journal of Rehabilitation Research and Development, 35,* 420–426.

Schick, F. L., & Schick, R. (1994). *Statistical handbook on aging Americans, 1994 Edition.* Phoenix, AZ: Oryx Press.

Shone, G., Altschuler, R. A., Miller, J. M., & Nuttall, A. L. (1991). The effect of noise exposure on the aging ear. *Hearing Research, 56,* 171–178.

Slawinski, E. B., Hartel, D. M., & Kline, D. W. (1993). Self-reported hearing problems in daily life throughout adulthood. *Psychology and Aging, 8,* 552–561.

Strawbridge, W. J., Wallhagen, M. I., Shema, S. J., & Kaplan, G. A. (2000). Negative consequences of hearing impairment in old age: A longitudinal analysis. *Gerontologist, 40,* 320–326.

Stypulkowski, P. H. (1990). Mechanisms of salicylate ototoxicity. *Hearing Research, 46,* 113–146.

Sweetow, R. W. (1996). Advising a new hearing aid candidate. In R. A. Goldenberg (Ed.), *Hearing aids: A manual for clinicians* (pp. 25–40). Philadelphia: Lippincott-Raven.

Sweetow, R. W. (2000). Hearing aid technology. *Current Opinion in Otolaryngology & Head and Neck Surgery, 8,* 426–430.

Taylor, K. S. (1993). Self-perceived and audiometric evaluations of hearing aid benefit in the elderly. *Ear and Hearing, 14,* 390–394.

Tinetti, M. E., Inouye, S. K., Gill, T. M., & Doucette, J. T. (1995). Shared risk factors for falls, incontinence, and functional dependence. Unifying the approach to geriatric syndromes. *Journal of the American Medical Association, 273,* 1348–1353.

Tolson, D. (1997). Age-related hearing loss: A case for nursing intervention. *Journal of Advanced Nursing, 26,* 1150–1157.

Tolson, D. (1999). Practice innovation: A methodological maze. *Journal of Advanced Nursing, 30,* 381–390.

Tolson, D., & McIntosh, J. (1997). Listening in the care environment—chaos or clarity for the hearing-impaired elderly person. *International Journal of Nursing Studies, 34,* 173–182.

Tolson, D., & Stephens, D. (1997). Age-related hearing loss in the dependent elderly population: A model for nursing care. *International Journal of Nursing Practice, 3,* 224–230.

Tolson, D., Swan, I. R., & McIntosh, J. (1995). Auditory rehabilitation: Needs and realities on long-stay wards for elderly people. *British Journal of Clinical Practice, 49*, 243–245.

United States Public Health Service. (1998). *The clinician's handbook of preventive services* (2nd ed.). McLean, VA: International Medical Publishing.

Ventry, I. M., & Weinstein, B. E. (1982). The Hearing Handicap Inventory for the Elderly: A new tool. *Ear and Hearing, 3*, 128–134.

Wallhagen, M. I., Strawbridge, W. J., Cohen, R. D., & Kaplan, G. A. (1997). An increasing prevalence of hearing impairment and associated risk factors over three decades of the Alameda County Study. *American Journal of Public Health, 87*, 440–442.

Wallhagen, M. I., Strawbridge, W. J., & Kaplan, G. A. (2001, April). Five-year impact of hearing impairment on physical functioning, mental health, and social relationships. *British Society of Audiology News*, Issue 32 (April), 9–11.

Weinstein, B. E., Richards, A. M., & Montano, J. (1995). Handicap versus impairment: An important distinction. *Journal of the American Academy of Audiology, 6*, 250–255.

Wiley, T. L., Cruickshanks, K. J., Nondahl, D. M., & Tweed, T. S. (2000). Self-reported hearing handicap and audiometric measures in older adults. *Journal of the American Academy of Audiology, 11*(2), 67–75.

Zhan, L. (2000). Cognitive adaptation and self-consistency in hearing impaired older persons: Testing Roy's Adaptation Model. *Nursing Science Quarterly, 13*, 158–165.

Chapter 13

Elder Mistreatment

TERRY FULMER

ABSTRACT

Elder mistreatment (EM) is a serious and prevalent syndrome that is estimated to affect between 500,000 to 1.2 million older adults in the United States annually (Pillemer & Finkelhor, 1988). This chapter reviews both the state of the published science and limitations in the knowledge base on the topic. The literature for this review was obtained through computer-assisted searches of PubMed (878 citations), the Cumulative Index of Nursing Research (CINAHL) (593 citations) and Psych-Info databases (443 citations). The search terms used were *elder mistreatment, elder neglect, elder abuse*, or *domestic abuse of the elderly*. No limit was placed on the age of publications because of the relative scarcity of research on the subject. Nonnursing articles were included because there are so few nurse researchers addressing this topic. The age limit for subjects in these studies was 65 years and older. Studies were limited to those conducted in the United States, and descriptive studies were included as they form the majority of the research to date. Findings indicate that frail, very old (over 75 years), older adults who have a diagnosis of depression or dementia are more likely to be mistreated (Dyer, Pavlik, Murphy, & Hyman, 2000; Coyne, Reichman, & Berbig, 1993; Fulmer & Gurland, 1996; Lachs & Pillemer, 1995; Lachs et al., 1997; Lachs, Williams, O'Brien, Pillemer, & Charlson, 1998; Lachs & Fulmer, 1993; Lachs, Berkman, Fulmer, & Horwitz, 1994). Those older adults who required assistance with activities of daily living had poor social networks and were at higher risk for EM (Lachs & Pillemer, 1995; Lachs et al., 1997; Lachs et al., 1998; Lachs & Fulmer, 1993; Lachs et al., 1994). Neglect, as a subcategory of EM, accounts for the majority of cases (Fulmer, Paveza, Abraham, & Fairchild, 2000; Pavlik, Hyman, Festa, & Bitondo Dyer, 2001; Fulmer & Gurland, 1996). There is still debate regarding the role of minority status, abuse in childhood, and the persons most likely to mistreat older adults. There is a critical need for replication studies and new research on this important topic. Problems with measurement, funding challenges, and the paucity of investigators conducting research on EM have left the field with several unanswered questions and some conflicting findings. This chapter summarizes the interdisciplinary literature and makes recommendations for future nursing research programs.

Keywords: elder mistreatment, elder neglect, elder abuse, domestic abuse

Elder mistreatment (EM) refers to serious, potentially fatal events or circumstances that occur with older adults and that are caused by others in the elder's environment. EM is the term generally used to refer to any action or inaction that causes harm or loss to an older individual, usually over 65 years of age. Specifically, EM covers the categories of abuse, neglect, exploitation, or abandonment, and American Medical Association guidelines have noted that "mistreatment of the elderly person may include physical, psychological, or financial abuse or neglect and it may be intentional or unintentional" (Aravanis et al., 1993). EM was first reported in the literature in the late 1970s (Walshe-Brennan, 1977; Illing, 1977). Walshe-Brennan used the term "granny-bashing" and discussed the subject anecdotally. The growth of interest in EM came from an increased awareness that older adults were also potential victims for domestic violence, and the development of the child abuse and battered spouse literature helped initiate work in the geriatric population.

Between 1980 and 1990, the majority of studies conducted on the topic were exploratory, descriptive studies (Hudson, 1986). Since that time, conceptual frameworks used for discussing EM have ranged from professional awareness models to law and order frameworks (Fulmer, 1982; Hall, 1989; Pratt, Koval, & Lloyd, 1983). For example, law and order frameworks have been used when EM is viewed from a perpetrator/victim perspective. Analysis of police records and court proceedings have provided one approach to understanding EM cases, an approach that continues today. The United States Department of Justice has supported several educational panels on the topic, and issued suggestions for further research (Reno, 1994; Office for Victims of Crime, 1993). Domestic violence models that screen for abusive partners have also been used, and there is some evidence to suggest that EM may be domestic violence "grown old" (Pillemer & Wolf, 1986). This latter model, however, is not able to account for other dyadic relationships in which there is EM, such as that between home attendants and older adults, daughters and older mothers, and older siblings. Risk assessment frameworks have also provided important clinical guidance for EM assessment (Lachs & Pillemer, 1995; Lachs & Fulmer, 1993). Risk assessment frameworks, frequently used in emergency departments, home health care agencies, and nursing homes, have helped practitioners become more sensitive and gain valuable skills in EM assessment and care planning, but have not had sufficient empirical validation.

Every state in the country has a procedure for reporting suspected elder mistreatment, and nurses, along with physicians and a wide array of allied health-care workers, are named as "responsible persons" for reporting suspected EM (Capezuti, Brush, & Lawson, 1997). Responsible reporting requires that "evidence" be scientifically based, and this can present a challenge given the multiple co-morbid conditions and resultant signs and symptoms which may be caused by medications or other therapies in older adults.

The EM field, after two decades, is at a critical juncture. There is general agreement that EM is a serious problem, but progress in knowledge generation is at a relative standstill. A literature and information synthesis is essential to help guide the field. There is a need to communicate to the scientific community EM data that are definitive, and gaps that must be addressed. The National Academies of Science (NAS) convened a panel on "Elder Abuse and Neglect" in the Spring of 2001 at the request of the National Institute on Aging (NIA), to help the field synthesize knowledge and make recommendations for research for all disciplines. Expert panels have previously convened and made recommendations, but a paucity of senior researchers in the field along with challenges in procuring research funds have stymied significant progress. These issues notwithstanding, momentum can only take place once the current science is well understood and clearly communicated.

The purpose of the chapter is to review the evidence base for EM and consider additional areas for research, which can enhance professional nursing practice for this serious syndrome. Specifically, the questions to be answered are:

1. What are the theoretical approaches used to study EM?
2. What are the strengths and limitations of measures designed to detect EM?
3. What are the incidence and the prevalence of EM?

4. What are risk factors for EM?
5. What is the nature of the EM problem?
6. How have data from reporting laws been used in research?
7. What is known from setting-specific studies on EM?

METHOD

The literature for this review, from 1977 through 2001, was obtained through computer-assisted searches of PubMed (878 citations), the Cumulative Index of Nursing Research (CINAHL) (593 citations), and Psych-Info databases (443 citations). The search terms used were *elder mistreatment, elder neglect, elder abuse*, or *domestic abuse of the elderly*. A total of 34 data-based studies, conducted in the United States, were used for this synthesis (Table 13.1). Review articles were not included. Studies were limited to those done in the United States. Studies of cultural differences in EM were not included in this review although this is an important area of work. No limit was placed on the age of the publication, because of the relative scarcity of research on the subject. Nonnursing articles were included because there are so few nurse researchers addressing this topic. Further, the issue of EM requires an interdisciplinary approach because of its complexity. The approach for this review necessarily took into consideration the historical context of the study (early pioneering work vs. later studies), as well as the disciplines of the researchers.

RESULTS AND DISCUSSION

What Are the Theoretical Approaches Used to Study EM?

Phillips (1986) has summarized conceptual approaches for research on the topic of EM, which include the situational model, social exchange theory, symbolic interactionism, and risk assessment conceptual frameworks. These theories and frameworks have begun to be tested; there is, however, a great need for replication of existing research. To date, epidemiologic studies have not used theoretical or conceptual frameworks to discuss approaches or findings.

TABLE 13.1   Summary of EM Studies

Study	Methods	Selected findings
Childs, H. W., Hayslip, B. Jr, Radika, L. M., & Reinberg, J. A. (2000)	Design: Descriptive Measure: (1) SVWS; (2) EAA BIS-R Sample: Nonrandom: 422 young and 201 middle-aged adults	• Middle-aged respondents viewed psychological behavior more harshly than younger respondents • Both middle-aged women and young men were less tolerant of middle-aged perpetrators • Data support relativistic nature of elder abuse
Coyne, A. C., Reichman, W. E., & Berbig, L. J. (1993)	Design: Descriptive survey Measure: Demographics; Zarit Burden interview; Zung Self-Rating Depression Scale Sample: 1000 caregivers who called a telephone help-line for dementia; 342 respondents	• Mean age of caregiver is 56.1; 54.5% were adult children caring for parents; 37.1% caring for spouses; 8.4% cared for other relatives • 11.9% reported they had been physically abusive toward dementia patients. • Abusers had been providing care for more years; patients functioned at a lower level; caregivers had higher burden and depression scores
Dyer, C. B., Pavlik, V. N., Murphy, K. P., & Hyman, D. J. (2000)	Design: Case control study Intervention: Comprehensive geriatric assessment Measure: Standard geriatric assessment tools Sample: 47 older persons referred for neglect and 97 referred for other reasons	• 45 cases of abuse or neglect identified • 37 were self-neglect • EM cases were more likely to be White and male • Higher prevalence of depression and dementia
Ertem, I. O., Leventhal, J. M., & Dobbs, S. (2000)	Design: Descriptive Method: Meta-analysis Sample: 10 studies	• Ten studies: 4 cohort, 1 cross-sectional, and 5 case control • The RR of maltreatment in children of abused parents were significantly increased in 4 studies (RR 4.75–37.8) • In three other studies the RR was less than 2 • Significant validity issues

(continued)

TABLE 13.1   *(continued)*

Study	Methods	Selected findings
Fulmer, T., & Gurland, B. (1996)	Design: Descriptive Measure: CTS, FRS and NMAP Survey, Beck Depression Scale, BDBS Sample: 125 elder-caregiver dyads; 51 dyads with cognitive impairment and 74 dyads with no cognitive impairment; mean age of the elder 78 years Theory: Risk and vulnerability	• Cognitive impairment risk factor for elder mistreatment • CTS higher for CI patients • FRS higher for CI patients • CI patients more dependent • CI patients had higher BDBS • CI patients had higher Zarit Burden scores
Fulmer, T., Ramirez, M., Fairchild, S., Holmes, D., Koren, M. J., & Teresi, J. (1999)	Design: Descriptive Method: Analysis of a probability sample of ADHC clients in New York State. Social workers served as informants Sample: Nine sites drawn through random sampling	• Prevalence of EM 12.3% • Apprehensive behavior was highest reported behavior; with this item removed, prevalence 3.6% • Social workers noted concern regarding elders who appeared frightened in the presence of their home caregiver
Fulmer, T., Paveza, G., Abraham, I., & Fairchild, S. (2000)	Design: Descriptive Measure: EAI, MMSE Sample: 180 emergency department patients over the age of 70 with an MMSE of 18 or greater	• 36 patients eligible for study • 7 patients screened positive for neglect • Nurses were able to screen for elder neglect with greater than 70% accuracy; true positive 71%, false positive 7%.
Huber, R., Borders, K., Netting, F. E., & Nelson, H. W. (2001)	Design: Descriptive Method: Analysis of cross-sectional 6-State ombudsman database Sample: 23,787 complaints	• Five most frequent complaints were 1) loss of dignity and respect; 2) accidents; 3) physical abuse; 4) call lights unanswered; 5) poor personal hygiene. • Race and gender differences noted

TABLE 13.1   *(continued)*

Study	Methods	Selected findings
Hudson, M. F. (1991)	Design: Descriptive Measure: 3-round Delphi survey Sample: 63 EM experts	• Agreement on a five-level taxonomy • 11 theoretical definitions proposed by panel
Hwalek, M. A., Neale, A. V., Goodrich, C. S., & Quinn, K. (1996)	Design: Descriptive Method: Database analysis Measure: Risk of Future Abuse instrument Sample: State of Illinois Abuse, Neglect and Exploitation Tracking System; 2,577 cases from October 1989 to December 1991. 552 substantiated reports used for this study	• Most victims were women, 73% • Mean age 77 (60–99) • Caucasian 73%; widowed 54%; living at home 76% • Caregiver substance abuse more likely to involve physical or emotional abuse
Jogerst, G. J., Dawson, J. D., Hartz, A. J., Ely, J. W., & Schweitzer, L. A. (2000)	Design: Descriptive Method: Analysis of county level data between 1984 to 1993 to test association between county characteristics and rates of elder abuse Sample: 99 counties in Iowa Analysis: univariate correlational analysis and stagewise linear regression	Community characteristics that had a positive association with rates of reported or substantiated EM were: (1) population density (2) children in poverty (3) reported child abuse
Jones, J. S., Veenstra, T. R., Seamon, J. P., & Krohmer, J. (1997)	Design: Descriptive Method: Random sample survey Sample: 3,000 members of the American College of the Emergency Physicians; 705 completed surveys (response rate 24%)	• 52% of respondents described EM as prevalent but less than spouse or child abuse • Respondents evaluated a mean of 4 ± 8 suspected cases of EM in last 12 months • 50% reported • Only 31% reported having a written protocol

(continued)

TABLE 13.1 *(continued)*

Study	Methods	Selected findings
Lachs, M. S., Berkman, L., Fulmer T., & Horwitz, R. J. (1994)	Design: Prospective cohort study Method: Case matching with adult protective service database Sample: 329 elders investigated in 1985 and 1986 Analysis: Relative risk calculations	• 68 (2.4%) of database cohort members received ombudsman investigation • Risk factors for EM investigation using logistic regression included requiring assistance with feeding, OR 3.5, being a minority elder, OR 2.3, over age 75 at cohort inception, OR 1.9, and poor social networks, OR 1.7
Lachs, M. S., Williams, C., O'Brien, S., Hurst, L., & Horwitz, R. I. (1997)	Design: Prospective cohort study Method: Case matching with adult protective service database Sample: 184 cohort members Analysis: Pooled logistic regression	• 47 cohort members were seen for EM (prevalence 1.6%) • Age, race, poverty, functional disability and cognitive impairment were identified as risk factors for reported EM, with ORs reported • The onset of new cognitive impairment was also associated with abuse and neglect • The influence of race and poverty is likely to be overestimated due to reporting bias
Lachs, M. S., Williams, C. S., O'Brien, S., Hurst, L., Kossack, A., Siegal, A., & Tinetti, M. E. (1997)	Design: Prospective cohort study Method: 7-year longitudinal database with identification of 182 victims of elder abuse Sample: 114 elders seen in 2 EDs	• 114 individuals accounted for 628 visits (median 3, range 1–46) • 30.6% resulted in hospital admission • 66% had at least one visit that resulted in an injury-related chief complaint

TABLE 13.1 *(continued)*

Study	Methods	Selected findings
Lachs, M. S., Williams, C. S., O'Brien, S., Pillemer, K. A., & Charlson, M. E. (1998)	Design: Prospective cohort study Measure: Outcome Measure: mortality among elders for whom protective services were used to corroborate EM and elderly persons for whom protective services were used for self-neglect Sample: 176 APS elders	• Cohort members seen for EM at any time during follow-up had poorer survival (9%) than others • Reported and corroborated EM and self-neglect are associated with shorter survival after adjusting for other factors associated with increased mortality in older adults
Moody, L. E., Voss, A., & Lengacher, C. A. (2000)	Design: Descriptive Measure: H-S/EAST Sample: 100 African American, Hispanic, and White elders living in public housing	• Principal components FA of 15 item instrument supported the three-factor structure for a total of ten items, explaining 38% of the variance • A discriminant function analysis showed that 6 items were as effective as the 9-item model in classifying cases as abused (71.4%)
The National Center on Elder Abuse at The American Public Human Services Association [Formerly the American Public Welfare Association] in collaboration with Westat, Inc. (1998)	Design: Descriptive Study Method: Incidence study using sentinel agency reports Sample: 20 counties in 15 states: nationally representative sample	• 551,000 EM cases in 1996 • Female elders are abused at higher rates than males • The oldest elders (80 years and older) are abused and neglected at 2–3 times their proportion in the elderly population • In almost 90% of EM cases, the perpetrator is a family member and 2/3 are adult children or spouses • Victims of self-neglect are usually depressed, confused or extremely frail

(continued)

TABLE 13.1 *(continued)*

Study	Methods	Selected findings
O'Malley, T. A., O'Malley, M. A., Everitt, D. E., & Sarson, D. (1984)	Design: Descriptive Measure: Case analysis using OARS Sample: 22 cases from primary care clinic	• Cases divided into three categories: (1) extremely impaired who receive care from individuals responsible for abuse and neglect ($N = 4$); (2) impaired elders who receive inadequate or intermittent care ($N = 9$); (3) involved independent elders whose only care needs resulted from threats or violence from relatives ($N = 11$)
Paveza, G. J., Cohen, D., Eisdorfer, C., Freels, S., Semla, T., Ashford, J. W., Gorelick, P., Hirschman, R., Luchins, D. J., & Levy, P. (1992)	Design: Descriptive Measure: CTS Sample: Purposive sample from Alzheimer's disease registry: 184 AD patients	• Severe family violence as measured by the CTS was a significant problem: overall prevalence 17.4% • 15.8% of patients had been violent since diagnosis • 5.4% of caregivers reported being violent toward the patient • Violence by the AD victim against the caregiver was serious problem.
Pavlik, V. N., Hyman, D. J., Festa, N. A., & Bitondo Dyer, C. (2001)	Design: Descriptive Method: Analysis of Texas Department of Protective and Regulatory Services-Adult Protective Services Sample: 62,258 allegations of EM in 1997	• Neglect accounted for 80% of allegations • The incidence of being reported to APS increased sharply after age 65 • The prevalence was 1,310 over $100,000 \geq 65$ years of age

TABLE 13.1   *(continued)*

Study	Methods	Selected findings
Phillips, L. R., & Rempusheski, V. F. (1985)	Design: Descriptive Method: Interviews with grounded theory analysis Sample: 29 health care providers (16 nurses and 13 social workers)	• A four-stage model describing decisions of health care providers about elder abuse • Model identifies three types of decisions: diagnostic, value, and intervention • Complexity of decision processes is revealed via 5 pathways
Phillips, L. R., Morrison, E. F., & Chae, Y. M. (1990a)	Design: Adaptation of the QUALPACS Method: Instrument development Sample: Piloted with 8 data collectors (4 in each of 2 sites) who interviewed 4 elder–caregiver dyads. A total of 29 elder-caregiver dyads were interviewed.	• QUALCARE Scale contains six subscales and 53 items • Included in 6 subscales: environmental, physical, medical maintenance, psychological, human rights, and financial
Phillips, L. R., Morrison, E. F., & Chae, Y. M. (1990b)	Design: Descriptive correlational study Measure: QUALCARE Sample: Convenience sample of 249 elder–caregiver dyads	• Interrater reliability: for 55 observations ranged from 79% to 88% • Internal consistency: alpha = .97 • Conceptual structure: confirmatory factor analysis indicated 6 significant factors accounting for 64.4% of the variance • Criterion validity: all correlations between criteria variables and QUALCARE were in correct direction and $p \leq 0.05$ level • Construct validity: 8 of 9 correlations in the predicted direction

(continued)

TABLE 13.1 *(continued)*

Study	Methods	Selected findings
Pillemer, K. A., & Finkelhor, D. (1988)	Design: Descriptive Method: Stratified random sample survey Sample: 2,020 community dwelling elders in metropolitan Boston	• 63 elder persons were mistreated • Rate of 32 per 1000 • 95% competence interval of 25–39 per 1,000 • No minority differences or age differences • Those in poor health were 3 to 4 times likely to be abused • Males were more likely to be abused than females
Pillemer, K. A., & Finkelhor, D. (1989)	Design: Descriptive Method: Case Control Sample: 46 abuse or neglect victims and 215 random controls	• Factors associated with EM included abuser factors of deviance, dependence on victim, and life stress. • Victim factors included court help, disability, dependence on abuser, and conflictual relationship (spouse only).
Pillemer, K. A., & Moore, D. W. (1989)	Design: Descriptive Measure: CTS Sample: 577 nursing personnel from 31 nursing homes in New Hampshire	• 36% of the sample had seen at least one incident of physical abuse in the preceding year • Most frequent abuse observed was excessive restraint • Second most frequent type was physical abuse • 81% observed at least one psychologically abusive incident in the preceding year • 10% of respondents reported committing physical abuse • 40% of respondents reported committing psychological abuse

TABLE 13.1   *(continued)*

Study	Methods	Selected findings
Pillemer, K. A., & Suitor, J. J. (1992)	Design: Descriptive Method: Analysis of quantitative and qualitative data Sample: 236 family caregivers for dementia victims	• Characteristics predictive of violent feelings in caregivers included: physical aggression by elder, disruptive behaviors, and a shared living situation. • Structural relationship and caregiver age were related to actual violence: spouses were more likely to be violent than other relatives, as were older individuals • Violence by elder was positively related to caregiver violence
Rosenblatt, D. E., Cho, K. H., & Durance, P. W. (1996)	Design: Descriptive Method: Analysis of State of Michigan records of reported cases of suspected elder abuse 1989–1993 Sample: 27,371 cases of possible EM	• 17,238 of cases were older than age 65 • Physicians reported only 2% of cases • Physician reporting rates did not increase over a 5-year period
Shaw, M. M. C. (1998)	Design: Descriptive Method: Grounded Theory Sample: 21 semistructured interviews conducted with six abuse investigators and 15 nursing home staff	• The two types of abusive nursing home staff were identified as reactive and sadistic.
Wolf, R. S. (1986)	Design: Descriptive Method: Analysis of cases from an EM intervention project Sample: 59 EM cases compared with 49 cases randomly selected from a nonabuse caseload	• Victims and nonabuse clients were similar in age, sex, and health status • Caretakers for both groups were similar in age and health status

(continued)

TABLE 13.1 *(continued)*

Study	Methods	Selected findings
		• More perpetrators were males • A majority of EM cases resided with family members versus nonabused persons living alone • Victims and perpetrators had more psychological and emotional health problems • Abused elders did not appear to be more dependent
Wolf, R. S., & Pillemer, K. A. (1997)	Design: Descriptive Measure: ADLs, IADLs, CTS Sample: 73 older women: 22 victimized by husbands and 51 victimized by adult children	• Wives more likely to be dependent on husbands for IADLs • Adult children more likely to be dependent on mothers for housing and finances • Husbands more likely to use physical violence against wives than adult children against mothers
Wolf, R. S., & Li, D. (1999)	Design: Descriptive Measure: DV was number of reports per 1,000 persons aged 60 years and older during 1994. Sample: 27 geographical areas in Massachusetts	• Rate of reports varied from a low of 2.41 per 1,000 through 9.31 per 1,000 • Higher rates of reporting were associated with lower SES, more community training, higher agency service rating scores, lower community agency relationship score

What Are the Strengths and Limitations of Measures Designed to Detect EM?

Measurement is a complex issue in EM research, and clinical researchers have used pathophysiologic signs and symptoms such as unexplained bruising, dehydration, urine burns, and fractures (Fulmer, 1984; Lachs &

Fulmer, 1993; Dyer, Pavlik, Murphy, & Hyman, 2000; Haviland & O'Brien, 1989; O'Brien, 1986). This approach is complicated, given the number of older individuals who might have these markers from other causes, such as a disease state or medication reaction. It also lends itself to false positive/false negative reports because of the subjective nature of the clinical interview and the lack of definitive biomarkers. Legal experts use case law to determine measurement outcomes, and social scientists most often use relevant instruments from the literature (Greenberg, Ramsey, Mitty, & Fulmer, 1999). These varied approaches can lead to confusion in findings reported in the literature.

In some instances, outcome measures of EM have been operationalized by using scales and cut scores from relevant screening instruments such as: (a) the Conflict Tactic Scale (CTS) (Straus, 1978), (b) the Elder Assessment Instrument (EAI) (Fulmer, 1984; Fulmer, Street, & Carr, 1984; Fulmer & Wetle, 1986), (c) the QUALCARE Scale (Phillips, Morrison, & Chae, 1990a; Phillips, Morrison, & Chae, 1990b), (d) the Hwalek-Sengstock Elder Abuse Screening Test (H-S/EAST) (Neale, Hwalek, Scott, Sengstock, & Stahl, 1991; Moody, Voss, & Lengacher, 2000), (e) the Fulmer Restriction Scale (FRS) (Fulmer & Gurland, 1996), and (f) Indicators of Abuse Screen (IOA) (Reis & Nahmiash, 1998) in order to attempt to measure domains of EM (Table 13.2). None of the instruments, except the CTS, are widely used, which may be because of (a) flaws in the instruments, (b) specific clinical instrument parameters which are irrelevant in other settings, or (c) a lack of awareness that these instruments exist.

Substantiated APS reports, which are reports received by public hotlines and state agencies and evaluated by adult protective services workers for confirmation, may result in anything from clinical services support or court proceedings (Tatara, 1993). Concerns related to this strategy include the subjective nature of reports, the subjective review by APS workers who may have little clinical background, and refusal by the older adult to have the report filed. Self-report of EM is another outcome measure, which has been demonstrated to be culturally influenced and also inherently subjective.

What Are the Incidence and the Prevalence of EM?

The National Elder Abuse Incidence Study (NEAIS) (The National Center on Elder Abuse at The American Public Human Services Association

TABLE 13.2 Review of EM Measures

Measure	Summary	Characteristics	Properties
Pathophysiological signs and symptoms Dyer, Pavlik, Murphy, & Hyman (2000); Fulmer (1984); Haviland & O'Brien (1989); Lachs & Fulmer (1993); O'Brien (1986)	Uses items such as: unexplained bruising, dehydration, urine burns, fractures	Subjective and objective clinical observations as documented by health care clinicians	Poor sensitivity and specificity
Conflict Tactic Scale (CTS) Straus (1978)	Perception of upsetting and injurious circumstances in a person's life	19 item self-report e.g., "Has anyone threatened you with a knife or gun?"	Chronbach's alpha Reliability: .88 Content validity .80 (available in Spanish)
Elder Assessment Instrument (EAI) Fulmer (1984)	Provides information to clinicians to better inform judgements about risk of EM	40-item screening tool with both subjective and objective items to determine if an older person should be referred for suspected EM.	Content validity .83 Interrater agreement .84 (available in Spanish)
The QUALCARE Scale Phillips, Morrison, & Chae (1990a, 1990b)	Assessment of six areas: physical, medical management, psychosocial, environmental, human rights, and financial	53-item observational rating scale designed to quantify and qualify family caregiving.	Extensive psychometrics reported Interrater agreement range: .79–.88 Chronbach's alpha: .81–.95 on 6 subscales

TABLE 13.2 *(continued)*

Measure	Summary	Characteristics	Properties
Hwalek-Sengstock Elder Abuse Screening Test (H-S/EAST) Neale, A., Hwalek, M., Scott, R., Sengstock, M., & Stahl, C. (1991)	Assessment of physical, financial, psychological, and neglectful situations	15-item assessment screen for detecting suspected elder abuse and neglect.	Discriminant function analysis: 9 items identified 94% of cases. Three conceptual domains: violation of personal rights, characteristics of vulnerability, and potentially abusive situations.
Fulmer Restriction Scale (FRS) Fulmer & Gurland (1996)	Assessment of physical, psychological, and financial restriction of older adults	34-item scale designed to elicit information regarding unnecessary restriction in the older adult.	Chronbach's alpha reliability: .78 Interrater agreement: .93 (available in Spanish)
Indicators of Abuse Screen (IOA) Reis & Nahmiash (1998)	Developed specifically for use by social service agency practitioners likely to visit the older adult in the home	29-item set of indicators for use by social service agency practitioners to identify EM.	Discriminant function analysis: 29 items identified 96.3% of cases. Factor analysis: no reliable pattern of variable clusters.
Adult Protective Service Reports (APS)	Intake forms used to document calls of suspected EM from public hotlines and state agencies.	No specific format.	No psychometrics available

385

[Formerly the American Public Welfare Association] in collaboration with Westat, Inc. 1998) has determined that in the U.S. approximately 450,000 older adults in domestic settings were abused and/or neglected during 1996. If older adults who experienced self-neglect were included, the number would be approximately 551,000 individuals. Findings from this study are summarized in Table 13.1. This groundbreaking research provides national incidence estimates using standardized definitions of EM. Prevalence information was best established in the Pillemer and Finkelhor study (1988).

What Are the Risk Factors for EM?

It is widely recognized that the best data on risk factors for EM have come from a prospective cohort analysis with case matching of an adult protective service EM database (Lachs & Pillemer, 1995; Lachs et al., 1997; Lachs et al., 1998; Lachs & Fulmer, 1993; Lachs et al., 1994) (Table 13.1). Using the Yale Health and Aging Database, this prospective cohort analysis was established as a part of the NIA's *Established Populations for Epidemiologic Studies of the Elderly* (EPESE) (Cornoni-Huntley et al., 1996). The excellent quality of the EPESE data enabled the researchers to utilize adult protective service data, which would have otherwise been impossible.

What Is the Nature of the EM Problem?

The study, "Major Findings From Three Model Projects on Elderly Abuse," was a significant contribution to the EM literature (Wolf, 1986). The primary purpose of the Model Projects was to provide casework services to abused and neglected elders and members of their families. Psychological abuse was the most prevalent form of EM reported in this project, followed by physical abuse, material abuse, and passive neglect. Active neglect was reported in less than one-fifth of the cases. This is in contrast to the data from other studies that have a much higher prevalence of neglect (The National Center on Elder Abuse at The American Public Human Services Association [Formerly the American Public Welfare Association] in collaboration with Westat, Inc. 1998; Pavlik et al., 2001). The investigators suggested that psychopathology, increased dependency, and stress might be important factors in the outcome of EM. Unfortunately, they note that limitations and methodology make it impossible to associate theory with causality. Findings from these data indicated that the victims were more likely to be female, about 75 years of age, and living in a household with family members. The perpetrator was more often a male and younger in age.

One study examined caregiver stress versus problem relatives in order to get at the theory that burden and stress may cause EM. Subanalysis of data from a larger study was examined in order to address this question. Of the 61 elderly persons identified as abuse or neglect victims, follow-up interviews were completed with 46 (76%). Out of 251 randomly selected controls, 215 (86%) agreed to be reinterviewed. It should be noted that the determination of caregiver stress was made by examining features and responses related to the older individual, not the caregiver directly. In fact, this may be an extremely appropriate approach, while data triangulation with input from both the caregiver and the older adult are seen as a higher standard. It was discovered that the abusers had a high prevalence of having been arrested, hospitalized for a psychiatric condition, involved in other violent behavior, or limited by some health problem (Pillemer, Hegeman, Albright, & Henderson, 1998). They were especially likely to be dependent on financial assistance, household repairs, transportation, and housing. Finally, they were more likely to have suffered life stresses in the previous year, for example, an illness or the death of a relative (Pillemer et al., 1998). In conclusion, there appears to be support for the belief that increased caregiver stress leads to elder mistreatment.

Violence and violent feelings in caregivers were examined by exploring 236 family caregivers of dementia victims. Independent variables included caregiver demands, interactional stressors, and caregiver characteristics and the caregiver context. The dependent variable, violence and violent feelings, was measured by a set of questions which embedded questions on violence, which progressed from less sensitive to most sensitive. Thirty-two caregivers feared that they might be violent, and 14 reported actually being violent with the elder (Pillemer & Suitor, 1992).

The association of elder abuse with substance abuse in the Illinois elder abuse system was reported from 2,557 cases of EM, using a subset of 552 cases of substantiated elder abuse in Illinois. Frequencies were reported from a risk assessment of future abuse. When the abuser was identified as having a substance abuse (SA) problem, the type of elder abuse substantiated was more likely to involve either physical or emotional abuse than neglect or financial exploitation. Elder abusers with SA problems were more frequently men and children of their victims, and less likely to be caregivers. Abuser SA was associated with victim SA. Cases involving abusers with SA problems were more likely to be evaluated by caseworkers as having a high potential risk for future abuse (Hwalek, Neale, Goodrich, & Quinn, 1996).

Wives and mothers have been compared as a way of examining older women who are victims of EM. The verbal aggression shown by adult children toward their mothers was perceived to be more serious than similar acts by husbands toward their wives. The authors suggest that shelters are one way of dealing with dependency of victims on mothers, but made no suggestions as to how one is to cope with abusive husbands (Wolf & Pillemer, 1997).

In another study, intergenerational continuity of child abuse was examined in order to determine if the widespread belief that those individuals who were physically abused during childhood are more likely to abuse their own children is true. This was not an EM study, but is included given the continuity concept (Ertem, Leventhal, & Dobbs, 2000).

How Have Data From Reporting Laws Been Used in Research?

Physician reporting of EM was studied using an analysis of a statewide record of reported cases of suspected EM for the years of 1989–1993 (Rosenblatt, Cho, & Durance, 1996). The investigators concluded that physicians report an average of only 2% of all reports of suspected EM, and increasing physician awareness of the problem could potentially increase appropriate reporting of EM (Anetzberger et al., 1993; Anetzberger, Dayton, & McMonagle, 1997).

A model intervention for elder abuse and dementia was conducted during a 2-year collaborative project in Cleveland, Ohio that sought to improve reporting and management of potential and suspected elder abuse involving persons with dementia. Educational curricula, screening tools, and referral protocols were developed and tested, and the success of the project was determined in three ways: (a) curricula materials were developed, (b) project goals were achieved with cross training and collaboration, and (c) APS reporting increased (Anetzberger et al., 2000).

In terms of reporting, there is some information about what factors affect the rate of EM reports to Adult Protective Services (Wolf & Li,

1999). In this study, every geographical area of Massachusetts ($n = 27$) served by Adult Protective Services was used to determine factors that influence EM reporting rates. The dependent variable was the number of reports per 1,000 persons age 60 years and older received during 1994.

In another analysis of a statewide database, the goal was to describe the universe of case reports received during 1 year in a centralized computer database maintained in the "Texas Department of Protective and Regulatory Services—Adult Protective Service Division." There were over 62,000 allegations of EM in 1997. Neglect accounted for 80% of the allegations (Pavlik et al., 2001).

A national survey of emergency-room physicians was undertaken to determine the perceived magnitude of EM and physician awareness. Most physicians were not certain, or did not believe, that a clear-cut medical definition of EM exists (74%). The authors suggest that practicing ED physicians are not competent to identify or report EM, although the response rate of 24% makes these data questionable (Jones, Veenstra, Seamon, & Krohmer, 1997).

What Is Known From Setting-Specific Studies on EM?

ED utilization is frequent for older EM victims. A study was conducted using a cohort analysis to determine ED utilization. The investigators noted that strategies to identify EM in a less acute setting will address needs earlier and improve the quality of life as well as result in substantial savings in health care expenditures for the older adult (Lachs et al., 1997).

Fulmer and colleagues used an emergency department setting to determine whether it was feasible for ED nurses to conduct accurate screening protocols for neglect in the context of a busy practice. During a 3-week period, 180 patients, older than 70 years (90% of all possible patients) were screened to determine if they met study criteria and could be enrolled in the protocol. This study confirmed that elder neglect protocols are feasible in busy emergency departments and that neglect can be accurately detected, but there is room for improved accuracy in this process (Fulmer, Paveza, Abraham, & Fairchild, 2000).

Abuse of patients in nursing homes has been addressed by data from a random sample survey of 577 nurses and nursing aides working in long-term care facilities. Although there is extensive MDS data on the topic of physical abuse in nursing homes, few articles have been written on this topic (Pillemer & Moore, 1989).

Huber, Borders, Netting, and Nelson (2001) have studied a long-term care ombudsman to collect resident demographics in order to discern implications of collecting such demographics. Data from long-term care ombudsmen programs from six states were analyzed to begin to understand the nature of such reports. A higher percentage of complaints lodged on behalf of racial minorities was verified, yet a lower percentage was fully resolved. The authors concluded that the ombudsman databases are a potential resource for identifying resident characteristics that increase their vulnerability in long-term care settings.

Elder mistreatment has been studied in adult day health care from interviews conducted with social workers at nine sites in New York State (Fulmer et al., 1999). Using random sampling, social workers from the nine sites were interviewed in order to discuss how they perceived elder mistreatment indicators in the ADHC. A major limitation of this work lies in the social worker's ability to interpret objective behaviors in AD clients as they relate to suspected EM.

Community characteristics associated with elder abuse have been examined through the analysis of 99 counties in Iowa. Residents age 65 or older who were eligible in the county level population of adjusted numbers of abused elderly served as the mechanism for counting cases. Lower substantiated elder abuse rates were associated with higher community rates of high-school dropouts, number of chiropractors, and number of nurse practitioners. The authors concluded that the strongest risk factor for reported elder abuse was reported child abuse, and that the risk factors may reflect conditions that influence the amount of elder abuse or the detection of existing abuse (Jogerst, Dawson, Hartz, Ely, & Schweitzer, 2000).

SUMMARY

In summary, EM research and knowledge has developed slowly over the past 20 years. This literature review and information synthesis reflects several immediate issues. There is a critical need for more investigators and, in particular, for nurse investigators to address the topic. Fewer than five nurse scientists have committed their program of research to the topic of elder mistreatment, and stayed with it for a significant period of their careers. Nursing, as a clinical, theoretical, and scientific profession, has much to offer with regard to approaches to this challenging topic. EM research requires an interdisciplinary approach, given the biopsychosocial context of EM events. Nurse scientists have led the field to date, and should seek out interested colleagues from other disciplines and fields to enhance the quality of their collective work. Synthesis across fields will not happen in the absence of interdisciplinary research teams. It may be that the paucity of research dollars, along with the difficulty in clearly defining a dependent variable in EM research, has discouraged nurse scientists. There is also a need to replicate studies to verify findings, and develop new questions from what is known. Replication studies are not popular, and it is highly speculative as to why this is true. Finally, there is a critical need for intervention studies on EM. The review of the literature reflects the grave paucity of databased studies, and intervention studies are arguably absent. Only Dyer claims to have an intervention study, and that consists of comprehensive geriatric assessment (CGA). Further, the way her study is described, CGA appears to be an assessment procedure more than an intervention. EM social interventions are well-described in the practice literature and it should be noted that they are expensive. It is estimated that over $20 million is spent annually on adult protective services for EM in the United States (E. Kutas, personal communication, May 24, 2001). However, there are no good data to explain what was paid for or whether it helped the older adult. Surely nursing has valuable contributions to make. The growing number of gerontological nurse scientists should be encouraged to explore the topic of EM. With strong nursing leadership, there is an opportunity to influence the practice of over 2.4 million nurses in this country who can help assess and intervene in EM cases. The National Academy of Sciences special panel is likely to have an important impact on the field, especially because the NIA has specifically requested an analysis of the EM science. Hopefully, funds will be forthcoming that can help recruit nurse investigators who have an interest in the topic. The demographic trends in this country mandate a better system for prevention and intervention in EM cases. The development of interventions based on sound conceptual and theoretical foundations can do much to improve the quality of life for older adults, both now and in the future.

REFERENCE

Anetzberger, G. J., Dayton, C., & McMonagle, P. (1997). A community dialogue series on ethics and elder abuse: Guidelines for decision making. *Journal of Elder Abuse and Neglect, 91*(1), 33–50.

Anetzberger, G. J., Lachs, M. S., O'Brien, J. G., O'Brien, S., Pillemer, K. A., & Tomita, S. K. (1993). Elder mistreatment: A call for help. *Patient Care, 27*(11), 93–95, 99–100.

Anetzberger, G. J., Palmisano, B. R., Sanders, M., Bass, D., Dayton, C., Eckert, S., & Schimer, M. R. (2000). A model intervention for elder abuse and dementia. *Gerontologist, 40,* 492–497.

Aravanis, S. C., Adelman, R. D., Breckman, R., Fulmer, T., Holder, E., Lachs, M. S., O'Brien, J. G., & Sanders, A. B. (1993). Diagnostic and treatment guidelines on elder abuse and neglect. *Archives of Family Medicine, 2*(4), 371–388.

Capezuti, E., Brush, B. L., & Lawson, W. T. (1997). Reporting elder mistreatment. *Journal of Gerontological Nursing, 23*(7), 24–32.

Childs, H. W., Hayslip, B., Jr., Radika, L. M., & Reinberg, J. A. (2000). Young and middle-aged adults' perceptions of elder abuse. *Gerontologist, 40*(1), 75–85.

Cornoni-Huntley, J., Brock, D., Ostfeld, A., Taylor, J., Wallace, R., & Lafferty, M. (Eds.). (1996). *Established Populations for Epidemiologic Studies of the Elderly [NIH#86-2443].* Washington, DC: National Institute on Aging.

Coyne, A. C., Reichman, W. E., & Berbig, L. J. (1993). The relationship between dementia and abuse. *American Journal of Psychiatry, 150,* 643–646.

Dyer, C. B., Pavlik, V. N., Murphy, K. P., & Hyman, D. J. (2000). The high prevalence of depression and dementia in elder abuse or neglect. *Journal of the American Geriatrics Society, 48*(2), 205–208.

Ertem, I. O., Leventhal, J. M., & Dobbs, S. (2000). Intergenerational continuity of child physical abuse: How good is the evidence? *Lancet, 356,* 814–819.

Fulmer, T. (1982). Elder abuse detection and reporting. *Mass Nurse, 51*(5), 10–12.

Fulmer, T. (1984). Elder abuse assessment tool. *Dimensions of Critical Care Nursing, 3,* 216–220.

Fulmer, T., & Gurland, B. (1996). Restriction as elder mistreatment: Differences between caregiver and elder perceptions. *Journal of Mental Health and Aging, 2,* 89–98.

Fulmer, T., Paveza, G., Abraham, I., & Fairchild, S. (2000). Elder neglect assessment in the emergency department. *Journal of Emergency Nursing, 26,* 436–443.

Fulmer, T., Ramirez, M., Fairchild, S., Holmes, D., Koren, M. J., & Teresi, J. (1999). Prevalence of elder mistreatment as reported by social workers in a probability sample of adult day health care clients. *Journal of Elder Abuse & Neglect, 11*(3), 25–36.

Fulmer, T., Street, S., & Carr, K. (1984). Abuse of the elderly: Screening and detection. *Journal of Emergency Nursing, 10,* 131–140.

Fulmer, T., & Wetle, T. (1986). Elder abuse screening and intervention. *Nurse Practitioner, 11*(5), 33–38.

Greenberg, S., Ramsey, G., Mitty, E., & Fulmer, T. (1999). Elder mistreatment: Case law and ethical issues in assessment, reporting and management. *Journal of Nursing Law, 6*(3), 7–20.

Hall, P. A. (1989). Elder maltreatment items, subgroups, and types: Policy and practice implications. *International Journal of Aging and Human Development, 28,* 191–205.

Haviland, S., & O'Brien, J. (1989). Physical abuse and neglect of the elderly: Assessment and intervention. *Orthopedic Nursing, 8*(4), 11–19.

Huber, R., Borders, K., Netting, F. E., & Nelson, H. W. (2001). Data from long-term care ombudsman programs in six states: The implications of collecting resident demographics. *Gerontologist, 41*(1), 61–68.

Hudson, M. (1986). Elder mistreatment: Current research. In K. A. Pillemer & R. S. Wolf, *Elder abuse: Conflict in the family* (pp. 125–166). Dover, MA: Auburn House.

Hudson, M. F. (1991). Elder mistreatment: A taxonomy with definitions by Delphi. *Journal of Elder Abuse and Neglect, 3*(2), 1–20.

Hwalek, M. A., Neale, A. V., Goodrich, C. S., & Quinn, K. (1996). The association of elder abuse and substance abuse in the Illinois Elder Abuse System. *Gerontologist, 36*, 694–700.

Illing, M. (1977). Granny bashing: Comment on how we can identify those at risk. *Nursing Mirror, 145*(25), 34.

Jogerst, G. J., Dawson, J. D., Hartz, A. J., Ely, J. W., & Schweitzer, L. A. (2000). Community characteristics associated with elder abuse. *Journal of the American Geriatrics Society, 48*, 513–518.

Jones, J. S., Veenstra, T. R., Seamon, J. P., & Krohmer, J. (1997). Elder mistreatment: National survey of emergency physicians. *Annals of Emergency Medicine, 30*, 473–479.

Lachs, M. S., Berkman, L., Fulmer, T., & Horwitz, R. (1994). A prospective community-based pilot study of risk factors for the investigation of elder mistreatment. *Journal of the American Geriatrics Society, 42*(2), 169–173.

Lachs, M. S., & Fulmer, T. (1993). Recognizing elder abuse and neglect. *Clinical Geriatric Medicine, 9*(3), 665–681.

Lachs, M. S., & Pillemer, K. A. (1995). Abuse and neglect of elderly persons. *New England Journal of Medicine, 332*, 437–443.

Lachs, M. S., Williams, C., O'Brien, S., Hurst, L., & Horwitz, R. I. (1997). Risk factors for reported elder abuse and neglect: A nine-year observational cohort study. *Gerontologist, 37*, 469–474.

Lachs, M. S., Williams, C. S., O'Brien, S., Hurst, L., Kossack, A., Siegal, A., & Tinetti, M. E. (1997). ED use by older victims of family violence. *Annals of Emergency Medicine, 30*, 448–454.

Lachs, M. S., Williams, C. S., O'Brien, S., Pillemer, K. A., & Charlson, M. E. (1998). The mortality of elder mistreatment. *Journal of the American Medical Association, 280*, 428–432.

Moody, L. E., Voss, A., & Lengacher, C. A. (2000). Assessing abuse among the elderly living in public housing. *Journal of Nursing Measurement, 8*(1), 61–70.

The National Center on Elder Abuse at The American Public Human Services Association [Formerly the American Public Welfare Association] in collaboration with Westat, Inc. (1998). *The National Elder Abuse Incidence Study, Final Report: September 1998*. Washington, DC: National Aging Information Center.

Neale, A., Hwalek, M., Scott, R., Sengstock, M., & Stahl, C. (1991). Validation of the Hwalek-Sengstock Elder Abuse Screening Test. *Journal of Applied Gerontology, 10*(4), 406–418.

O'Brien, J. G. (1986). Elder abuse and the physician. *Michigan Medicine, 85*, 618, 620.

Office for Victims of Crime. (1993). *Improving the police response to domestic elder abuse, instructor training manual & participant training manual* (NCJ 147558 ed.). Washington, DC: U.S. Department of Justice.

O'Malley, T. A., O'Malley, H. C., Everitt, D. E., & Sarson, D. (1984). Categories of family-mediated abuse and neglect of elderly persons. *Journal of the American Geriatrics Society, 32*, 362–369.

Paveza, G. J., Cohen, D., Eisdorfer, C., Freels, S., Semla, T., Ashford, J. W., Gorelick, P., Hirschman, R., Luchins, D. J., & Levy, P. (1992). Severe family violence and Alzheimer's disease: Prevalence and risk factors. *Gerontologist, 32,* 493–497.

Pavlik, V. N., Hyman, D. J., Festa, N. A., & Bitondo Dyer, C. (2001). Quantifying the problem of abuse and neglect in adults—analysis of a statewide database. *Journal of the American Geriatrics Society, 49*(1), 45–48.

Phillips, L. R. (1986). Theoretical explanations of elder abuse: Competing hypotheses and unresolved issues. In K. A. Pillemer & R. S. Wolf, *Elder abuse: Conflict in the family* (pp. 197–217). Dover, MA: Auburn House.

Phillips, L. R., Morrison, E. F., & Chae, Y. M. (1990a). The QUALCARE Scale: Developing an instrument to measure quality of home care. *International Journal of Nursing Studies, 27*(1), 61–75.

Phillips, L. R., Morrison, E. F., & Chae, Y. M. (1990b). The QUALCARE Scale: Testing of a measurement instrument for clinical practice. *International Journal of Nursing Studies, 27*(1), 77–91.

Phillips, L. R., & Rempusheski, V. F. (1985). A decision-making model for diagnosing and intervening in elder abuse and neglect. *Nursing Research, 34,* 134–139.

Pillemer, K. A., & Finkelhor, D. (1988). The prevalence of elder abuse: A random sample survey. *Gerontologist, 28*(1), 51–57.

Pillemer, K. A., & Finkelhor, D. (1989). Causes of elder abuse: Caregiver stress versus problem relatives. *American Journal of Orthopsychiatry, 59,* 179–187.

Pillemer, K. A., Hegeman, C. R., Albright, B., & Henderson, C. (1998). Practice concepts. Building bridges between families and nursing home staff: The Partners in Caregiving program. *Gerontologist, 38,* 499–503.

Pillemer, K. A., & Moore, D. W. (1989). Abuse of patients in nursing homes: Findings from a survey of staff. *Gerontologist, 29,* 314–320.

Pillemer, K. A., & Suitor, J. J. (1992). Violence and violent feelings: What causes them among family caregivers? *Journal of Gerontological Nursing, 47*(4), S165–S172.

Pillemer, K. A., & Wolf, R. S. (1986). *Elder abuse: Conflict in the family.* Dover, MA: Auburn House.

Pratt, C. C., Koval, J., & Lloyd, S. (1983). Service workers' responses to abuse of the elderly. *Social Casework, 64,* 147–153.

Reis, M., & Nahmiash, D. (1998). Validation of the indicators of abuse (IOA) screen. *Gerontologist, 38,* 471–480.

Reno, J. (1994). Keynote Address. Sponsored by the *National Conference on Family Violence: Health and Justice* (pp. 115–120). Chicago: American Medical Association.

Rosenblatt, D. E., Cho, K. H., & Durance, P. W. (1996). Reporting mistreatment of older adults: The role of physicians. *Journal of the American Geriatrics Society, 44*(1), 65–70.

Shaw, M. M. C. (1998). Nursing home resident abuse by staff: Exploring the dynamics. *Journal of Elder Abuse and Neglect, 9*(4), 1–21.

Straus, M. A. (1978). The Conflict Tactic Scale. In J. Touliatos, B. Perlmutter, & M. Straus, *Handbook of family measurement techniques.* Newbury Park, CA: Sage.

Tatara, T. (1993). Understanding the nature and scope of domestic elder abuse with the use of state aggregate data: Summaries of key findings of a national survey of state APS and aging agencies. *Journal of Elder Abuse and Neglect, 5,* 35–57.

Walshe-Brennan, K. (1977). Granny bashing. *Nursing Mirror, 145*, 32–34.

Wolf, R. S. (1986). Major Findings From Three Model Projects on Elderly Abuse. In K. A. Pillemer & R. S. Wolf (Eds.), *Elder abuse: Conflict in the family* (pp. 218–238). Dover, MA: Auburn House.

Wolf, R. S., & Li, D. (1999). Factors affecting the rate of elder abuse reporting to a state protective services program. *Gerontologist, 39*, 222–228.

Wolf, R. S., & Pillemer, K. A. (1997). The older battered woman: Wives and mothers compared. *Journal of Mental Health & Aging, 3*, 325–336.

Index

AACN, *see* American Association of Colleges of Nursing
Abuse of elders, 369–394
  Adult Protective Service Reports, 385
  Conflict Tactic Scale, 383, 384
  Elder Assessment Instrument, 383, 384
  Fulmer Restriction Scale, 383, 385
  Hwalek-Sengstock Elder Abuse Screening Test, 383, 385
  incidence, 383–386
  Indicators of Abuse Screen, 383, 385
  laws, reporting, data from, 388–389
  National Academies of Science, 371
  National Center on Elder Abuse at American Public Human Services Association, 386
  National Elder Abuse Incidence Study, 383
  National Institute on Aging, 371
  QUALCARE scale, 383, 384
  risk factors for, 386
  State of Illinois Abuse, Neglect and Exploitation Tracking System, 375
  State of Michigan records of reported cases of suspected elder abuse 1989–1993, 381
  Texas Department of Protective and Regulatory Services-Adult Protective Services, 378
  Zarit Burden interview, 373
  Zung Self-Rating Depression Scale, 373

ACCESS, regional databases in, tele-health, 300
ACP, *see* Advance care planning
Acquired immunodeficiency syndrome, dementia related, 91
Activities of daily living, 3–34
  Arthritis Impact Measurement Scales 2, 12
  Beck Dressing Performance Scale, 19
  behavior therapy, 6
  Cleveland Scale for Activities of Daily Living, 9
  conceptualization of, 7–8
  disability evaluation, 6
  Duke Activity Status Index, 13
  exercise, 6
  factors associated with poor physical function, 10–16
  geriatric assessment, 6
  Instrumental Activities of Daily Living, 4
  interventions, maintaining, improving physical function, 17–25
  measurement of, 8–10
  nurse–patient relations, 6
  nursing assessment, 6
  nursing care, effect on physical function, 16–17
  Physical Self-Maintenance Scale, 23
  Pulmonary Functional Status Scale, 13, 14
  World Health Association, Assessment of Functional Capacity, 11

Adult Protective Service Reports, 385
Advance directives, 231–265
  advance care planning, 234
  Agency on Aging, Web site, 234
  communication, at end of life,
      235–241
  facility characteristics, influencing
      care services delivery,
      248–250
  Kolcaba Model of Comfort Care, 259
  Mixed Model of Eventually Fatal ill-
      ness, 259
  in nursing home, assisted living facil-
      ity, 234
  symptom assessment, management,
      241–248
Agency on Aging, Web site, 234
AIDS, see Acquired immunodeficiency
    syndrome
AIMS2, see Arthritis Impact Measure-
    ment Scales 2
Alcohol-related brain damage, 91
Alzheimer's disease, 89–125, 150; see
    also Dementia
  behavioral symptoms, 100–104
  cognitive performance, interventions,
      95–96
  continuation of self, interventions pro-
      moting, 110–111
  depression, reduction of, 98–99
  elimination, 108
  engagement
    increasing, 97–98
    interventions promoting, 110–111
  family caregiver, 149–181
    case management, 169
    counseling, 167–168
    education, 165–166
    interventions, testing of, 151–165
    multicomponent interventions,
        169–170
    respite care, 168–169
    support, 166–167
  functional abilities, independence in,
      104–105

  general functioning, 99–100
  memory, interventions, 96–97
  mild to early-moderate dementia,
      94–100
  moderate to severe dementia,
      100–106
  nursing interventions, 92–94
  nutritional needs, 106–108
  Progressively Lowered Stress Thresh-
      old, 92
  progressive supranuclear palsy, 91
  quality of life, 99–100
  skin integrity, 108
  staging, 94
  therapeutic activities, 105–106
  vegetative disease stages, 106–111
  vocalizations, problematic, 108–110
American Association of Colleges of
    Nursing, 333
American Nurses Association and Inter-
    national Society of Nurses in
    Genetics, 330
Amplification systems, for hearing im-
    pairment, 361
APS, see Adult Protective Service
    Reports
Arthritis Impact Measurement Scales 2,
    12
Assessment of Functional Capacity,
    World Health Association, 11
Assistive devices, for hearing impair-
    ment, 361
Attachments for telephone, for hearing
    impairment, 361

Beck Depression Inventory, 353
Beck Dressing Performance Scale, 19
Bedsores, 35–63
  incidence, 36–38
  management, 45
    comprehensive, 47–51
    healing
      adjunctive therapies in, 51–53
      instruments to monitor, 46

Pressure Sore Status Tool, 46
Pressure Ulcer Scale for Healing, 47
staging, 45–46
prediction of, instruments for, 40–41
prevalence of, 36–38
prevention, 39–45
mechanical loading, 42–43
program for, implementation of, 44–45
risk factors, 39–40
skin care, 41–42
support surfaces, 43–44
Behavior therapy, 6
Behavioral symptoms, dementia, 100–104
Beliefs about pain, 74–75

Case management
assistance for family caregiver of dementia patient, 169
in transitional care, 129
CCU, see Coronary care unit
Checklist of Nonverbal Pain Indicators, 72
CHF, see Congestive heart failure
Chronic Musculoskeletal Pain and Depressive symptoms in National Health and Nutrition Examination I, epidemiologic follow-up study, 68
Chronic obstructive pulmonary disease, home care, 284
Cleveland Scale for Activities of Daily Living, 9
CNPI, see Checklist of Nonverbal Pain Indicators
Cognitive impairment, 89–125
AIDS-related dementia, 91
alcohol-related brain damage, 91
Alzheimer's disease, 91, 149–181
behavioral symptoms, 100–104
cognitive performance, interventions, 95–96

continuation of self, interventions promoting, 110–111
Creutzfeld-Jacob disease, 91
depression, reduction of, 98–99
elimination, 108
engagement, increasing, 97–98
family caregiver, 149–181
case management, 169
counseling, 167–168
education, 165–166
interventions, testing of, 151–165
multicomponent interventions, 169–170
respite care, 168–169
support, 166–167
functional abilities, independence in, 104–105
Huntington's disease, 91
lead poisoning, 91
Lewy body, 91
memory, interventions, 96–97
mild to early–moderate dementia, 94–100
moderate to severe dementia, 100–106
multiple sclerosis, 91
neurosyphilis, 91
nursing interventions, 92–94
nutritional needs, 106–108
Parkinson's disease, 91
Progressively Lowered Stress Threshold, 92
progressive supranuclear palsy, 91
quality of life, 99–100
staging, 94
therapeutic activities, 105–106
vegetative disease stages, 106–111
vocalizations, problematic, 108–110
Wilson's disease, 91
Cognitive performance, interventions, dementia, 95–96
Communication, at end of life, 235–241
Community based care, 280
Computer–mediated communication, telehealth, 293–322

Computer–mediated communication, telehealth *(continued)*
acceptance of by elders, 313–314
analysis, 301
congestive heart failure, 297
cost, face-to-face assessments, compared, 314
data collection, 296
evaluation, 296–301
face-to-face assessments, compared, 311–313
mini-mental state exam, 313
problem formulation, 295–296
regional databases in ACCESS, 300
as substitute for face-to-face nursing care, 301–311
Conflict Tactic Scale, 383, 384
Congestive heart failure, telehealth, 297
Continuation of self, interventions promoting, with dementia, 110–111
Continuity of care, 127–148
care coordination, 129
case management, 129
discharge planning, 129
evaluation, 136–139
implementation, 134–136
needs assessment, 130–132
planning, 132–134
transitional care and, 129
COPD, *see* Chronic obstructive pulmonary disease
Coping skills training, for hearing loss, 358–360
Coronary intensive care unit, 181–232
Counseling, for family caregiver of dementia patient, 167–168
Creutzfeld-Jacob disease, 91
Critical care unit, 181–231
decision making
at end of life, 201–215
improving, 217–218
do not resuscitate order, 185, 192, 196

families, end-of-life decision making, 213–215
families of dying patients, 195–198
health care providers, 196–201
end-of-life decision making, 210–213
hospital, characteristics of, 184–189
ICU patient experience, 190
improving care, 217–218
intervention studies, 216–218
limitation-of-treatment decisions, 202–209
Society of Critical Care Medicine Ethics Committee, 210
Study to Understand Prognoses and Preferences for Outcomes and Risks of Treatments, 185, 191, 193, 211, 218
CTS, *see* Conflict Tactic Scale

Data collection by telephone, 293–322
acceptance of by elders, 313–314
analysis, 301
congestive heart failure, 297
cost, face-to-face assessments, compared, 314
data collection, 296
evaluation, 296–301
face-to-face assessments, compared, 311–313
mini-mental state exam, 313
problem formulation, 295–296
regional databases in ACCESS, 300
as substitute for face-to-face nursing care, 301–311
Deafness, 341–368
amplification systems, 361
assessment of, 346–350
assistive devices, 361
attachments for telephone, 361
Beck Depression Inventory, 353
changes in hearing, 343–344
culture influences, 361
dyadic experience of, 360

factors influencing, 344–345
Five Minute Hearing Test, 357
impact of, 351–356
  family, 355
  friends, 355
  physical functioning, 351–355
  psychological functioning, 351–355
interventions, 356–360
  coping skills training, 358–360
  sensory aids, 356–357
    with environmental manipula-
      tion, 357–358
measures of, 347–348
medications, long-term use of, 362
Mental Status Questionnaire, 353
microphones, 361
National Council on Aging, 357
Quantified Denver Scale of Communication, 354
Rosenberg Global Self-Esteem Scale,
  355
Rosow-Breslau function, 352
Self Evaluation of Life Function, 353
telecommunicating device, 361
telephones, 361
UCLA Loneliness Scale, 355
Ventry-Weinstein Scale, 347
warning devices, 361
Whispered Voice, 348
Decubitus ulcer, 35–63
incidence, 36–38
management, 45
  comprehensive, 47–51
  healing
    adjunctive therapies in, 51–53
    instruments to monitor, 46
    Pressure Sore Status Tool, 46
    Pressure Ulcer Scale for Healing,
      47
  staging, 45–46
prediction of, instruments for, 40–41
prevalence of, 36–38
prevention, 39–45
  mechanical loading, 42–43

program for, implementation of,
  44–45
risk factors, 39–40
skin care, 41–42
support surfaces, 43–44
Dementia, 150
family caregiver, 149–181
  case management, 169
  counseling, 167–168
  education, 165–166
  interventions, testing of, 151–165
  multicomponent interventions,
    169–170
  respite care, 168–169
  support, 166–167
irreversible, 89–125
  AIDS-related dementia, 91
  alcohol-related brain damage, 91
  Alzheimer's disease, 91
  behavioral symptoms, 100–104
  cognitive performance, interven-
    tions, 95–96
  continuation of self, interventions
    promoting, 110–111
  Creutzfeld-Jacob disease, 91
  depression, reduction of, 98–99
  elimination, 108
  engagement
    increasing, 97–98
    interventions promoting,
      110–111
  functional abilities, independence
    in, 104–105
  general functioning, 99–100
  Huntington's disease, 91
  lead poisoning, 91
  Lewy body, 91
  memory, interventions, 96–97
  mild to early–moderate dementia,
    94–100
  moderate to severe dementia,
    100–106
  multiple sclerosis, 91
  neurosyphilis, 91

Dementia *(continued)*
    nursing interventions, 92–94
    nutritional needs, 106–108
    Parkinson's disease, 91
    Progressively Lowered Stress
        Threshold, 92
    progressive supranuclear palsy, 91
    quality of life, 99–100
    skin integrity, 108
    stages of, 95
    staging, 94
    therapeutic activities, 105–106
    vegetative disease stages, 106–111
    vocalizations, problematic,
        108–110
    Wilson's disease, 91
Depression in dementia, reduction of,
    98–99
Discharge planning, transitional care
    and, 129
Discomfort Scale for Patients with De-
    mentia of Alzheimer's Type,
    71
DNR order, *see* Do not resuscitate order
Domestic abuse of elderly, 369–394
    Adult Protective Service Reports, 385
    Conflict Tactic Scale, 383, 384
    Elder Assessment Instrument, 383,
        384
    Fulmer Restriction Scale, 383, 385
    Hwalek-Sengstock Elder Abuse
        Screening Test, 383, 385
    incidence, 383–386
    Indicators of Abuse Screen, 383, 385
    laws, reporting, data from, 388–389
    National Academies of Science, 371
    National Center on Elder Abuse at
        American Public Human Ser-
        vices Association, 386
    National Elder Abuse Incidence
        Study, 383
    National Institute on Aging, 371
    QUALCARE scale, 383, 384
    risk factors for, 386

    State of Illinois Abuse, Neglect and
        Exploitation Tracking Sys-
        tem, 375
    State of Michigan records of reported
        cases of suspected elder
        abuse 1989–1993, 381
    Texas Department of Protective and
        Regulatory Services-Adult
        Protective Services, 378
    Zarit Burden interview, 373
    Zung Self-Rating Depression Scale,
        373
Do not resuscitate order, 185, 192, 196
DS-DAT, *see* Discomfort Scale for pa-
    tients with Dementia of Alz-
    heimer's Type
Duke Activity Status Index, 13

EAI, *see* Elder Assessment Instrument
Education, for family caregiver of de-
    mentia patient, 165–166
Elder Assessment Instrument, 383, 384
Elder mistreatment, 369–394
    Adult Protective Service Reports, 385
    Conflict Tactic Scale, 383, 384
    Elder Assessment Instrument, 383,
        384
    Fulmer Restriction Scale, 383, 385
    Hwalek-Sengstock Elder Abuse
        Screening Test, 383, 385
    incidence, 383–386
    Indicators of Abuse Screen, 383, 385
    laws, reporting, data from, 388–389
    National Academies of Science, 371
    National Center on Elder Abuse at
        American Public Human Ser-
        vices Association, 386
    National Elder Abuse Incidence
        Study, 383
    National Institute on Aging, 371
    QUALCARE scale, 383, 384
    risk factors for, 386
    State of Illinois Abuse, Neglect and
        Exploitation Tracking Sys-
        tem, 375

State of Michigan records of reported cases of suspected elder abuse 1989-1993, 381
Texas Department of Protective and Regulatory Services-Adult Protective Services, 378
Zarit Burden interview, 373
Zung Self-Rating Depression Scale, 373
Elimination, maintenance of, 108
ELSI Program, see Ethical, Legal, and Social Implications Program
End-of-life care
decision making, improving, 217–218
intensive care unit, 181–231
decision making, at end of life, 201–215
do not resuscitate order, 185, 192, 196
families, end-of-life decision making, 213–215
families of dying patients, 195–198
health care providers, 196–201
end-of-life decision making, 210–213
hospital, characteristics of, 184–189
ICU patient experience, 190
improving care, 217–218
intervention studies, 216–218
limitation-of-treatment decisions, 202–209
Society of Critical Care Medicine Ethics Committee, 210
Study to Understand Prognoses and Preferences for Outcomes and Risks of Treatments, 185, 191, 193, 211, 218
in nursing home, assisted living facility, 231–265
advance care planning, 234
Agency on Aging, Web site, 234
communication, at end of life, 235–241

facility characteristics, influencing care services delivery, 248–250
Kolcaba Model of Comfort Care, 259
Mixed Model of Eventually Fatal illness, 259
symptom assessment, management, 241–248
Engagement in life, interventions promoting, 97–98, 110–111
Epidemiologic Analysis of Pain in Elderly: Iowa 65+ Rural Health Study, 1994, 68
Ethical, Legal, and Social Implications Program, 330
Ethical issues, genetics, 323–339
Exercise, physical function and, 6

Faces Pain Scale, 70
Face-to-face assessments, telehealth, compared, 311–313
cost, 314
Face-to-face nursing care, telehealth, compared, 301–311
Facility characteristics, influencing care services delivery, 248–250
Families, of dying patients, 195–198
end-of-life decision making, 213–215
Family caregiver, dementia patient, 149–181
case management, 169
counseling, 167–168
education, 165–166
interventions, testing of, 151–165
multicomponent interventions, 169–170
respite care, 168–169
support, 166–167
Five Minute Hearing Test, 357
FMHT, see Five Minute Hearing Test
FPS, see Faces Pain Scale
Free Voice, see Whispered Voice
FRS, see Fulmer Restriction Scale

Fulmer Restriction Scale, 383, 385
Functional abilities, independence in,
    with dementia, 104–105
Functional physical status, 3–34
    Arthritis Impact Measurement Scales
        2, 12
    Beck Dressing Performance Scale, 19
    behavior therapy, 6
    Cleveland Scale for Activities of
        Daily Living, 9
    conceptualization of, 7–8
    disability evaluation, 6
    Duke Activity Status Index, 13
    exercise, 6
    factors associated with, 10–16
    geriatric assessment, 6
    Instrumental Activities of Daily Liv-
        ing, 4
    interventions, maintaining, improving
        physical function, 17–25
    measurement of, 8–10
    nurse-patient relations, 6
    nursing assessment, 6
    nursing care, effect on physical func-
        tion, 16–17
    Physical Self-Maintenance Scale, 23
    Pulmonary Functional Status Scale,
        13, 14
    World Health Association, Assess-
        ment of Functional Capacity,
        11

Genetics, 323–339
    advocacy, 329–331
    American Association of Colleges of
        Nursing, 333
    American Nurses Association and In-
        ternational Society of Nurses
        in Genetics, 330
    behavioral research, 325
    complex care management, 327
    counseling, 326
    disease prevention, 326–327
    Ethical, Legal, and Social Implica-
        tions Program, 330
    Gerontological Society of America
        Scientific Meeting, 330
    health assessment, 325–326
    health education, 326
    health promotion, 326–327
    Human Genome Project, 330
    International Society of Nurses in Ge-
        netics, 333
    medication monitoring, 327–329
    National Coalition for Health Profes-
        sional Education in Genetics,
        333
    National Human Genome Research In-
        stitute, 333
        2000, 330
    Partners Center for Human Genetics,
        331
    psychological model, 325
    public health curriculum, 325
    social science research, 325
Geriatric Pain Measure, 71
Gerontological Society of America Sci-
        entific Meeting, 330
GPM, see Geriatric Pain Measure

Healing, of pressure ulcer
    adjunctive therapies in, 51–53
    instruments to monitor, 46
Health care providers, end-of-life deci-
        sion making, 210–213
Hearing impairment, 341–368
    amplification systems, 361
    assessment of, 346–350
    assistive devices, 361
    attachments for telephone, 361
    Beck Depression Inventory, 353
    changes in hearing, 343–344
    culture influences, 361
    dyadic experience of, 360
    factors influencing, 344–345
    Five Minute Hearing Test, 357
    impact of, 351–356
        family, 355
        friends, 355

physical functioning, 351–355
psychological functioning, 351–355
interventions, 356–360
    coping skills training, 358–360
    sensory aids, 356–357
        with environmental manipula-
        tion, 357–358
measures of, 347–348
medications, long-term use of, 362
Mental Status Questionnaire, 353
microphones, 361
National Council on Aging, 357
Quantified Denver Scale of Communi-
    cation, 354
Rosenberg Global Self-Esteem Scale,
    355
Rosow-Breslau function, 352
Self Evaluation of Life Function, 353
telecommunicating device, 361
telephones, 361
UCLA Loneliness Scale, 355
Ventry-Weinstein Scale, 347
warning devices, 361
Whispered Voice, 348
HGP, see Human Genome Project
Hip fracture, home care of, 284
Hip replacement, home care, 284
Home health care, 267–293, 293–322
    chronic obstructive pulmonary dis-
        ease, 284
    community based care, 280
    defining, 272–275
    hip fracture, 284
    hip replacement, 284
    individual factors, 275–278
    organizational factors, 278–279
    outcomes of, 280–284
    patient outcomes, 282–284
    policy factors, 279–280
    research needed, 284–286
    resource use
        defining, 272–273
        trajectories, 273–275
    service utilization outcomes, 280–282

stroke, 284
telehealth, 293–322
    acceptance of by elders, 313–314
    analysis, 301
    congestive heart failure, 297
    cost, face-to-face assessments, com-
        pared, 314
    data collection, 296
    evaluation, 296–301
    face-to-face assessments, com-
        pared, 311–313
    mini-mental state exam, 313
    problem formulation, 295–296
    regional databases in ACCESS,
        300
    as substitute for face-to-face nurs-
        ing care, 301–311
    theoretical framework, for study of,
        270–271
Hospice, 231–265
    advance care planning, 234
    Agency on Aging, Web site, 234
    communication, at end of life,
        235–241
    facility characteristics, influencing
        care services delivery,
        248–250
    Kolcaba Model of Comfort Care, 259
    Mixed Model of Eventually Fatal ill-
        ness, 259
    symptom assessment, management,
        241–248
H-S/EAST, see Hwalek-Sengstock Elder
    Abuse Screening Test
Human Genome Project, 330
Huntington's disease, 91
Hwalek-Sengstock Elder Abuse Screen-
    ing Test, 383, 385

IADL, see Instrumental Activities of
    Daily Living
ICU, see Intensive care unit
Illinois Abuse, Neglect and Exploitation
    Tracking System, 375

Impact of hearing loss, 351–356
  on family, 355
  on friends, 355
  on physical functioning, 351–355
  on psychological functioning,
      351–355
Indicators of Abuse Screen, 383, 385
Informatics, 293–322
  acceptance of by elders, 313–314
  analysis, 301
  congestive heart failure, 297
  cost, face-to-face assessments, com-
      pared, 314
  data collection, 296
  evaluation, 296–301
  face-to-face assessments, compared,
      311–313
  mini-mental state exam, 313
  problem formulation, 295–296
  regional databases in ACCESS, 300
  as substitute for face-to-face nursing
      care, 301–311
Innovative transitional care, 139–140
Instrumental Activities of Daily Living,
    4
Intensive care unit, end-of-life care, 232
  decision making
    at end of life, 201–215
    improving, 217–218
  do not resuscitate order, 185, 192,
      196
  families, end-of-life decision making,
      213–215
  families of dying patients, 195–198
  health care providers, 196–201
    end-of-life decision making,
        210–213
  hospital, characteristics of, 184–189
  ICU patient experience, 190
  improving care, 217–218
  intervention studies, 216–218
  limitation-of-treatment decisions,
      202–209
  Society of Critical Care Medicine Eth-
      ics Committee, 210

Study to Understand Prognoses and
    Preferences for Outcomes
    and Risks of Treatments,
    185, 191, 193, 211, 218
International Society of Nurses in Genet-
    ics, 333
IOA, see Indicators of Abuse Screen
Irreversible dementia, 89–125
  AIDS-related dementia, 91
  alcohol-related brain damage, 91
  Alzheimer's disease, 91
  behavioral symptoms, 100–104
  cognitive performance, interventions,
      95–96
  continuation of self, interventions pro-
      moting, 110–111
  Creutzfeld-Jacob disease, 91
  depression, reduction of, 98–99
  elimination, 108
  engagement
    increasing, 97–98
    interventions promoting, 110–111
  functional abilities, independence in,
      104–105
  general functioning, 99–100
  Huntington's disease, 91
  lead poisoning, 91
  Lewy body, 91
  memory, interventions, 96–97
  mild to early-moderate dementia,
      94–100
  moderate to severe dementia,
      100–106
  multiple sclerosis, 91
  neurosyphilis, 91
  nursing interventions, 92–94
  nutritional needs, 106–108
  Parkinson's disease, 91
  Progressively Lowered Stress Thresh-
      old, 92
  progressive supranuclear palsy, 91
  quality of life, 99–100
  skin integrity, 108
  stages of, 95

staging, 94
therapeutic activities, 105–106
vegetative disease stages, 106–111
vocalizations, problematic, 108–110
Wilson's disease, 91
ISONG, *see* International Society of
      Nurses in Genetics

Kolcaba Model of Comfort Care, 259

Laws, reporting of elder abuse, data
      from, 388–389
Lead poisoning, 91
Lewy body, in dementia, 91
Life support care, 181–232
   decision making
      at end of life, 201–215
      improving, 217–218
   do not resuscitate order, 185, 192,
      196
   families, end-of-life decision making,
      213–215
   families of dying patients, 195–198
   health care providers, 196–201
      end-of-life decision making,
         210–213
   hospital, characteristics of, 184–189
   ICU patient experience, 190
   improving care, 217–218
   intervention studies, 216–218
   limitation-of-treatment decisions,
         202–209
   Society of Critical Care Medicine Eth-
      ics Committee, 210
   Study to Understand Prognoses and
      Preferences for Outcomes
      and Risks of Treatments,
      185, 191, 193, 211, 218
Limitation-of-treatment decisions,
      202–209
Loading, mechanical, pressure ulcer,
      42–43

Mechanical loading, pressure ulcer,
      42–43

Medical intensive care unit, 181–231
   decision making
      at end of life, 201–215
      improving, 217–218
   do not resuscitate order, 185, 192,
      196
   families, end-of-life decision making,
      213–215
   families of dying patients, 195–198
   health care providers, 196–201
      end-of-life decision making,
         210–213
   hospital, characteristics of, 184–189
   ICU patient experience, 190
   improving care, 217–218
   intervention studies, 216–218
   limitation-of-treatment decisions,
         202–209
   Society of Critical Care Medicine Eth-
      ics Committee, 210
   Study to Understand Prognoses and
      Preferences for Outcomes
      and Risks of Treatments,
      185, 191, 193, 211, 218
Medications, long-term use of, deafness
      and, 362
Memory; *see also* Dementia
   interventions for, 96–97
Mental Status Questionnaire, 353
Michigan records of reported cases of
      suspected elder abuse, 381
Microphones, with hearing impairment,
      361
MICU, *see* Medical intensive care unit
Mild to early–moderate dementia,
      94–100
Mini-mental state exam, telehealth, 313
Mixed Model of Eventually Fatal ill-
      ness, 259
MMSE, *see* Mini-mental state exam
Moderate to severe dementia, 100–106
Multicomponent interventions, for fam-
      ily caregiver of dementia pa-
      tient, 169–170

Multiple sclerosis, 91
Musculoskeletal Complaints and Associ-
     ated Consequences in Elderly
     Chinese age 70 years and
     over, 68

NAS, *see* National Academies of
     Science
National Academies of Science, 371
National Center on Elder Abuse at
     American Public Human Ser-
     vices Association, 386
National Coalition for Health Profes-
     sional Education in Genetics,
     333
National Council on Aging, 357
National Elder Abuse Incidence Study,
     383
National Human Genome Research Insti-
     tute, 333
  2000, 330
National Institute on Aging, 371
NCHPEG, *see* National Coalition for
     Health Professional Educa-
     tion in Genetics
NCOA, *see* National Council on Aging
NEAIS, *see* National Elder Abuse Inci-
     dence Study
Neglect, of elder, 369–394
  Adult Protective Service Reports, 385
  Conflict Tactic Scale, 383, 384
  Elder Assessment Instrument, 383,
       384
  Fulmer Restriction Scale, 383, 385
  Hwalek-Sengstock Elder Abuse
       Screening Test, 383, 385
  incidence, 383–386
  Indicators of Abuse Screen, 383, 385
  laws, reporting, data from, 388–389
  National Academies of Science, 371
  National Center on Elder Abuse at
       American Public Human Ser-
       vices Association, 386
  National Elder Abuse Incidence
       Study, 383

  National Institute on Aging, 371
  QUALCARE scale, 383, 384
  risk factors for, 386
  State of Illinois Abuse, Neglect and
       Exploitation Tracking Sys-
       tem, 375
  State of Michigan records of reported
       cases of suspected elder
       abuse 1989–1993, 381
  Texas Department of Protective and
       Regulatory Services-Adult
       Protective Services, 378
  Zarit Burden interview, 373
  Zung Self-Rating Depression Scale,
       373
Neurosyphilis, 91
NIA, *see* National Institute on Aging
Nutrition, dementia and, 106–108

Pain, 63–88
  adequacy of treatment, 75–79
  attitudes about pain, 74–75
  beliefs about, 74–75
  Checklist of Nonverbal Pain Indica-
       tors, 72
  Chronic Musculoskeletal Pain and De-
       pressive Symptoms in Na-
       tional Health and Nutrition
       Examination I, epidemiologic
       follow-up study, 68
  Discomfort Scale for Patients with De-
       mentia of Alzheimer's Type,
       71
  Epidemiologic Analysis of Pain in El-
       derly: Iowa 65+ Rural Health
       Study, 1994, 68
  evidence on pain, 81–82
    limitations of, 82–84
  Faces Pain Scale, 70
  Geriatric Pain Measure, 71
  incidence of, 66–68
  measurement, 70–74
  Musculoskeletal Complaints and Asso-
       ciated Consequences in El-

derly Chinese Age 70 Years and Over, 68
Pain and Suffering in Seriously Ill Hospitalized Patients, study, 67
Pain in Nursing Home, study, 67
Population-based Study of Pain in Elderly People: A Descriptive Study, 66
prevalence, 66–68
Prevalence of Pain in General Population: Results of Postal Survey in County in Sweden, 66
treatments, 74–75, 79–81
variation across population groups, 65–70
Pain and Suffering in Seriously Ill Hospitalized Patients, study, 67
Pain in Nursing Home Study, 67
Palliative care, 181–231, 231–265
advance care planning, 234
Agency on Aging, Web site, 234
communication, at end of life, 235–241
decision making
at end of life, 201–215
improving, 217–218
do-not-resuscitate order, 185, 192, 196
facility characteristics, influencing care services delivery, 248–250
families, end-of-life decision making, 213–215
families of dying patients, 195–198
health care providers, 196–201
end-of-life decision making, 210–213
hospital, characteristics of, 184–189
ICU patient experience, 190
improving care, 217–218
intervention studies, 216–218
Kolcaba Model of Comfort Care, 259
limitation-of-treatment decisions, 202–209

Mixed Model of Eventually Fatal illness, 259
Society of Critical Care Medicine Ethics Committee, 210
Study to Understand Prognoses and Preferences for Outcomes and Risks of Treatments, 185, 191, 193, 211, 218
symptom assessment, management, 241–248
Palsy, progressive supranuclear, 91
Parkinson's disease, 91
Partners Center for Human Genetics, 331
Patient assessment, 129
Pharmacogenetics, 323–339
advocacy, 329–331
American Association of Colleges of Nursing, 333
American Nurses Association and International Society of Nurses in Genetics, 330
behavioral research, 325
complex care management, 327
counseling, 326
disease prevention, 326–327
Ethical, Legal, and Social Implications Program, 330
Gerontological Society of America Scientific Meeting, 330
health assessment, 325–326
health education, 326
health promotion, 326–327
Human Genome Project, 330
International Society of Nurses in Genetics, 333
medication monitoring, 327–329
National Coalition for Health Professional Education in Genetics, 333
National Human Genome Research Institute, 333
2000, 330
Partners Center for Human Genetics, 331

Pharmacogenetics *(continued)*
  psychological model, 325
  public health curriculum, 325
  social science research, 325
Physical function, 3–34
  Arthritis Impact Measurement Scales
    2, 12
  Beck Dressing Performance Scale, 19
  behavior therapy, 6
  Cleveland Scale for Activities of
    Daily Living, 9
  conceptualization of, 7–8
  disability evaluation, 6
  Duke Activity Status Index, 13
  exercise, 6
  factors associated with poor physical
    function, 10–16
  geriatric assessment, 6
  Instrumental Activities of Daily Liv-
    ing, 4
  interventions, maintaining, improving
    physical function, 17–25
  measurement of, 8–10
  nurse–patient relations, 6
  nursing assessment, 6
  nursing care, effect on physical func-
    tion, 16–17
  Physical Self-Maintenance Scale, 23
  Pulmonary Functional Status Scale,
    13, 14
  World Health Association, Assess-
    ment of Functional Capacity,
    11
Physical Self-Maintenance Scale, 23
PLST, *see* Progressively Lowered Stress
    Threshold
Poisoning, lead, 91
Population-based Study of Pain in El-
    derly People: A Descriptive
    Study, 66
Postdischarge follow-up, 129
Pressure Sore Status Tool, 46
Pressure ulcer, 35–63
  incidence, 36–38

management, 45
  comprehensive, 47–51
  healing
    adjunctive therapies in, 51–53
    instruments to monitor, 46
    Pressure Sore Status Tool, 46
    Pressure Ulcer Scale for Healing,
      47
  staging, 45–46
  prediction of, instruments for, 40–41
  prevalence of, 36–38
  prevention, 39–45
    mechanical loading, 42–43
    program for, implementation of,
      44–45
    risk factors, 39–40
    skin care, 41–42
    support surfaces, 43–44
Pressure Ulcer Scale for Healing, 47
Prevalence of Pain in General Popula-
    tion: Results of Postal Survey
    in County in Sweden, 66
Progressively Lowered Stress Thresh-
    old, 92
Progressive supranuclear palsy, 91
Pulmonary Functional Status Scale, 13,
    14
PUSH, *see* Pressure Ulcer Scale for
    Healing

QDS, *see* Quantified Denver Scale of
    Communication
QUALCARE scale, elder abuse, 383,
    384
Quantified Denver Scale of Communica-
    tion, 354

Referrals, transitional care and, 129
Regional databases in ACCESS, tele-
    health, 300
Reporting of elder abuse, laws regard-
    ing, data from, 388–389
Respite care, with family caregiver of
    dementia patient, 168–169
Risk factors, pressure ulcer, 39–40

Rosenberg Global Self-Esteem Scale, 355
Rosow-Breslau function, 352

SELF, *see* Self Evaluation of Life Function
Self Evaluation of Life Function, 353
Sensory aids, for hearing loss, 356–357
  with environmental manipulation, 357–358
Settings for care
  end-of-life care, in nursing home, assisted living facility, 231–265
  family caregiver, dementia patient, 149–181
  intensive care unit, end-of-life care, 232
  transitional care, 127–148
Shared decision making, at end of life, 235–240
SICU, *see* Surgical intensive care unit
Skin care, pressure ulcers and, 41–42
Skin integrity, 108
Society of Critical Care Medicine Ethics Committee, 210
Stages of dementia, 95
State of Illinois Abuse, Neglect and Exploitation Tracking System, 375
State of Michigan records of reported cases of suspected elder abuse, 381
Stroke, home health care, 284
Study to Understand Prognoses and Preferences for Outcomes and Risks of Treatments, 185, 191, 193, 211, 218
SUPPORT, *see* Study to Understand Prognoses and Preferences for Outcomes and Risks of Treatments
Support, for family caregiver of dementia patient, 166–167
Support surfaces, pressure ulcers and, 43–44

Supranuclear palsy, progressive, 91
Surgical intensive care unit, 181–232
  decision making
    at end of life, 201–215
    improving, 217–218
  do not resuscitate order, 185, 192, 196
  families, end-of-life decision making, 213–215
  families of dying patients, 195–198
  health care providers, 196–201
    end-of-life decision making, 210–213
  hospital, characteristics of, 184–189
  ICU patient experience, 190
  improving care, 217–218
  intervention studies, 216–218
  limitation-of-treatment decisions, 202–209
  Society of Critical Care Medicine Ethics Committee, 210
  Study to Understand Prognoses and Preferences for Outcomes and Risks of Treatments, 185, 191, 193, 211, 218

TDD, *see* Telecommunicating device
Telecommunicating device, with hearing impairment, 361
Telehealth, 293–322
  acceptance of by elders, 313–314
  analysis, 301
  congestive heart failure, 297
  cost, face-to-face assessments, compared, 314
  data collection, 296
  evaluation, 296–301
  face-to-face assessments, compared, 311–313
  mini-mental state exam, 313
  problem formulation, 295–296
  regional databases in ACCESS, 300
Telehealth *(continued)*
  as substitute for face-to-face nursing care, 301–311

Telephones, with hearing impairment, 361
Terminal care, 231–265
  advance care planning, 234
  Agency on Aging, Web site, 234
  communication, at end of life, 235–241
  decision making, improving, 217–218
  facility characteristics, influencing care services delivery, 248–250
  intensive care unit, 181–232
    decision making
      at end of life, 201–215
      improving, 217–218
    do not resuscitate order, 185, 192, 196
    families, end-of-life decision making, 213–215
    families of dying patients, 195–198
    health care providers, 196–201
      end-of-life decision making, 210–213
    hospital, characteristics of, 184–189
    ICU patient experience, 190
    improving care, 217–218
    intervention studies, 216–218
    limitation-of-treatment decisions, 202–209
    Society of Critical Care Medicine Ethics Committee, 210
    Study to Understand Prognoses and Preferences for Outcomes and Risks of Treatments, 185, 191, 193, 211, 218
  Kolcaba Model of Comfort Care, 259
  Mixed Model of Eventually Fatal illness, 259
  in nursing home, assisted living facility, 231–265
    advance care planning, 234
    Agency on Aging, Web site, 234
    communication, at end of life, 235–241

facility characteristics, influencing care services delivery, 248–250
    Kolcaba Model of Comfort Care, 259
    Mixed Model of Eventually Fatal illness, 259
    symptom assessment, management, 241–248
    symptom assessment, management, 241–248
Texas Department of Protective and Regulatory Services-Adult Protective Services, 378
Transitional care, 127–148
  care coordination, 129
  case management, 129
  continuity of care, 129
  discharge planning, 129
  effectiveness of, 139–140
  evaluation, 136–139
  implementation, 134–136
  innovative, 139–140
  needs assessment, 130–132
  patient assessment, 129
  planning, 132–134
  postdischarge follow-up, 129
  referrals, 129

UCLA Loneliness Scale, 355
Ulcer, pressure, 35–63
  incidence, 36–38
  management, 45
    comprehensive, 47–51
    healing
      adjunctive therapies in, 51–53
      instruments to monitor, 46
      Pressure Sore Status Tool, 46
      Pressure Ulcer Scale for Healing, 47
    staging, 45–46
  prediction of, instruments for, 40–41
  prevalence of, 36–38
  prevention, 39–45

mechanical loading, 42–43
program for, implementation of,
     44–45
risk factors, 39–40
skin care, 41–42
support surfaces, 43–44

Vegetative disease stages, 106–111
Ventry-Weinstein Scale, 347
Vocalizations, problematic, with demen-
     tia, 108–110

Warning devices, with hearing impair-
     ment, 361
Whispered Voice, 348
WHO, *see* World Health Association
Wilson's disease, 91
World Health Association, Assessment
     of Functional Capacity, 11

Zarit Burden interview, 373
Zung Self-Rating Depression Scale, 373

Contents of Previous Volumes

VOLUME I

Part I. Research on Nursing Practice
1. Nursing Research Related to Infants and Young Children   KATHRYN E. BARNARD
2. Nursing Research Related to School-Age Children and Adolescents   MARY J. DENYES
3. Adulthood: A Promising Focus for Future Research   JOANNE SABOL STEVENSON
4. Clinical Geriatric Nursing Research   MARY OPAL WOLANIN
5. Nursing Research on Death, Dying, and Terminal Illness: Development, Present State, and Prospects   JEANNE QUINT BENOLIEL

Part II. Research on Nursing Care Delivery
6. Nursing Staff Turnover, Stress, and Satisfaction: Models, Measures, and Management   ADA SUE HINSHAW AND JAN R. ATWOOD
7. Interorganizational Relations Research in Nursing Care Delivery Systems   JANELLE C. KRUEGER

Part III. Research on the Profession of Nursing
8. Socialization and Roles in Nursing   MARY E. CONWAY

Part IV. Other Research
9. Philosophic Inquiry   ROSEMARY ELLIS

VOLUME II

Part I. Research on Nursing Practice
1. Family Research: Issues and Directions for Nursing   SUZANNE L. FEETHAM

2. Anxiety and Conflict in Pregnancy: Relationship to
    Maternal Health Status   REGINA P. LEDERMAN
3. The Experience of Being a Parent   ANGELA BARRON MCBRIDE
4. Health Promotion and Illness Prevention   NOLA J. PENDER
5. Coping with Elective Surgery   JEAN E. JOHNSON

    Part II. Research on Nursing Care Delivery
6. Assessment of Quality of Nursing Care   NORMA M. LANG AND
    JACQUELINE F. CLINTON
7. Public Health Nursing Evaluation, Education, and
    Professional Issues, 1977 to 1981   MARION E. HIGHRITER

    Part III. Research on Nursing Education
8. Research on the Teaching-Learning Process in
    Nursing Education   RHEBA DE TORNYAY
9. Research on Nursing Students   PATRICIA M. SCHWIRIAN
10. Curricular Research in Nursing   MARILYN L. STEMBER

    Part IV. Research on the Profession of Nursing
11. Information Processing in Nursing Practice   MARGARET R. GRIER

    Part V. Other Research
12. Nursing Research and the Study of Health Policy   NANCY MILIO
13. Nursing Research in Scotland: A Critical Review   LISBETH HOCKEY
    AND MARGARET O. CLARK

VOLUME III

    Part I. Research on Nursing Practice
1. The Community as a Field of Inquiry in Nursing   GRAYCE M. SILLS
    AND JEAN GOEPPINGER
2. School Nursing   SHU-PI C. CHEN AND JUDITH A. SULLIVAN
3. Teenage Pregnancy as a Community Problem   RAMONA T. MERCER
4. Cross-Cultural Nursing Research   TONI TRIPP-REIMER AND MOLLY C.
    DOUGHERTY

    Part II. Research on Nursing Care Delivery
5. Nurse Practitioners and Primary Care Research:
    Promises and Pitfalls   SHERRY L. SHAMANSKY
6. Nursing Diagnosis   MARJORY GORDON

Part III. Research on Nursing Education

7. Research on Continuing Education in Nursing   ALICE M. KURAMOTO
8. Doctoral Education of Nurses: Historical Development,
    Programs, and Graduates   JUANITA F. MURPHY

Part IV. Research on the Profession of Nursing

9. Ethical Inquiry   SUSAN R. GORTNER
10. Cost-Effectiveness Analysis in Nursing Research   CLAIRE M. FAGIN
    AND BARBARA S. JACOBSEN

Part V. Other Research

11. Philosophy of Science and the Development of Nursing
    Theory   FREDERICK SUPPE AND ADA K. JACOX

VOLUME IV

Part I. Research on Nursing Practice

1. Maternal Anxiety in Pregnancy: Relationship to Fetal and
    Newborn Health Status   REGINA PLACZEK LEDERMAN
2. Preschool Children   JUANITA W. FLEMING
3. Menopause   ANN M. VODA AND THERESA GEORGE
4. Aging: Gerontological Nursing Research   MARY ADAMS
5. Bereavement   ALICE STERNER DEMI AND MARGARET SHANDOR MILES

Part II. Research on Nursing Care Delivery

6. Evaluation of Primary Nursing   PHYLLIS GIOVANNETTI
7. Nurse-Midwifery Care: 1925 to 1984   JOYCE E. THOMPSON

Part III. Research on Nursing Education

8. Faculty Productivity   KATHLEEN G. ANDREOLI AND LEIGH ANNE
    MUSSER
9. Nontraditional Nursing Education   CARRIE B. LENBURG
10. Computer-Aided Instruction in Nursing Education   BETTY L. CHANG

Part IV. Research on the Profession of Nursing

11. Nursing's Heritage   IRENE SABELBERG PALMER

Part V. Other Research

12. Nursing Education Research in Canada   MARGARET M. ALLEMANG
    AND MARGARET C. CAHOON

VOLUME V

Part I. Research on Nursing Practice
1. Stress   BRENDA L. LYON AND JOAN STEHLE WERNER
2. Pain   ANN GILL TAYLOR
3. Human Biologic Rhythms   GERALDENE FELTON
4. Physiologic Responses in Health and Illness: An Overview   MI JA KIM

Part II. Research on Nursing Care Delivery
5. Critical Care Nursing   KATHLEEN DRACUP

Part III. Research on Nursing Education
6. Faculty Practice   GRACE H. CHICKADONZ
7. Teaching Clinical Judgment   CHRISTINE A. TANNER

Part IV. Research on the Profession of Nursing
8. Leadership in Nursing   JOANNE COMI MCCLOSKEY AND MARILYN T. MOLEN

Part V. Other Research
9. International Nursing Research   AFAF IBRAHIM MELEIS
10. Conceptual Models of Nursing   MARY CIPRIANO SILVA

VOLUME VI

Part I. Research on Nursing Practice
1. Touch   SANDRA J. WEISS
2. Patient Education   CAROL A. LINDEMAN
3. The Physical Environment and Patient Care   MARGARET A. WILLIAMS
4. Social Support   JANE S. NORBECK
5. Relaxation   MARIAH SNYDER

Part II. Research on Nursing Care Delivery
6. Variable Costs of Nursing Care in Hospitals   MARGARET D. SOVIE

Part III. Research on Nursing Education
7. Psychiatric-Mental Health Nursing Education   MAXINE E. LOOMIS
8. Community Health Nursing Education   BEVERLY C. FLYNN

Part IV. Research on the Profession of Nursing
9.   Men in Nursing   LUTHER P. CHRISTMAN

Part V. Other Research
10.   Women's Health   NANCY FUGATE WOODS
11.   Human Information Processing   SISTER CALLISTA ROY
12.   Nursing Research in the Philippines   PHOEBE DAUZ WILLIAMS

VOLUME VII

Part I. Research on Nursing Practice
1.   Neurologic Nursing Research   L. CLAIRE PARSONS AND
       PAMELA STINSON KIDD
2.   Endotracheal Suctioning   KATHLEEN S. STONE AND BARBARA TURNER
3.   Physiological Response to Stress   WILLA M. DOSWELL
4.   Sleep   JOAN L. F. SHAVER AND ELIZABETH C. GIBLIN
5.   Infection Control   ELAINE L. LARSON

Part II. Research on Nursing Care Delivery
6.   Nursing Diagnosis   MI JA KIM
7.   Patient Contracting   SUSAN BOEHM

Part III. Research on Nursing Education
8.   Parent-Child Nursing Education   CHERYL S. ALEXANDER AND KARIN
       E. JOHNSON

Part IV. Research on the Profession of Nursing
9.   Moral Reasoning and Ethical Practice   SHAKÉ KETEFIAN

Part V. Other Research
10.   Patient Education: Part II   CAROL A. LINDEMAN

VOLUME VIII

Part I. Research on Nursing Practice
1.   Cardiovascular Nursing Research   MARIE J. COWAN
2.   Prevention of Pressure Sores   CAROLYN E. CARLSON AND ROSEMARIE
       B. KING
3.   The Effects of Stress During the Brain Growth Spurt   ELIZABETH M.
       BURNS

4.   Smoking Cessation: Research on Relapse Crises   KATHLEEN A. O'CONNELL

Part II. Research on Nursing Care Delivery
5.   Home Health Care   VIOLET H. BARKAUSKAS
6.   Nursing Administration Research, Part One: Pluralities of Persons   PHYLLIS R. SCHULZ AND KAREN L. MILLER

Part III. Research on Nursing Education
7.   Education for Critical Care Nursing   MARGUERITE R. KINNEY
8.   Nursing Research Education   JOANN S. JAMANN-RILEY

Part IV. Research on the Profession of Nursing
9.   Acquired Immunodeficiency Syndrome   JOAN G. TURNER

Part V. Other Research
10. Interpersonal Communication between Nurses and Patients   BONNIE J. GARVIN AND CAROL W. KENNEDY

VOLUME IX

Part I. Research on Nursing Practice
1.   Arthritis   VICKIE A. LAMBERT
2.   Alzheimer's Disease   MERIDEAN L. MAAS AND KATHLEEN C. BUCKWALTER
3.   Human Responses to Catastrophe   SHIRLEY A. MURPHY
4.   Family Caregiving for the Elderly   BARBARA A. GIVEN AND CHARLES W. GIVEN
5.   Family Adaptation to a Child's Chronic Illness   JOAN KESSNER AUSTIN

Part II. Research on Nursing Care Delivery
6.   Disaster Nursing   PAULINE KOMNENICH AND CAROLYN FELLER
7.   Nurse Anesthesia Care   MATTILOU CATCHPOLE

Part III. Research on Nursing Education
8.   Occupational Health Nursing Education   BONNIE ROGERS

Part IV. Research on the Profession of Nursing
9.   Mentorship   CONNIE NICODEMUS VANCE AND ROBERTA KNICKREHM OLSON

Part V. Other Research

10. Nutritional Studies in Nursing   NONI L. BODKIN AND BARBARA
    C. HANSEN
11. Health Conceptualizations   MARGARET A. NEWMAN

VOLUME X

1. Review of the First Decade of the *Annual Review of Nursing
   Research*   JOANNE SABOL STEVENSON

Part I. Research on Nursing Practice

2. Urinary Incontinence in Older Adults   KATHLEEN A. MCCORMICK
   AND MARY H. PALMER
3. Diabetes Mellitus   EDNA HAMERA
4. Battered Women and Their Children   JACQUELYN C. CAMPBELL AND
   BARBARA PARKER
5. Chronic Mental Illness   JEANNE C. FOX
6. Alcohol and Drug Abuse in Nurses   ELEANOR J. SULLIVAN AND
   SANDRA M. HANDLEY
7. Childhood and Adolescent Bereavement   NANCY D. OPIE

Part II. Research on Nursing Care Delivery

8. Nursing Centers   SUSAN K. RIESCH

Part III. Research on Nursing Education

9. Nursing Administration Education   RUTH A. ANDERSON

Part IV. Research on the Profession of Nursing

10. The Staff Nurse Role   NORMA L. CHASKA

Part V. Other Research

11. International Nursing Research   BEVERLY M. HENRY AND JEAN M.
    NAGELKERK

VOLUME XI

Part I. Research on Nursing Practice

1. Acute Confusion in the Elderly   MARQUIS D. FOREMAN
2. The Shivering Response   BARBARA J. HOLTZCLAW
3. Chronic Fatigue   KATHLEEN M. POTEMPA
4. Side Effects of Cancer Chemotherapy   MARYLIN J. DODD
5. Pain in Children   NANCY O. KESTER

Part II. Research on Nursing Care Delivery

6. Patient Care Outcomes Related to Management
    of Symptoms   SUE T. HEGYVARY
7. The Role of Nurse Researchers Employed
    in Clinical Settings   KARIN T. KIRCHHOFF

Part III. Research on Nursing Education

8. Nurse-Midwifery Education   CLARE M. ANDREWS AND CAROL
    E. DAVIS

Part IV. Research on the Profession of Nursing

9. AIDS-related Knowledge, Attitudes, and Risk for
    HIV Infection Among Nurses   JOAN G. TURNER

Part V. Other Research

10. Family Unit-Focused Research: 1984–1991   ANN L. WHALL AND
    CAROL J. LOVELAND-CHERRY
11. Opiate Abuse in Pregnancy   CATHY STRACHAN LINDENBERG AND
    ANNE B. KEITH
12. Alcohol and Drug Abuse   ELEANOR J. SULLIVAN AND SANDRA
    M. HANDLEY
13. Nursing Research on Patient Falls in Health Care
    Institutions   JANICE M. MORSE

VOLUME XII

Part I. Research on Nursing Practice

1. Psychogenic Pain in Children   NANCY M. RYAN-WENGER
2. Fatigue During the Childbearing Period   RENÉE MILLIGAN AND
    LINDA C. PUGH
3. Elder Mistreatment   TERRY T. FULMER
4. Rural Health and Health-Seeking Behaviors   CLARANN WEINERT,
    S. C. AND MARY BURMAN

Part II. Research on Nursing Care Delivery

5. Nursing Workload Measurement Systems   SANDRA R. EDWARDSON
    AND PHYLLIS B. GIOVANNETTI
6. Dying Well: Symptom Control Within Hospice Care   INGE B.
    CORLESS

Part III. Research on Nursing Education

7. Research on the Baccalaureate Completion Process for RNs   MARY
    BETH MATHEWS AND LUCILLE L. TRAVIS

Part IV. Research on the Profession of Nursing
8. Minorities in Nursing   DIANA L. MORRIS AND MAY L. WYKLE

Part V. Other Research
9. Native American Health   SHAROL F. JACOBSON
10. Nursing Research in Korea   ELIZABETH C. CHOI

VOLUME XIII

Part I. Research on Nursing Practice
1. Quality of Life and the Spectrum of HIV Infection   WILLIAM L. HOLZEMER AND HOLLY SKODOL WILSON
2. Physical Health of Homeless Adults   ADA M. LINDSEY
3. Child Sexual Abuse: Initial Effects   SUSAN J. KELLEY
4. The Neurobehavioral Effects of Childhood Lead Exposure   HEIDI vonKOSS KROWCHUK

Part II. Research on Nursing Care Delivery
5. Case Management   GERRI S. LAMB
6. Technology and Home Care   CAROL E. SMITH
7. Nursing Minimum Data Set   POLLY RYAN AND CONNIE DELANEY
8. Pediatric Hospice Nursing   IDA M. MARTINSON

Part III. Research on Nursing Education
9. Faculty Practice: Interest, Issues, and Impact   PATRICIA HINTON WALKER

Part IV. Research on the Profession of Nursing
10. The Professionalization of Nurse Practitioners   BONNIE BULLOUGH
11. Feminism and Nursing   PEGGY L. CHINN

Part V. Other Research
12. Health Risk Behaviors for Hispanic Women   SARA TORRES AND ANTONIA M. VILLARRUEL

VOLUME XIV

Part I: Research on Nursing Practice
1. Blood Pressure   SUE A. THOMAS AND FREDA DeKEYSER
2. Psychoneuroimmunological Studies in HIV Disease   NANCY L. McCAIN AND JANICE M. ZELLER

3. Delirium Intervention Research in Acute Care Settings   DIANE
    CRONIN-STUBBS
4. Smoking Cessation Interventions in Chronic Illness   MARY ELLEN
    WEWERS AND KAREN L. AHIJEVYCH
5. Quality of Life and Caregiving in Technological Home Care   CAROL
    E. SMITH

    Part II: Research on Nursing Care Delivery
6. Organizational Redesign: Effect on Institutional and Consumer
    Outcomes   GAIL L. INGERSOLL
7. Organizational Culture   BARBARA A. MARK

    Part III: Research on Nursing Education
8. Oncology Nursing Education   M. LINDA WORKMAN

    Part IV: Research on the Profession of Nursing
9. Moral Competency   VIRGINIA R. CASSIDY

    Part V: Other Research
10. Nursing Research in Israel   HAVA GOLANDER AND TAMAR KRULIK
11. The Evolution of Nursing Research in Brazil   ISABEL AMÉLIA COSTA
    MENDES AND MARIA AUXILIADORA TREVIZAN

VOLUME XV

    Part I: Research on Nursing Practice
1. Parenting the Prematurely Born Child   DIANE HOLDITCH-DAVIS
    AND MARGARET SHANDOR MILES
2. Interventions for Cognitive Impairment and Neurobehavioral
    Disturbances of Older Adults   DIANE CRONIN-STUBBS
3. Uncertainty in Acute Illness   MERLE H. MISHEL
4. Violence in the Workplace   JEANNE BEAUCHAMP HEWITT AND PAMELA
    F. LEVIN
5. Interventions to Reduce the Impact of Chronic Disease: Community-
    Based Arthritis Patient Education   JEAN GOEPPINGER AND KATE
    LORIG
6. Parent–Adolescent Communication in Nondistressed Families   SUSAN
    K. RIESCH
7. Adherence to Therapy in Tuberculosis   FELISSA L. COHEN

    Part II: Research on Nursing Care Delivery
8. Health Promotion and Disease Prevention in the Worksite   SALLY
    LECHLITNER LUSK

Part III: Other Research
9. Nursing at War: Catalyst for Change   QUINCEALEA BRUNK
10. Long-Term Vascular Access Devices   JANET S. FULTON
11. Nursing Research in Taiwan   SHYANG-YUN PAMELA KOONG SHIAO
    AND YU-MEI YU CHAO

VOLUME XVI

Part I: Health Promotion Across the Life Span
1. Childhood Nutrition   CHRISTINE M. KENNEDY
2. Health Care for the School-Age Child   KATHLEEN ANN LONG AND
    DAVID WILLIAMS
3. Childhood Diabetes: Behavioral Research   PATRICIA BRANDT
4. Prevention of Mental Health Problems in Adolescence   SUSAN
    KOOLS
5. The Development of Sexual Risk Taking in Adolescence   ROSEMARY
    A. JADACK AND MARY L. KELLER
6. Motivation for Physical Activity Among Children and Adolescents
    NOLA J. PENDER
7. Health Promotion in Old Age   SUSAN M. HEIDRICH
8. Health Promotion for Family Caregivers of Chronically Ill Elders
    BARBARA A. GIVEN AND CHARLES W. GIVEN

Part II: Research on Care Delivery
9. Prenatal and Parenting Programs for Adolescent Mothers   PAULETTE
    J. PERRONE HOYER

Part III: Other Research
10. Chronic Obstructive Pulmonary Disease: Strategies to Improve
    Functional Status   JANET L. LARSON AND NANCY KLINE LEIDY
11. Schizophrenia   JEANNE C. FOX AND CATHERINE F. KANE

VOLUME XVII

Part I: Complementary Therapies
1. Music Therapy   MARIAH SNYDER AND LINDA CHLAN
2. Sleep Promotion in Adults   JUDITH A. FLOYD
3. Guided Imagery Interventions for Symptom Management   LUCILLE
    SANZERO ELLER
4. Patient-Centered Communication   SARAH JO BROWN

Part II: Pain
5. Acute Pain   MARION GOOD
6. The Chronobiology, Chronopharmacology, and Chronotherapeutics of Pain   SUSAN E. AUVIL-NOVAK
7. Chronic Low Back Pain: Early Interventions   JULIA FAUCETT

Part III: Other Research
8. Wandering in Dementia   DONNA L. ALGASE
9. Cognitive Interventions Among Older Adults   GRAHAM J. MCDOUGALL, JR.
10. Primary Health Care   BEVERLY J. MCELMURRY AND GWEN BRUMBAUGH KEENEY
11. Uncertainty in Chronic Illness   MERLE H. MISHEL
12. Nursing Research in Italy   RENZO ZANOTTI

VOLUME XVIII

Part I: Research in Chronic Illness
1. Two Decades of Insider Research: What We Know and Don't Know About Chronic Illness Experience   SALLY E. THORNE AND BARBARA L. PATERSON
2. Children with Epilepsy: Quality of Life and Psychosocial Needs   JOAN K. AUSTIN AND DAVID W. DUNN
3. Adherence in Chronic Disease   JACQUELINE DUNBAR-JACOBS, JUDITH A. ERLEN, ELIZABETH A. SCHLENK, CHRISTOPHER M. RYAN, SUSAN M. SEREIKA, AND WILLA M. DOSWELL
4. Heart Failure Management: Optimal Health Care Delivery Programs   DEBRA K. MOSER
5. Cancer Care: Impact of Interventions on Caregiver Outcomes   JEANNIE V. PASACRETA AND RUTH MCCORKLE
6. Interventions for Children with Diabetes and Their Families   MARGARET GREY
7. Management of Urinary Incontinence in Adult Ambulatory Care Populations   JEAN F. WYMAN
8. Family Interventions to Prevent Substance Abuse: Children and Adolescents   CAROL J. LOVELAND-CHERRY
9. School-Based Interventions for Primary Prevention of Cardiovascular Disease: Evidence of Effects for Minority Populations   JANET C. MEININGER

Part II: Milestones in Nursing Research
10. Breakthroughs in Scientific Research: The Discipline of Nursing, 1960–1999   SUE K. DONALDSON

VOLUME XIX

Part I: Introduction

1   What We Know and How We Know It: Contributions from Nursing to Women's Health Research and Scholarship   DIANA TAYLOR AND NANCY WOODS

2   Conceptual Models for Women's Health Research: Reclaiming Menopause As an Exemplar of Nursing's Contributions to Feminist Scholarship   LINDA C. ANDRIST AND KATHLEEN I. MACPHERSON

Part II: Research on Women's Social Roles and Health

3   Women As Mothers and Grandmothers   ANGELA BARRON MCBRIDE AND CHERYL PROHASKA SHORE

4   Women and Employment: A Decade Review   MARCIA GRUIS KILLIEN

5   Interventions for Women As Family Caregivers   MARGARET J. BULL

Part III: Research on Diversity and Women's Health

6   Lesbian Health and Health Care   LINDA A. BERNHARD

7   Immigrant Women and Their Health   KAREN J. AROIAN

Part IV: Research on Women's Health and Illness Issues

8   Women and Stress   CHERYL A. CAHILL

9   Sleep and Fatigue   KATHRYN A. LEE

10   Intimate Partner Violence Against Women   JANICE HUMPHREYS, BARBARA PARKER, AND JACQUELYN C. CAMPBELL

11   Health Decisions and Decision Support for Women   MARILYN L. ROTHERT AND ANNETTE M. O'CONNOR

12   Female Troubles: An Analysis of Menstrual Cycle Research in the NINR Portfolio As a Model for Science Development in Women's Health   NANCY KING REAME